Vision, Brain, and Behavior in Birds

Vision, Brain, and Behavior in Birds

edited by H. Philip Zeigler and
Hans-Joachim Bischof

A Bradford Book
The MIT Press
Cambridge, Massachusetts
London, England

This book was set in Palatino by DEKR Corporation and was printed and bound in the United States of America.

Library of Congress Cataloging-in-Publication Data

Vision, brain, and behavior in birds / [edited by] H. Philip Zeigler
and Hans-Joachim Bischof.
  p.   cm.
  "A Bradford book."
  Includes bibliographical references and index.
  ISBN 0-262-24036-X
  1. Birds—Physiology. 2. Visual pathways. 3. Eye. 4. Brain.
I. Zeigler, H. Philip (Harris Philip), 1931–   . II. Bischof, Hans
-Joachim.
QL698.V57   1993
598.2′1823 — dc20   93-22353
                                                  CIP

Dedicated, with affection, to Susannah Bloch and Carlos Martinoya

In Memoriam

Monika Remy (1949–1992)

Students of avian vision share a sense of community that makes the loss of one of its members an occasion for communal mourning. Thus, our pleasure at the publication of this book is shadowed by the loss of one of its contributors, Monika Remy. Monika will be missed by a large circle of friends and colleagues on four continents. Over the last few years this circle had expanded as her work brought her to new laboratories and new scientific approaches. Monika's research was frequently interdisciplinary, combining an interest in vision and behavior with anatomy and physiology.

Monika started science late in life at the Ruhr-Universät Bochum, where she received her Diplom degree in biology. She acquired an interest in avian vision while working with Jacky Emmerton in the psychology department, and the association with Jacky continued when she began her doctorate in psychology. The final stages of her disser-

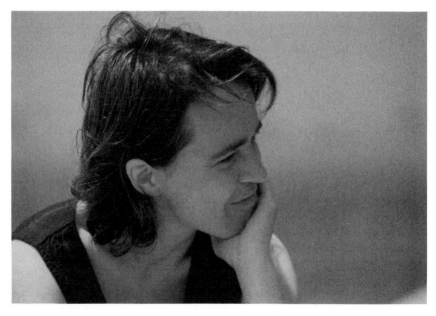

Monika Remy (1949–1992)

tation were completed in the psychology department at the Universität Konstanz, to which she moved from Bochum with Juan Delius's "Mannschaft." In her doctoral research, on functional aspects of pigeon's retinal organization, Monika showed her patience and skill, not only in applying anatomical techniques, but also in using complex behavioral techniques to coax from her subjects precise data on the organization of retinal fields in pigeon.

After receiving her doctorate (Dr. rer. nat.), Monika moved to New York in 1990 to work with Phil Zeigler's group at Hunter College. Characteristically, she combined behavioral work on classical conditioning of jaw movement with electrophysiological studies of the pigeon's oromotor system. This was an especially happy year for Monika, during which she wrote friends and family about the pleasures of New York and her feelings of being at home there. Then, having been awarded a Fellowship from the Deutsche Forschungsgemeinschaft, she took a train across the United States to join Harvey Karten and his colleagues at the University of California, San Diego. There, despite what she used to call the oppressively sunny climate, she worked cheerfully on the anatomy of retinal development. Her return to Germany, to Klaus-Peter Hoffman's zoology and neurobiology department in Bochum, was the start of a new venture, the study of visually guided eye movements and psychophysics in primates (including the human variety). It was shortly after Monika began this new project that her illness was diagnosed, and she continued her work for as long as health permitted.

Those of us who worked with Monika will not forget her good humor, her uncanny psychological intuitions, or the quiet determination and effort she put into making things succeed. She brought this positive attitude into coping with her final illness, supported in the effort by her friends and family, especially her daughter Anke and her son Jan. For what she gave us, we are grateful, regretting only that she did not live to tease us about our mistakes in this book, and then to proceed to ventures beyond it.

MONIKA REMY: A BIBLIOGRAPHY

Remy, M., and Emmerton, J. Behavioral spectral sensitivities of different retinal areas in pigeon. *Behav. Neurosci.* 103 (1989), 170–177.

Remy, M., and Emmerton, J. Directional dependence of intraocular transfer of stimulus detection in pigeons (*Columbia livia*). *Behav. Neurosci.* 105 (1991), 647–652.

Remy, M., and Güntürkün, O. Retinal afferents to the tectum opticum and the nucleus opticus principalis thalami in the pigeon. *J. Comp. Neurol.* 304 (1991), 1–14.

Bermejo, R., Remy, M., and Zeigler, H. P. Jaw movement kinematics and jaw muscle (EMG) activity during drinking in the pigeon (*Columbia livia*). *J. Comp. Physiol.* A 170 (1992), 303–309.

Remy, M., and Zeigler, H. P. Classical conditioning of jaw movements in the pigeon: Acquisition and response topography. *Animal Learn. Behav.* 21 (1993), 131–137.

Contents

Contributors

Patrice Adret
School of Biological and Medical
Sciences
University of St. Andrews
St. Andrews, Fife, Scotland

Robert W. Allan
Department of Psychology
Lafayette College
Easton, Pennsylvania

R. J. Andrew
School of Biological Sciences
University of Sussex
Brighton, England

Paola Bagnoli
Department of Environmental
Sciences
University of Tuscia
Viterbo, Italy

Verner P. Bingman
Department of Psychology
Bowling Green State University
Bowling Green, Ohio

Hans-Joachim Bischof
Department of Behavioral
Physiology
University of Bielefeld
Bielefeld, Germany

Giovanni Casini
Departments of Anatomy and
Cell Biology and Medicine
UCLA School of Medicine and
VAMC-West Los Angeles
Los Angeles, California

Andrea Ciocchetti
Department of Environmental
Sciences
University of Tuscia
Viterbo, Italy

Juan D. Delius
Department of Psychology
University of Konstanz
Konstanz, Germany

M. Dharmaretnam
School of Biological Sciences
University of Sussex
Brighton, England

Winand Dittrich
Department of Psychology
University of Exeter
Exeter, England

Jacky Emmerton
Department of Psychology
Purdue University
West Lafayette, Indiana

Jürgen Engelage
Department of Behavioral
Physiology
University of Bielefeld
Bielefeld, Germany

Gigliola Fontanesi
Department of Physiology and
Biochemistry
University of Pisa
Pisa, Italy

Timothy H. Goldsmith
Department of Biology
Yale University
New Haven, Connecticut

Onur Güntürkün
Faculty of Psychology
Ruhr University
Bochum, Germany

Kathrin Hermann
Laboratory of Neurophysiology
National Institutes of Health
Poolesville, Maryland

William Hodos
Department of Psychology
University of Maryland
College Park, Maryland

Ralf Jäger
Department of Psychology
University of Konstanz
Konstanz, Germany

Harvey J. Karten
Department of Neurosciences
University of California,
San Diego
San Diego, California

Gadi Katzir
Department of Biology
University of Haifa, Oranim
Haifa, Israel

Stephen E. G. Lea
Department of Psychology
University of Exeter
Exeter, England

Juan-Carlos Letelier
Department of Biology
City College,
City University of New York
New York, New York

Graham R. Martin
School of Biological Sciences and
Continuing Studies
University of Birmingham
Birmingham, England

Sally A. McFadden
Department of Psychology
University of Newcastle
Newcastle, NSW, Australia

Jörg Mey
Department of Ophthalmology
University of Tübingen School of
Medicine
Tübingen, Germany

Dom Miceli
Department of Psychology
University of Québec at Trois-
Rivières
Trois-Rivières, Québec, Canada

Hans-Ortwin Nalbach
Max Planck Institute for
Biological Cybernetics
University of Tübingen
Tübingen, Germany

Adrian G. Palacios
Department of Biology
Yale University
New Haven, Connecticut

Monika Remy†
Department of Zoology and
Neurobiology
Ruhr University
Bochum, Germany

Lesley J. Rogers
Department of Physiology
University of New England
Armidale, NSW, Australia

Toru Shimizu
Department of Psychology
University of South Florida
Tampa, Florida

Solon Thanos
Department of Ophthalmology
University of Tübingen
School of Medicine
Tübingen, Germany

Francisco J. Varela
Institute of Neurosciences
University of Paris
Paris, France

Josh Wallman
Department of Biology
City College,
City University of New York
New York, New York

Masami Watanabe
Department of Physiology
Institute for Developmental
Research
Kasugai, Japan

Shigeru Watanabe
Department of Psychology
Keio University
Tokyo, Japan

† Deceased

Friederike Wolf-Oberhollenzer
Max Planck Institute for
Biological Cybernetics
University of Tübingen
Tübingen, Germany

H. Philip Zeigler
Biopsychology Program
Hunter College, City University
of New York
New York, New York

Preface

The behavior of birds is characterized by a unique mixture of stereotypy and plasticity that has fascinated and delighted both amateur bird lovers and professional ornithologists. For the ethologist, avian behavior is the source of a wide variety of species-typical "fixed-action patterns" and the study of these patterns has helped to clarify our understanding of the complex interaction between heredity and environment. For the experimental psychologist, pigeons are the subjects of choice in studies of psychophysics, learning, perception, and cognitive processes. Indeed, the pigeon's pecking response may well be the most exhaustively studied behavior in contemporary psychology. For the neurobiologist, bird behavior and the avian brain have provided "model systems" for the analysis of neural mechanisms of sensation, movement, orientation and navigation, vocalization, and hormonal mechanisms of reproduction. For all these reasons, research on the avian brain and bird behavior occupies an increasingly important place in contemporary behavioral and neural biology.

Because the visual capacities of birds rival, and in some cases exceed those of primates, much of this research has been focused on the avian visual system. During the past decade there has been considerable progress in the analysis of the optics of the avian eye, the morphology of the retina, the anatomy of the visual system, and the functional organization of the avian brain. However, there is currently no up-to-date and comprehensive review of this work.

The present volume is designed to provide such a review. It brings together contributions by researchers from a variety of countries (Australia, Canada, England, France, Germany, Israel, Italy, Japan, and the United States) with expertise across a range of disciplines including ornithology, ethology, experimental psychology, anatomy, neurophysiology, and developmental neurobiology. Each of the contributors is an internationally recognized authority (in some cases *the* authority) on some aspect of the avian visual system, the avian brain, or bird behavior. However, their contributions are broadly focused, providing an introduction to a problem area, its central questions, its methodology, and the current status of research in the area. The chapters are organized into sections, each dealing with a general problem: retinal mechanisms, visual psychophysics, anatomy and physiology, visuomotor mechanisms, vision and cognition, and development and plasticity. Each section is preceded by a general introduction providing background material and placing the chapter within a broader perspective.

This organizational strategy should help to integrate disparate materials and increase the utility of the volume for both the specialist and the general reader. It should also make the book useful for teaching purposes and as a comprehensive reference source for workers in behavioral, developmental, and neural biology, comparative neuroanatomy, ornithology, and psychology.

We would like to acknowledge the generous support of the following organizations, institutions, and individuals: Stiftung Volkswagen, Deutsche Forschungsgemeinschaft, Minister für Wissenschaft und Forschung des Landes Nordrhein-Westfalen, and University of Bielefeld. Fiona Stevens, our editor at MIT Press, was enthusiastic, helpful, and patient throughout.

H. P. Z.
H.-J. B.

Introduction

BIRDS AND VISION

Despite its apparently parochial nature, a collection of essays on avian vision and behavior should be of interest to all students of visual function. The visual system of vertebrates has probably evolved only once, so that its operation in any vertebrate class is likely to reflect a set of principles—a *bauplan*—common to all classes. It is becoming increasingly clear, for example, that the apparently striking differences in the morphology of avian and mammalian visual systems mask an extraordinary degree of similarity (see the chapter by Shimizu and Karten). Moreover, birds, like humans, are a diurnal species, and their sensory world is more "visual" and far more intuitively accessible to us than those of most mammalian species. Yet our choice of preparations for the study of visual processes is oddly unbalanced. We seem to have eschewed the visual world of birds in favor of that of cats, crepuscular, afoveate creatures with their peculiar color vision and a disinclination to report to us their visual perceptions. Perhaps this collection of papers on avian vision and behavior will help to restore that balance by providing an opportunity to explore the operation of the visual system in a class in which that system is dominant, a class with not just one, but often two foveae, and many species that, if properly trained, can, like primates, tell us a great deal about what they see.

For the student of visual function, birds offer an unusual combination of behavioral complexity and experimental utility. The avian eye provides a rich array of environmental inputs, and avian visuomotor mechanisms exercise relatively precise control over effectors like the beak or foot. These characteristics are well exemplified in the pigeon, a relatively unspecialized bird with a highly sophisticated visual system, linked to a prehensile effector organ (the beak), and susceptible of experimental control by conditioning paradigms. These paradigms, when combined with psychophysical techniques, make it possible for us to define the parameters of the bird's visual world with a degree of precision not always matched with human and nonhuman primates. It is these characteristics, combined with its low cost and ease of maintenance, that has made the pigeon's pecking behavior perhaps the most exhaustively utilized indicator response in behavioral science (Abs, 1983). Not surprisingly, it is an ubiquitous subject in studies of visual psychophysics, visual physiology, and visuomotor and cognitive mechanisms cited in this volume.

However, this book also reflects the fact that avian visual and visuomotor mechanisms represent a wide range of solutions to ecological problems. These are evident in the variety of sensory and motor specializations of birds, e.g., the extraordinary development of color vision, the range of eye positions from lateral to "frontal," the presence of two foveae and the possibility of independent movements of each eye, the diversity of feeding behaviors, from pecking at grain to tracking moving fish underwater (see chapters by Martin, Nalbach et al., Katzir, and Wallman and Letelier). By providing a variety of "natural experiments," this diversity has made possible a comparative analysis of mechanisms for the processing of visual information and the control of visually guided behaviors. Birds have comparable advantages for the study of development, since they exhibit a relatively brief developmental period and a range of developmental modes from extremely precocial to altricial, all of which share the advantages of extrauterine development. Finally, some of the visually guided behaviors of birds bear a striking resemblance to what, in primates, are designated as "cognitive" processes.

AVIAN BRAIN AND BEHAVIOR

The relationship between the brain and behavior of birds was the focus of considerable attention by the physiologists and comparative anatomists of the late nineteenth and early twentieth centuries (Flourens, Wallenberg, Ten Cate, etc.). However, for almost half a century thereafter, neurobehavioral studies of birds were rare, while this same period witnessed an extraordinary increase in the study of bird behavior by both ethologists and behavioral psychologists. This development becomes less paradoxical if we recall that for ethologists, like Lorenz, neurobehavioral experiments were incompatible with their conception of the experimenter–subject relationship, while for behaviorists like Skinner, they were a distraction from the central task of analyzing mechanisms of behavioral control.

The contemporary renaissance in avian brain-behavior studies has both conceptual and empirical origins. The publication of seminal papers on comparative neuroanatomy (Karten, 1969; Hodos and Campbell, 1969) clarified some critical misconceptions about brain evolution, suggested a number of putative homologies between the avian and mammalian brain, and provided a scientific rationale for the use of avian neurobehavioral preparations as "model systems" in behavioral neuroscience. The availability of a stereotaxic atlas of the pigeon brain

(Karten and Hodos, 1967) facilitated the initiation of neurobehavioral research programs focusing, inter alia, on visual psychophysics (Hodos, 1976) and feeding behavior (Zeigler, 1976). In the decades that followed, the study of the avian brain and visual behavior has flourished.

This volume attempts to provide a systematic account of the current status of behavioral and brain mechanisms of avian vision. Its central chapters deal with the anatomy, physiology, and development of the avian visual system. They are flanked, on one side by chapters on optics and visual psychophysics, and on the other by chapters on visuomotor and cognitive behaviors. In all cases the emphasis is on the delineation of persistent problems and a current review of our attempts at their solution.

Part I (The Avian Eye View) begins on the input side, with a consideration of the physical parameters of the avian eye, including the adaptation of those parameters to the ecological constraints under which different species operate (Martin). This is followed by a review of retinal mechanisms which transform the optical image into a pattern of neural excitation in the retina, preparatory to further processing by brain structures (Nalbach, Wolf-Oberhollenzer, and Remy). The problem of how a three-dimensional world is constructed from two-dimensional inputs is discussed in the chapter on binocular vision (McFadden). The last two chapters provide reviews of avian visual psychophysics in general (Hodos), and on retinal mechanisms and avian color vision (Varela, Palacios, and Goldsmith). Part II (Functional Anatomy of the Avian Visual System) reviews what is known about the anatomical organization of the central visual systems in birds. The plural form is chosen advisedly, since several functionally distinct visual systems have been identified in birds. The opening chapter, by Shimizu and Karten, considers the arguments for homologies between the avian and mammalian visual systems and their implications for the evolution of the neocortex. There follow reviews of the anatomy and physiology of thalamofugal (Güntürkün, Miceli, and Watanabe) and tectofugal (Engelage and Bischof) pathways, with some discussion of the problem of their differential visual functions. Finally, since much work on central visual pathways has used lateral-eyed birds like the pigeon, the section concludes with a brief review of data from frontal-eyed birds like owls (Casini, Fontanesi, and Bagnoli).

Developmental processes and their relationship to plasticity are the special focus of Part III (Development of the Avian Visual System). It begins with an analysis of the development of the chick retinotectal projection, a "model system" for the study of the ontogeny of patterning in the nervous system (Mey and Thanos). The next two chapters both deal with the role of external input in controlling the development of avian visual structures. The chapter by Fontanesi et al. focuses on the development of neurotransmitters and that by Herrmann and Bischof on the role of visual stimulation in the development of the tectofugal system. The final chapter (Rogers and Adret) reviews an elegant series of developmental studies bearing on the origins of central lateralization in the control of some visually guided behaviors.

Part IV (Visuomotor Mechanisms) moves to the output side of the visual system. It begins with two chapters that review mechanisms mediating specific behaviors, beginning with the relatively simple movements of the eye (Wallman and Letelier) and proceeding to pecking/grasping behavior in pigeons (Zeigler, Jäger, and Palacios). A methodological chapter by Allen describing the use of conditioning techniques for the analysis of visuomotor behaviors follows. The section concludes with an analysis of the coordinated eye, head, and body movements required for prey capture behavior by water birds (Katzir). Part V (Vision and Cognition) takes us beyond sensorimotor mechanisms and explores more complex "cognitive" manipulations of visual inputs. The chapter by Andrew and Dharmaretnam uses a variety of simple but revealing experimental tasks to introduce the notion of "viewing strategies," while Remy and Watanabe examine mechanisms related to processing of a continuous flow of inputs to the two eyes. The chapters on concept formation (Watanabe, Lea, and Dittrich) and on visual cognition (Emmerton and Delius) deal with behaviors that are not explicable in terms of immediately present external visual stimuli but seem to demand the postulation of some form of internal "representation." The final chapter on avian spatial behavior (Bingman) attempts to bridge the gap between laboratory studies of spatial discrimination and the complex processing of spatial information used to guide avian homing behavior.

In surveying the current state of neurobehavioral research on avian vision several conclusions emerge. First, it is clear that the functional characterization of the various visual systems remains a persistent problem. Little or nothing is known about the function of the isthmo-optic (centrifugal) system, nor do we have any clear idea as to the differential contributions of the thalamofugal and tectofugal systems. Recent research indicates that in pigeon, the two systems process inputs from different parts of the visual field (Remy and Güntürkün, 1991) and Hodos (Part I) suggests that the placement of stimuli in neurobehavioral experiments should reflect that fact. Second, it is clear that our restriction of experimental preparations to a few, well-studied species may obscure some general principles that can be elucidated only by comparative studies. In this respect, comparison of visual functioning in lateral-eyed and frontal-eyed birds has proven quite enlightening. Finally, the study of avian visual physiology (both retinal and central) continues to be a relatively neglected research area. Despite these caveats, the present volume reflects a healthy and continuing interest in the study of vision, brain and behavior in birds.

REFERENCES

Abs, M. *Physiology and Behavior of the Pigeon*. London: Academic Press, 1983.

Hodos, W. Vision and the visual system: A bird's-eye view. In J. M. Sprague and A. N. Epstein (Eds.), *Progress in Psychobiology and Physiological Psychology*, Vol. 6. New York: Academic Press, 1976, pp. 29–62.

Hodos, W., and Campbell, C. B. G. *Scala Naturae*: Why there is no theory in comparative psychology. *Psychol. Rev.* 76 (1969), 337–350.

Karten, H. J. The organization of the avian telencephalon and some speculations on the phylogeny of the amniote telencephalon. *Ann. N.Y. Acad. Sci.* 167 (1969), 46–179.

Karten, H. J., and Hodos, W. *A Stereotaxic Atlas of the Brain of the Pigeon (Columbia livia)*. Baltimore, MD: Johns Hopkins University Press, 1967.

Remy, M., and Güntürkün, O. Retinal afferents to the tectum opticum and the nucleus opticus principalis thalami in the pigeon. *J. Comp. Neurol.* 304 (1991), 1–14.

Zeigler, H. P. Feeding behavior of the pigeon. In J. S. Rosenblatt, R. A. Hinde, E. Shaw, and C. Beer (Eds.), *Advances in the study of behavior*, Vol. 7. New York: Academic Press, 1976, pp. 286–390.

I   The Avian Eye View

Introduction

Sally A. McFadden

Of all the vertebrates, birds are one of the most visually dependent classes. Their visual systems have evolved independently of the primate line, and reveal a degree of sophistication and complexity for which, in many respects, our own visual experience provides little intuitive appreciation. The basic design of the avian visual system is similar to other vertebrate classes in that it is constrained to a certain extent by physiological optics and neural processing limitations of a biological visual system. However, because of the wide variety in avian habitats, from land, water, and air, subtle variations in design abound. These variations provide a rich source of information to unravel the intricacies of visual system design. In addition to this ecological approach, much research has also concentrated on just a few species (especially the pigeon) that are easily studied in the laboratory setting. Such within-species comparisons complement the ecological approach, as the questions asked can build on an enhanced understanding of particular aspects of the visual system.

The fundamental question of "how can birds see?" is addressed in this first series of chapters. Vision is traditionally thought of as beginning with a physical registration of light on the photoreceptors of the eye. This process is influenced by the position and shape of the eye and its elements. Information regarding the amount, position, and the wavelength of light is separately extracted at this early stage. The quality of this raw image is affected by the subsequent retinal processing and varies in its fundamental qualities in different parts of the retina. This retinal variation is in turn related to a particular bird's behavioral repertoire.

It will be seen in chapter 1 that there are many subtle variations in the optical design of avian eyes. Some basic factors in eye design, such as eye size, can be related to light sensitivity and thus are also related to niche characteristics such as nocturnal and diurnal habitat. However, when other individual parts of eye design are examined, such as refractive power of the cornea, it is clear that a complexity of factors is involved and a simple relationship to niche is not so apparent. Of prime importance in determining what images a particular bird will register is the position of the eyes in the head and the type and variety of eye movements. Together, these two factors govern the quality and range of space that are visually relevant to a particular avian species.

Within a particular eye design and visual field shape, one also finds regional variation in visual capacity. Chapter 2 shows that this variation is evident in many aspects of the retinal topography, including the photoreceptor distribution, the organization of the retinal cells, and the degree of convergence from one cell layer to the next. Variation in visual perceptual capacity in different parts of the visual field mirror some of these physical differences, and provide insight into what role particular features may play. These differing features subserving different parts of visual space indicate that there may be multiple modes of viewing in birds. Thus, we find that birds make maximum use of the whole of their visual space by specializing the corresponding optical and retinal regional design. In addition, the multiple viewing modes potentially allow for a fast attention switch that does not have to necessarily rely on eye movements to explore visual space. This is not to say that birds do not have an extensive array of eye movements. One finds an enormous diversity in different avian species, with the dependence on eye movements inversely related to the static size of the visual field (see chapter 14, by Wallman and Letelier).

In birds, eye movements can be quite independent in each eye. This contrasts with the yoked system of primates and mammals. It has the advantage that attention may be mediated separately with each eye. In addition, within a binocular mode of viewing, eye movements can also be coordinated between the two eyes. Chapter 3 explains how such eye movements can underlie the perception of the position of objects in space, so that the third dimension can be used to guide visual perception.

Visual perception is based on a number of channels of processing including luminance and contrast, orientation, color, and spatial and temporal coding. The sophistication of the avian system is reinforced when one examines the capacity of the avian visual system to resolve the fine details within these different channels (chapter 4). For example, the visual acuity of the common pigeon approaches our own while that of the hawks and eagles is an order of magnitude greater.

It is within the avian color system that one can appreciate how birds have exploited the visual domain in a way beyond competition of other vertebrates. Evidence is presented in chapter 5 for a tetrachromatic or possibly pentachromatic color system. It is even possible that color may serve as a major affective dimension in the cognition of perceptual categories in birds.

Despite all we know about how birds produce, explore, reconstruct, and perceive an image, there are still many unanswered questions, particularly in relation to how different brain pathways may mediate avian visual perception. These unanswered questions need to be addressed by studying the avian visual system at both the molecular and systems levels, and relating it to the ecological and behavioral world of a variety of different species. In the following five chapters, the reader will find that the avian visual system is complex and sophisticated, but more often than not, the biological design is beautifully adapted to the behavioral needs, both within and between different avian species.

1 Producing the Image

Graham R. Martin

Optically, a bird's eye performs a simple function: the projection of an image of the bird's environment on its retina. This is achieved by an optical system employing just two principal refractive elements, lens and cornea. While this basic optical design is simple, interspecific comparisons show that it has been the subject of many subtle modifications. Furthermore, the absolute size of bird eyes, their position, and amplitude of movements in the skull also differ markedly between species. These interspecific variations mean that the view of the environment made available for analysis by the brain, and hence providing visual guidance for behavior, must differ markedly between species. Understanding these variations in the image producing mechanisms and visual fields of bird eyes is the theme of this section.

Probably the most useful basis for elucidating the overall optical function of an eye is the construction of a schematic eye model (Martin, 1983, 1985; Hughes, 1986). This is a mathematical description of the eye's optical system that represents an hypothetical average eye for the species and is a useful tool for interspecific comparisons of optical design. Drawings of schematic eye models in four bird species are shown in figure 1.1 and are used to illustrate general points throughout this chapter.

EYE SIZE

In absolute terms, bird eyes show a wide interspecific variation in size and figure 1.1 shows a group of eyes whose axial length varies over a range between 8 and 28.5 mm. The largest eyes of any land vertebrates are those of ostriches *Struthio camelus* (body weight 63–104 kg), with an axial length of 50 mm. Even the much smaller tawny owl *Strix aluco* (body weight approx. 450 g) has an eye whose axial length is approximately 4.5 mm greater than that of the human eye (Hughes, 1977).

Optically the most important parameter associated with eye size is the anterior focal length (or posterior nodal distance, PND) since this determines the size of the retinal area over which the image of an object

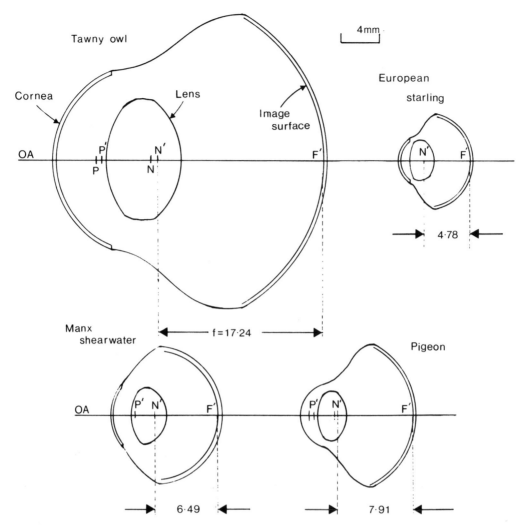

Figure 1.1 Scaled diagrams of the schematic eye models of Manx shearwaters *Puffinus puffinus*, European starlings *Sturnus vulgaris*, tawny owls *Strix aluco*, and pigeons *Columba livia*. Also shown is the overall shape of each eye in an approximately horizontal plane. OA, optic axis; P and P′, anterior and posterior principal points; N and N′, anterior and posterior nodal points; F′ posterior focal point. The focal length (posterior nodal distance) of each eye is also shown. All numerical values are in millimeters (Manx shearwaters, Martin and Brooke, 1991; European starlings, Martin 1986b; tawny owls, Martin, 1982; pigeons, Marshall et al., 1973; Martin and Brooke, 1991.)

is spread. Miller (1979) demonstrated that a large PND is essential if the eye is to achieve the maximum theoretical limit of visual resolution. This is because there exists a finite limit on the minimum size and packing density of the retinal photoreceptors that sample the retinal image. If PND is increased, spreading the image over more photoreceptors, then the amount of detail that can be resolved at a given receptor density will increase. However, this process cannot be continued ad infinitum since diffraction effects and aberrations within the optical system (Miller, 1979) will set limits to image resolution.

Martin (1982) has argued that a large PND is also essential if an eye is to function adequately throughout the complete range of naturally occurring luminance levels, which in terrestrial habitats can vary over approximately 11 orders of magnitude (Martin, 1990a). This is because for the optimal extraction of information from the retinal image at lower light levels large and widely spaced receptors are required. At high light levels small, densely packed receptors are necessary (Snyder et al. 1977). Thus, both the effective size and density of photoreceptors must alter with luminance level to maximize the amount of information which can be extracted from a retinal image. Snyder et al. (1977) suggest that this flexibility of image sampling can be achieved by pooling photo-receptor outputs at the retinal bipolar cells to achieve increasingly large "effective receptors" as light levels decrease. The degree of flexibility that potentially can be achieved by pooling receptor outputs will be greater if the image is spread over many photoreceptors whose outputs can be summed in various ways by the nervous system.

Thus the large eyes of owls can perhaps be regarded not simply as nocturnal eyes (designed to function only within a narrow range of lower light levels), but as eyes of arrhythmic species that function adequately throughout the full range of naturally occurring day-time, twilight, and night-time light levels (Martin, 1982, 1990a). Indeed there is evidence that although tawny owls usually adopt a strictly nocturnal life-style (Martin, 1990a), their visual system functions adequately by both day and night, yielding acuity at high light levels very similar to that of strictly diurnal pigeons (Martin, 1986a). However, species such as warblers (Parulidae, Sylviidae), finches (Fringillidae), and European starlings *Sturnus vulgaris*, which are strictly diurnal, except perhaps on migration (Martin, 1990b), may be restricted to their diurnal life-style by the small size of their eyes, which are 6–8 mm in axial length (Walls, 1942; Rochon-Duvigneaud, 1943; Donner, 1951, and fig. 1.1). Because of the problems of optimally sampling the retinal image at various luminance levels, eyes of this size cannot function adequately over a wide luminance range, but can function optimally within the relatively narrow (four orders of magnitude) luminance range that occurs between sunrise and sunset. Within this range, the required variation in receptor pooling for maximizing the extraction of information from the retinal image is relatively small.

It seems that as light levels fall, these birds must roost, since their eye design prohibits the extraction of enough information from the visual environment to mediate flight safely under low-light conditions. During nocturnal migratory flights, such birds may collide with even well lit objects such as lighthouses, oil platforms, and office blocks (Martin, 1990b).

The possession of eyes designed to function close to the theoretical limit of spatial resolution at high light levels, such as those of the diurnal birds-of-prey (Falconiformes), may also restrict their visually guided behavior to a narrow range of light levels. This is because to achieve high acuity the image must not only be large but it must be analyzed by a retina that is dominated by photoreceptors whose inputs are not pooled (Snyder et al., 1977). This does indeed seem to be the case in diurnal raptors and there is evidence that in these birds spatial resolution and sensitivity deteriorate rapidly with decreasing light levels (Fox et al., 1976; Reymond and Wolfe, 1981; Hirsch, 1982; Reymond, 1985).

Theoretically, however, for species living in habitats with only very low light levels, there is no selective advantage in the possession of large eyes. Thus although the eyes of nocturnal, flightless kiwis (Apterygidae) are small relative to their body size (axial length approx. 8 mm) they may be regarded, like those of rats (axial length approx. 5 mm), as designed to function optimally in the narrow range of low light levels that occur at night below a forest canopy (Reid and Williams, 1975, Martin, 1982).

EYE SHAPE

Walls (1942) divided bird eyes into three broad categories: flat, globose, and tubular, with none approximating the typically spherical shape of the mammalian eye (fig. 1.1). The main differences between these eye categories lies in the ratio of their axial to equatorial diameters, and complete gradation may exist between the flat and globose types. Shape, however, is not independent of absolute size, the tubular shape being typically found only in species with the largest eyes including owls and some eagles (Accipitriformes) (figure 1.1).

It seems unlikely that these eye shapes are concerned directly with optical function although they do influence the extent of the functional visual field (see section on Eye Position and Visual Fields, below). Given the importance of weight considerations in birds (King and King, 1980), the different shapes may simply reflect solutions to the problems of placing a relatively large, heavy, fluid-filled object within a small aviform skull, especially at one extremity of the body, where it can influence balance during flight. While the eyes of tawny owls have a similar axial length and similar optical structure to human eyes (see section on Optical Design below), their tubular shape encloses a smaller volume and hence they will weigh less than human eyes. Thus the tubular and flat shapes may be viewed as spheres with sections trimmed away to facilitate both placement in the skull and to reduce weight.

Many, possibly all, bird eyes are asymmetrical. Typically there is a marked nasal-temporal asymmetry in the distance between the corneoscleral junction and the equator, but there is less asymmetry about a ventrodorsal axis. This "nasad-asymmetry" results in the retina being arranged asymmetrically about the optical axis, and this is manifest in complex asymmetry of the retinal visual field (see section on Eye Position and Visual Fields). It may also be related to variations in the degree of myopia in different parts of the visual field (see p. 14).

OPTICAL DESIGN

Figure 1.1 (see also table 1.1) shows that there are marked interspecific differences in the optical structure of bird eyes with the total refractive power of each eye being achieved by a quite different combination of lens and corneal powers. The most obvious parameter that characterizes these differences in optical design is the ratio of lens:corneal refractive power (FL:FC). The eyes of pigeons and Manx shearwaters, for example, are of near identical axial length but differ in optical design. These eyes also differ from those of owls and starlings. Thus in pigeons the cornea provides the bulk of the eye's total refractive power (FL:FC = 0.40) while in shearwaters the lens is the more powerful refractive element (FL:FC = 1.60). On the other hand this ratio is approximately identical in tawny owl and starling eyes indicating that although these eyes differ in size by a factor of 3.6 their optical systems are in fact scaled versions of a common form.

The result of these differences in the relative contributions of lens and cornea to total refractive power is not trivial. Thus, although pigeon and shearwater eyes are of a very similar size they differ in total refractive power by 28 diopters (D) and hence have different PNDs. The relatively more powerful cornea brings the nodal points of the optical system nearer to the cornea in pigeon eyes than in shearwaters. This means that the retinal image is larger in pigeons, so although these two bird eyes are the same size, pigeons have the potential for higher visual acuity under the same viewing conditions.

Table 1.1. Certain Eye Parameters in European Starlings, Manx Shearwaters, Pigeons, and Tawny Owls

	F_{eye} (D)	PND (mm)	F_{lens} (D)	F_{cornea} (D)	Ratio F_{lens}: F_{cornea}	Axial length (mm)	Ratio PND: axial length
Starling	209	4.78	112.5	124.6	0.90	7.92	0.60
Shearwater	154	6.49	108.6	68.1	1.60	11.82	0.55
Pigeon	126	7.91	38.7	95.9	0.40	11.62	0.68
Tawny owl	58	17.24	29.9	35.7	0.84	28.50	0.60

Refractive powers are in diopters (D) (the reciprocal of the focal length in meters). PND is the posterior nodal distance (or anterior focal length) of the eye. All data are from schematic eye models as referenced in figure 1.1.

Optical Structure and Ecological Factors

Differences in eye structure may be associated with habitat or behavioral differences such as nocturnal versus diurnal activity, and foraging below water versus foraging in air.

Nocturnal and Diurnal Habits Manx shearwaters are regularly active by both night and day. They enter and leave their breeding colonies at night when vision is probably used to locate individual nest burrows (Brooke, 1990). Tawny owls are strictly nocturnal (Martin, 1990a), while pigeons and starlings are strictly diurnal and are rarely active after dusk, although starlings sometimes migrate at night (Feare, 1984). Figure 1.2 shows the ratio FL:FC as a function of axial length in a range of diurnal and nocturnally active species for which schematic eye data are available. The straight line is the linear regression of data points for nocturnal forms and indicates that among nocturnal species lens power becomes relatively greater as eye size decreases. No such relationship seems to exist among the few diurnally active species, for which we have data.

Hughes (1977) suggested that the ratio of posterior nodal distance:axial length (PND:AL) in bird eyes is approximately constant across species at about 0.6, while Pettigrew et al. (1988) suggested that this ratio differs between vertebrate eyes designed to function primarily under nocturnal and diurnal conditions. However, figure 1.3 shows

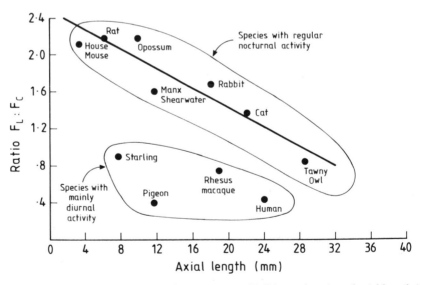

Figure 1.2 Ratio of lens:cornea refractive powers (F_L:F_C) as a function of axial length in the schematic eye models of seven species of mammals and four species of birds. The straight line is the linear regression of the data points for species that exhibit regular nocturnal activity. Data from the same sources as figure 1.1 plus rats (Hughes, 1979), house mice (Remtulla and Hallet, 1985), opossums (Oswaldo-Cruz et al., 1979), cats (Vakkur and Bishop, 1963), humans, rabbits, and Rhesus macaque (Hughes, 1977).

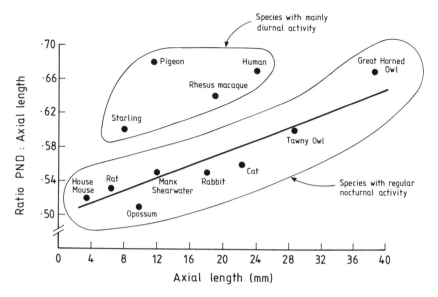

Figure 1.3 The ratio of posterior nodal distance:axial length (PND:AL) as a function of axial length in the eyes of five species of birds and seven species of mammals. The straight line is the linear regression of the data points for species that exhibit regular nocturnal activity. All data are based on schematic eye models from the same sources as listed in figure 1.2 plus data for the great horned owl (Murphy et al., 1985).

that this ratio is not simply a function of nocturnal–diurnal habits but is also a function of eye size. In small nocturnal eyes PND:AL is approximately 0.52, whereas in the largest owl eyes it is about 0.65. However, no such relationship is apparent in diurnal species although Schaeffel and Howland (1988) showed that in the developing chicken eye the ratio remained at approximately 0.6 over a wide range of axial lengths.

Amphibious Habitats   Sivak (1976) has argued that an eye designed for emmetropic vision in both air and water would benefit from a relatively flat cornea. This is because, on immersion, the refractive power of the cornea is abolished, and lost refractive power must be compensated for by increasing the power of the lens. The lower the refractive power of the cornea in air, the less compensation is required on immersion. Such an optical design is found in the eyes of penguins, where the cornea is relatively flat and consequently of low refractive power (Sivak, 1976; Martin and Young, 1984; Sivak et al., 1987). Although the refractive power of the cornea in Manx shearwaters is low compared with that in both starlings and pigeons (table 1.1), it is still approximately twice that in penguins [refractive power of the cornea in Humboldt penguins *Spheniscus humboldti* is 29.4 D (Martin and Young, 1984) compared with 68.08 D in the shearwater]. Whether the relatively less powerful cornea of shearwaters is more correctly viewed as an amphibious feature (shearwaters catch prey at the sea surface and a meter, perhaps more, below), rather than a result of optical adaptations concerned with nocturnality, is not clear. If the regression lines of figures 1.2 and 1.3 do indicate general features in the optical design of vertebrate eyes adapted for use at night, then a relatively low powered cornea would be expected for an eye with an axial length similar to that in Manx shearwaters. That the amphibious and nocturnal features of shearwater eyes cannot be easily separated illustrates the complexity of factors which underlie the apparently simple optics of bird eyes (see chapter by Katzir, this volume).

INFLUENCE OF THE IRIS

Although not a refractive component the iris controls the pupil aperture and five important functions have been ascribed to it: (1) control image brightness and prepare the eye for dark adaptation (Woodhouse and Campbell, 1975), (2) protect the eye from photic and thermal damage (Marshall et al., 1973), (3) control image quality (Denton, 1958; Campbell and Gregory, 1960, Miller, 1979), (4) control depth of focus (Miller, 1979; Martin 1983), and (5) function as part of an accommodatory mechanism (Levy and Sivak, 1980) (see section on Accommodation below). Thus the iris may serve more than one function simultaneously and factors that influence its aperture in any one circumstance will be complex. Although these factors are understood in theoretical terms data are only available concerning the first of these functions in birds eyes.

Pupil Size and Image Brightness

The brightness of the retinal image (when viewing an extended, as opposed to a point, source of light) is inversely related to the square of the f-number (Kirschfeld, 1974). [f-number = anterior focal length (PND)/entrance pupil diameter.] The smaller the f-number the relatively brighter the image.

Figure 1.4 shows maximum retinal image brightness as a function of axial length in the eyes of various species of birds and mammals. Three species—starlings, pigeons, and humans—may be regarded as primarily diurnal in their habits, while all other species are strictly nocturnal or regularly active at night. It can be seen that in both diurnal and nocturnal groups maximum retinal image brightness increases as eye size decreases. The average difference between the two groups is such that maximum image brightness appears to differ by 4- to 5-fold between nocturnal and diurnal eyes of the same size. This difference is clearly insufficient to account for the known 100-fold difference in absolute visual sensitivity between pigeons and tawny owls (Martin, 1982). It can be suggested therefore that this difference in visual sensitivity between nocturnal and diurnal birds should be attributed to differences

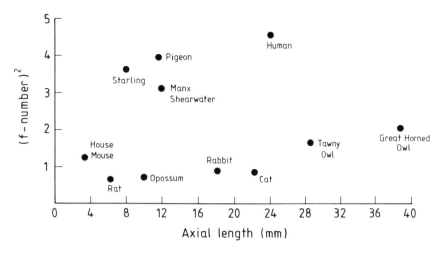

Figure 1.4 Relative maximum image brightness (f-number)^2 as a function of axial length in the eyes of six species of mammal and five species of birds. All values for (f-number)^2 are based on data from schematic eye models from the same sources as listed in figures 1.2 and 1.3.

in retinal sensitivity. However, the difference in maximum image brightness between humans and tawny owls does appear just sufficient to account for the difference in absolute visual threshold between these species (Martin, 1977) and thus suggests that their retinas are of equal sensitivity.

The difference between maximum and minimum pupil size in eyes with circular pupils produces a relatively small change in image brightness [approximately 16-fold in pigeons (Marshall et al., 1973] compared with the total range of luminance levels to which an eye can be exposed in the natural environment (approximately 11 orders of magnitude). Thus variations in pupil size cannot function to equalize image brightness over other than a small range of natural luminances.

Within a particular habitat, however, natural luminance levels usually change slowly and often by only a small amount. For example, when clouds quickly cover the sun, luminance levels change by a maximum of only 10-fold. Pupil size changes could therefore be sufficient to equalize retinal illuminance as ambient light levels change throughout the day. Thus it has been proposed that a variable pupil may function to keep the retina, even under bright-light conditions, in a partially dark-adapted state (Woodhouse and Campbell, 1975). This would be of adaptive value, since the retinal mechanisms of dark adaptation are relatively slow. With a fixed pupil a rapid diminution of ambient light level would result in the eye being inadequately dark adapted for a number of minutes. However, a partially closed mobile pupil can be rapidly opened thus increasing image luminance and so maintain optimal retinal adaptation to the new, lower, light level.

Only three species of birds, the Skimmers (Rhynchopidae), have pupils that are not circular (Zusi and Bridge, 1981). The function of the vertically oriented slit-shaped pupils in these birds is not fully understood. Slit-shaped pupils are relatively common in mammals where their function (as, for example, in the cat) has been associated with the presence of a relatively rod-rich retina, that is, a retina designed to function under the lower naturally occurring light conditions. Slit pupils can be closed to a smaller aperture than circular pupils of the same maximum aperture. Their particular function may be viewed as serving to protect such retinas from excessive bleaching of rod visual pigment, thereby enhancing the level of partial dark adaptation.

The slit pupils of the Skimmers may be viewed as well suited to such a function since in their natural habitats these birds bask in bright tropical sunlight or forage in flight low over smooth water surfaces (Zusi and Bridge, 1981). While this explanation may be true it is not known if the retinas of Skimmers are particularly rod-rich. However, these birds are noted for crepuscular and nocturnal foraging although at these times prey detection is thought to depend primarily on tactile cues from the bill rather than visual cues (Zusi and Bridge, 1981). Furthermore, it is not clear why other birds that frequent similar habitats and that may even nest in the same colonies, such as some populations of Common Terns (*Sterna hirundo*), do not also have slit pupils (Zusi and Bridge, 1981).

ACCOMMODATION

This is the process that allows the eye to bring into clear focus objects at varying distances, using a mechanism that may involve changing the refractive power of the lens and/or cornea. The range of accommodation possible in the eyes of different species is usually quantified by the change (in diopters) in the refractive power of the whole eye (a diopter is the reciprocal of the focal length in meters of the optical system). Much of the data on accommodative range is conflicting, perhaps because of differences in investigative techniques. Maximum accommodatory range for chickens are variously reported as 15–17 D (Schaeffel et al., 1986), 8–12 D (Walls, 1942), and 10–15 D (Suburo and Marcantoni, 1983); in pigeons accommodation of 8–12 D (Hess, 1910), 5 D (Levy and Sivak, 1980), 17 D (Gundlach et al., 1945), and 9 D (Schaeffel and Howland, 1987) are recorded while a study of Murphy and Howland (1983) in 15 owl (Strigiformes) species found that it ranged from 0.6 to more than 10 D. Accommodation of up to 50 D has been reported to occur in a number of amphibious species, including cormorants *Phalacrocorax carbo* (Hess, 1910), dippers *Cinclus mexicanus* (Goodge, 1960), hooded mergansers *Mergus cucullatus*, and redheads *Aythya americana* (Levy and Sivak, 1980). It is argued that such an extremely large range is necessary in these amphibious species to overcome the refractive error produced in an aerial emmetropic eye when the power of the cornea is negated by entry into water.

Another indication of the accommodatory range of an eye is given by the "near point of accommodation," i.e. the closest distance at which an object is presumed to be clearly focused upon the retina, and this will vary with luminance level. At high light levels, pigeons begin the ballistic phase of their pecks, which is thought to indicate the closest distance of accommodation, at between 55 and 66 mm from the target (Goodale, 1983; Macko and Hodos, 1985), compared with the distance of approximately 35 mm at which European starlings apparently inspect objects lying at the tips of their bills (Martin, 1986b).

Dynamic Accommodation Mechanisms

Beer (1893) presented evidence that accommodation in birds (pigeons, chickens, ducks, hawks, and owls) involves the cornea as well as the lens. This view was supported by Gundlach et al. (1945) in pigeons, but corneal accommodation was not confirmed in either owls (Steinbach and Money, 1973) or ducks (Levy and Sivak, 1980). Further support for corneal and lenticular accommodation in both chickens and pigeons has recently been provided (Troilo and Wallman, 1987; Schaeffel and Howland, 1987). Corneal accommodation is brought about by a change in the corneal radius of curvature, and in pigeons it accounts for most, if not all, of natural accommodation (up to approximately 9 D). In chickens, corneal accommodation is combined with lenticular accommodation, the two components contributing approximately equally to the total accommodatory range (15–17 D). Accommodation in chickens is completely independent in each eye (Schaeffel et al., 1986).

Accommodation in birds is probably mediated by the striated ciliary muscles. However, there is conflicting opinion about the number of these muscles, their mode of action, and the ways that they can influence the refractive power of both the cornea and lens. A wide variety of mechanisms has been proposed including active squeezing of the lens by the posterior ciliary muscle (Meyer, 1977), moving the lens forward (Slonaker, 1918), and changes in the hydrostatic pressure gradient between the vitreous body, lens, and anterior chamber, mediated primarily by the control of the flow of aqueous humour from the anterior chamber (Suburo and Marcantoni, 1983; see also Levy and Sivak, 1980; Coleman, 1986). To account for the high magnitude lenticular accommodation of some amphibious birds it has been suggested that the iris can form a rigid disk onto which the malleable lens is pushed and this produces a highly curved protuberance on the lens front surface where it bulges through the pupil (Hess, 1910; Levy and Sivak, 1980).

All these dynamic accommodation mechanisms involve the increase of refractive power in order to bring close objects into clear focus on the retina. However, decreases of up to 6 D in accommodatory power have also been found in chicken (Schaeffel et al., 1986) and the eye of the Humboldt penguin may require considerable loss of refractive power (26 D) in order to focus clearly in air and water (Martin and Young, 1984; Sivak et al., 1987) but the mechanisms involved are not known.

Static Accommodation Mechanisms

Although accommodation usually involves changing the refractive power of the eye to bring into focus images of objects at different distances, in some birds, objects at different distances can be simultaneously in focus even if the optical system itself has a shallow depth of focus. This is achieved by asymmetries in the eye's optical structure, such that the eye is emmetropic in some parts of the visual field and myopic in others. Initial studies in pigeons suggested that its eye was myopic in the frontal plane and emmetropic laterally (Millodot and Blough, 1971; Nye, 1973).

Further analysis has shown that this asymmetry of refraction within pigeons' visual fields is far from simple. Thus, the lateral visual field along a horizontal viewing direction and in the upper lateral visual field receives a well-focused image of distant objects. However, the lower lateral visual field and the lower binocular fields are myopic but the degree of myopia is not constant (Fitzke et al., 1985; McFadden, personal communication). The eye becomes progressively more myopic with decreasing elevation and this progressive change in myopic state seems sufficient to keep an image of the ground, at various distances from the standing bird, in sharp focus simultaneously. This refractive asymmetry should therefore enable pigeons to monitor the activities of conspecifics, scan for predators, or note celestial cues while foraging for nearby objects on the ground. This static accommodatory mechanism is not unique to pigeons but is also found in quails, chickens, and sandhill cranes *Grus canadensis* with the degree of lower field myopia related to the average height of the bird's eye (when walking in an upright posture) above the ground (Hodos and Erichsen, 1990). The optical mechanisms responsible for these changes in accommodation across the visual field are not clear, but could involve asymmetry of the cornea, asymmetry of the lens and cornea about an optical axis, or asymmetry of the retina about the optic axis (see Martin, 1986b).

EYE POSITION AND VISUAL FIELDS

The visual field of a bird defines that portion of space about it in which visual control of behavior may be possible. Head movements can allow a bird to scan all segments of space but we are concerned here with the portion of space that can be viewed instantaneously without head movements. This functional visual field is not identical with the optical field of view, i.e., the angular segment of space that is imaged by the optical system. Indeed, in all known bird eyes the functional retinal visual field of the eye has been found to be narrower than the optical visual field. This is because, although the eye may image a given segment of space, the extent of the retina may mean that not all of this image is analyzed by the visual system. The eyes of all birds are placed laterally in the skull and, even in so-called "frontally eyed" birds (like owls) the eyes do not face directly forward, parallel to each other (Martin, 1984). Functional analysis of visual fields is further confounded by the fact that in many species they can be altered considerably by eye movements that in birds are not necessarily conjugate (Nye, 1969).

Monocular, Binocular, and Panoramic Visual Fields

The optical visual field of an eye will vary between species depending on the precise relationship between the refractive powers and positions of lens and cornea (Martin, 1983). In the bird species so far examined, the functional monocular visual fields served by the retina (the retinal visual field) are highly asymmetric with respect to the optic axis. In some species (e.g., tawny owl; Martin, 1984) this has been shown to be due in part to marked asymmetries of the retina with respect to the optic axis. In all species the nasal hemifield (the portion of the visual field in a horizontal plane between the optic axis and the beak) is smallest while the temporal hemifield is always the largest (table 1.2). This seems surprising since, because of the lateral placement of the eyes, it is the nasal portion of the monocular fields that serves binocular vision and thus binocular field width would appear not to be maximized.

One possible explanation of this failure to use the full potential nasal visual field may be the need for a high quality optical image in frontal vision, which is invariably used to guide motion. Using the full width of the available optical field in the temporal quadrant may not be re-

Table 1.2. Monocular Retinal Field Widths (Degrees) in an Approximately Horizontal Plane that Contains the Optic Axes of Both Eyes in Five Species of Birds

Species	Total	Nasal	Temporal	Nasal:temporal
Pigeon	169	77	92	0.84
Mallard duck	191	92	99	0.93
Tawny owl	124	51	73	0.70
European starling	161	70	91	0.77
Manx shearwater	148	65	83	0.78

Data from the same sources as Figure 1.1 plus pigeons (Martin and Young, 1983 and mallards (Martin, 1986c).

stricted in this way because this portion of the visual field is not used for the control of behavior with respect to the critical detail of objects, but rather to simply detect the presence of objects that are then scrutinized by the frontal or central portions of the retinal visual fields. The assumption in such an analysis, however, is that image quality necessarily deteriorates with increasing eccentricity from the optic axis. While this assumption may be true for man-made optical systems, there is evidence that poor image quality in the periphery is not a necessary property of the vertebrate eye (Hughes and Vaney, 1978; Murphy and Howland, 1983).

The extent of the binocular and panoramic visual fields is determined by the position and movement of eyes in the skull. These fields are complex three-dimensional structures but some idea of the diversity of field shapes can be gained from figure 1.5, which presents the visual fields of four species in an approximately horizontal plane when the eyes have adopted a resting position. (Figure 1.6 presents the frontal retinal fields of tawny owls and Manx shearwaters.)

In pigeons, shearwaters, and starlings the line of the bill projects approximately at the center of this long binocular field (figure 1.6) and this can probably be correlated with the use of visual cues to control bill direction with respect to food items during foraging. This view is reinforced by comparative data from species in which bill position does not seem to be critically controlled by vision during foraging. Thus, in owls, the projection of the bill falls outside of the visual field (figure 1.6). This may be correlated with owl's habit of using its feet to catch prey, swinging them forward to lie within the region of the binocular field just prior to prey capture (Martin, 1984, 1990a). In mallard ducks, shovelers, and woodcocks (*Scolopax rusticola*), the bill falls on the periphery of their visual fields (Martin, 1986c and personal observation). This may be related to the fact that their foraging can be guided by tactile, rather than visual, cues (Gottschaldt, 1985). In these birds the eyes are placed so far back in the skull that there is a binocular field that extends from the bill through 180° to directly behind the head (Martin, 1986c and personal observation). Thus these birds have no blind area and can see the whole of the celestial hemisphere while the eyes are in their resting position.

Similar visual coverage of the world above and behind the head can almost be achieved in starlings by virtue of eye movements. In these birds the eyes can be swung forward and downward to achieve a binocular field about the bill as wide as that of owls, but the eyes can also be swung backward and upward to give the birds almost complete coverage of the celestial hemisphere, but at the same time abolishing the frontal binocular field (Martin, 1986b). Eye movements have their largest amplitude in a plane that passes approximately 20° below the bill. These alterations of the panoramic and binocular fields may enable starlings to use a large binocular field when searching for prey at or

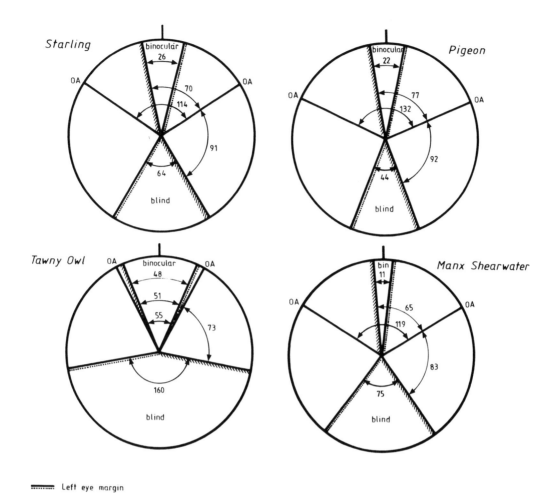

=========== Left eye margin

～～～～ Right eye margin

Figure 1.5 Diagrammatic representation of the retinal visual fields of Manx shearwaters, European starlings, pigeons, and tawny owls in an approximately horizontal plane containing the optic axes (OA). The bar at the top of each diagram indicates the direction of the bill. All numerical values are in degrees (expressed with reference to a hypothetical projection center, which lies at the center of the bird's skull midway between the nodal points of the eyes) and show the width of the binocular field, the width of the blind area behind the head, the divergence of the optic axes, and the width of the nasal and temporal hemifields of each eye. Data for starlings refer to the position of the eyes adopted post mortem (Martin, 1986b), whereas those for the other three species refer to the visual fields measured in sedated birds (Martin, 1984; Martin and Brooke, 1991).

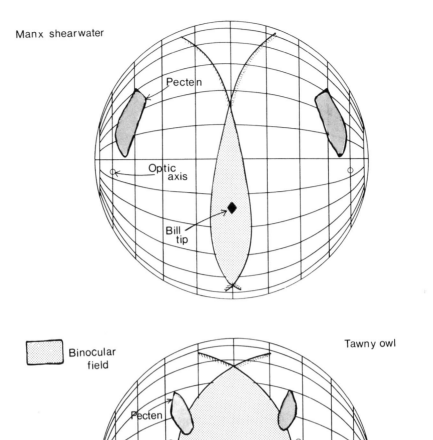

Manx shearwater

Pecten

Optic axis

Bill tip

Binocular field

Tawny owl

Pecten

Optic axis

Right eye Margin

Bill tip

Left eye Margin

Figure 1.6 Projection of the mean retinal field margins of the Manx shearwaters and tawny owls. In shearwaters the visual field is that determined when the eyes have adopted their presumed resting position. Eye movements are absent in owls (Steinbach and Money, 1973). The mean visual projections of the optic axes, pectens, and bill tip are also shown. The data are presented as though drawn on the projected surface of a sphere centered on the bird's head. The bird may be envisaged as facing the reader from the center of the diagram. The coordinate system follows that of conventional latitude and longitude, but with the poles opposite each eye and the equator (which falls within the bird's median sagittal plane) aligned vertically. All numerical values are in degrees (Martin, 1984; Martin and Brooke, 1991).

near the bill tips, while momentarily being able to scan the celestial hemisphere for conspecifics (starlings are highly sociable) and/or predators. Furthermore, extensive visual coverage of the celestial hemisphere could be of particular importance in the detection of navigational and orientational cues, in such migratory birds (Martin, 1990b). Wallman and Pettigrew (1985) showed how the eye movements of Tawny Frogmouths *Podargus strigoides* could also provide this bird with extensive visual coverage of the lateral visual field or a large frontal binocular field. Nalbach et al. (1990; see chapter 2) have described in detail the full extent of eye movements in pigeons and have shown how these rotations of the globe, as in starlings, can greatly enlarge the region of binocular overlap below the bill and also bring specialized areas of the retina to view particular portions of visual space about the bird.

Clearly eye movements can potentially alter the visual fields of birds in complex ways that are likely to be of considerable importance in an individual species' life style. Teasing out the important parameters of visual fields and how they are altered by eye movements requires further comparative data and detailed study of how vision is used in the control of key behaviors, especially, orientation and navigation, foraging, and surveillance for predators.

REFERENCES

Beer, T. Studien uber die Akkommodation des Vogelauges. *Pflugers Arch.* 53 (1893), 175–237.

Brooke, M. *The Manx Shearwater*. T and A D Poyser, London, 1990.

Campbell, F. W., and Gregory, A. H. Effect of size of pupil on visual acuity. *Nature (London)* 187 (1960), 1121–1123.

Coleman, D. J. On the unified suspension theory of accommodation. *Trans. Am. Ophthal. Soc.* 84 (1986), 846–868.

Denton, E. J. The response of the pupil of the gekko to external light stimulus. *J. Gen. Physiol.* 40 (1958), 201–218.

Donner, K. O. The visual acuity of some passerine birds. *Acta Zool. Fenn.* 66 (1951), 1–40.

Feare, C. J. *The Starling*, Oxford University Press, Oxford, 1984.

Fitzke, F. W., Hayes, B. P., Hodos, W., Holden, A. L., and Low, J. C. Refractive sectors in the visual field of the pigeon eye. *J. Physiol. London* 369 (1985), 33–44.

Fox, R., Lehmkuhle, S. W., and Westendorf, D. H. Falcon visual acuity. *Science, Wash., D.C.* 192 (1976), 263–265.

Goodale, M. A. Visually guided pecking in the pigeon. *Brain Behav. Evol.* 2 (1983), 22–41.

Goodge, W. R. Adaptations for amphibious vision in the Dipper (*Cinclus mexicanus*). *J. Morphol.* 107 (1960), 79–91.

Gottschaldt, K.-M. Structure and function of avian somatosensory receptors. In A. S. King and J. McLelland (Eds.), *Form and Function in Birds*, Vol III. Academic Press, London (1985).

Gundlach, R. H., Chard, R. D., and Skahen, J. R. The mechanism of accommodation in pigeons. *J. Comp. Psychol.* 38 (1945), 27–42.

Hess, C. Die Akkommodation bei Tauchervogeln. *Arch. Vergl. Ophthalmol.* 1 (1910), 153–164.

Hirsch, J. Falcon visual sensitivity to grating contrasts. *Nature (London)* 300 (1982), 57–58.

Hodos, W., and Erichsen, J. T. Lower-field myopia in birds; An adaptation that keeps the ground in focus. *Vision Res.* 30 (1990), 653–657.

Hughes, A. The topography of vision in mammals of contrasting life style: Comparative optics and retinal organisation. In F. Cresitelli (Ed.), *Handbook of Sensory Physiology*, Vol. VII/5 Springer, Berlin, 1977.

Hughes, A. A schematic eye for the rat. *Vision Res.* 19 (1979), 569–588.

Hughes, A. The schematic eye comes of age. In J. Pettigrew, K. J. Sanderson and W. R. Levick (Eds.), *Visual Neuroscience*. Cambridge University Press, Cambridge, 1986.

Hughes, A., and Vaney, D. I. The refractive state of the rabbit eye: variation with eccentricity and correction of oblique astigmatism. *Vision Res.* 18 (1978), 1351–1355.

King, A. S., and King, D. Z. Avian morphology: General principles, In A. S. King and J. McLelland (Eds.), *Form and Function in Birds*. Vol. 1. Academic Press, London, 1980.

Kirschfeld, K. Absolute sensitivity of lens and compound eyes. *Z. Naturforsch* 29c (1974), 592–596.

Levy, B., and Sivak, J. G. Mechanisms of accommodation in the bird eye. *J. Comp. Physiol.* 137 (1980), 267–272.

Macko, K. A., and Hodos, W. Near point of accommodation in pigeons. *Vision Res.* 25 (1985), 1529–1530.

Marshall, J., Mellerio, J., and Palmer, D. A. A schematic eye for the pigeon (*Columba livia*). *Vision Res.* 13 (1973), 2449–2453.

Martin, G. R. Absolute visual threshold and scotopic spectral sensitivity in the tawny owl. *Strix aluco, Nature (London)* 268 (1977), 636–638.

Martin, G. R. An owl's eye: schematic optics and visual performance in *Strix aluco* L., *J. Comp. Physiol.* 145 (1982), 341–349.

Martin, G. R. Schematic eye models in vertebrates. In D. Ottoson (Ed.), *Progress in Sensory Physiology*, Vol. 4. Springer, Berlin, 1983.

Martin, G. R. The visual fields of the tawny owl (*Strix aluco*). *Vision Res.* 24 (1984), 1739–1751.

Martin, G. R. Eye. In A. S. King and J. McLelland, *Form and Function in Birds*, Vol. III. Academic Press, London, 1985.

Martin, G. R. Sensory capacities and the nocturnal habit in owls. *Ibis* 128 (1986a), 266–277.

Martin, G. R. The eye of a passeriform bird, the European starling (*Sturnus vulgaris*): Eye movement amplitude, visual fields and schematic optics. *J. Comp. Physiol.* 159 (1986b), 545–557.

Martin, G. R. Total panoramic vision in the mallard duck, *Anas platyrhynchos. Vision Res.* 26 (1986c), 1303–1305.

Martin, G. R. *Birds by Night*. T and A D Poyser, London (1990a).

Martin, G. R. The visual problems of nocturnal migration. In E. Gwinner (Ed.), *Bird Migration: Physiology and Ecophysiology*. Springer-Verlag, Berlin (1990b).

Martin, G. R., and Brooke, M. The eye of a Procellariiform seabird, the Manx shearwater, *Puffinus puffinus*: Visual fields and optical structure, *Brain Behav. Evol.* 37 (1991), 65–78.

Martin, G. R., and Young, S. R. The retinal binocular field of the pigeon (*Columba livia*): English racing homer. *Vision Res.* 23 (1983), 911–915.

Martin, G. R., and Young, S. R. The eye of the Humboldt penguin *Spheniscus humboldti*: Visual fields and schematic optics. *Proc. R. Soc. London Ser. B* 223 (1984), 197–222.

Martinoya, C., Rey, J., and Bloch, S. Limits of the pigeon's binocular field and direction for best binocular viewing. *Vision Res.* 21 (1981), 1197–1200.

Meyer, D. B. C. The avian eye and its adaptations. In F. Crescitelli (Ed.), *Handbook of Sensory Physiology*, Vol. VII/5. Springer-Verlag, Berlin (1977).

Miller, W. H. Ocular optical filtering. In H. Autrum (Ed.), *Handbook of Sensory Physiology*, Vol. VII/6A. Springer-Verlag, Berlin (1979).

Millodot, M., and Blough, P. The refractive condition of the pigeon eye. *Vision Res.* 11 (1971), 1019–1022.

Murphy, C. J., and Howland, H. C. Owl eyes: Accommodation, corneal curvature and refractive state. *J. Comp. Physiol.* 151 (1983), 277–284.

Murphy, C. H., Evans, H. E., and Howland, H. C. Towards a schematic eye for the great horned owl. *Fortsch. Zool.* 30 (1985), 703–706.

Nalbach, H-O., Wolf-Oberhollenzer, F., and Kirschfeld, K. The pigeon's eye viewed through an ophthalmoscopic microscope: Orientation of retinal landmarks and significance of eye movements. *Vision Res.* 30 (1990), 529–540.

Nye, P. W. The monocular eye movements of the pigeon. *Vision Res.* 9 (1969), 133–144.

Nye, P. W. On the functional differences between frontal and lateral visual fields of the pigeon. *Vision Res.* 13 (1973), 559–574.

Oswaldo-Cruz, E., Hokoc, J. N., and Sousa, A. P. B. A schematic eye for the opossum. *Vision Res.* 19 (1979), 263–278.

Pettigrew, J. D., Dreher, B., Hopkins, C. S., McCall, M. J., and Brown, M. Peak density and distribution of ganglion cells in the retinae of microchiropteran bats: implications for visual acuity. *Brain, Behav. Evol.* 32 (1988), 39–56.

Reid, B., and Williams, G. R. The Kiwi. In G. Kuschell (Ed.), *Biogeography and Ecology in New Zealand*. Junk, The Hague (1975).

Remtulla, S., and Hallett, P. E. A schematic eye for the mouse, and comparisons with the rat. *Vision Res.* 25 (1985), 21–31.

Reymond, L. Spatial visual acuity of the eagle *Aquila audax*: A behavioural, optical and anatomical investigation. *Vision Res.* 25 (1985), 1477–1491.

Reymond, L., and Wolfe, J. Behavioural determination of the contrast sensitivity function of the eagle *Aquila audax*. *Vision Res.* 21 (1981), 263–271.

Rochon-Duvigneaud, A. *Les yeux et la vision des vertebres*. Masson, Paris (1943).

Schaeffel, F., and Howland, H. C. Corneal accommodation in chick and pigeon. *J. Comp. Physiol.* 160 (1987), 375–384.

Schaeffel, F., and Howland, H. C. Visual optics in normal and ametropic chickens. *Clin. Vision Sci.* 3 (1988), 83–98.

Schaeffel, F., Howland, H. C., and Farkas, L. Natural accommodation in the growing chicken. *Vision Res.* 26 (1986), 1977–1993.

Schaeffel, F., Glasser, A., and Howland, H. C. Accommodation, refractive error and eye growth in chickens. *Vision Res.* 28 (1988), 639–657.

Sivak, J. G. The role of a flat cornea in the amphibious behaviour of the blackfoot penguin (*Spheniscus demersus*). *Can. J. Zool.* 54 (1976), 1341–1346.

Sivak, J. G., and Howland, H. C. Refractive state of the eye of the brown kiwi (*Apteryx australis*). *Can. J. Zool.* 65 (1987), 2833–2835.

Sivak, J., Howland, H. C., and McGill-Harelstad, P. Vision of the Humboldt penguin (*Spheniscus humboldti*) in air and water. *Proc. R. Soc. London Ser. B* 229 (1987), 467–472.

Slonaker, J. R. A physiological study of the anatomy of the eye and its accessory parts of the English Sparrow (*Passer domesticus*). *J. Morphol.* 31 (1918), 351–359.

Snyder, A. W., Laughlin, S. B., and Stavenga, D. G. Information capacity of eyes. *Vision Res.* 17 (1977), 1163–1175.

Steinbach, M. J., and Money, K. E. Eye movements of the owl. *Vision Res.* 13 (1973), 889–891.

Suburo, A. M., and Marcantoni, M. The structural basis of ocular accommodation in the chick. *Rev. Can. Biol. Exp.* 42 (1983), 131–137.

Troilo, D., and Wallman, J. Changes in corneal curvature during accommodation in chicks. *Vision Res.* 27 (1987), 241–247.

Vakkur, G. J., and Bishop, P. O. The schematic eye in the cat. *Vision Res.* 3 (1963), 357–381.

Wallman, J., and Pettigrew, J. Conjugate and disjunctive saccades in two avian species with contrasting oculomotor strategies. *J. Neurosci.* 5 (1985), 1418–1428.

Walls, G. L. *The Vertebrate Eye and Its Adaptive Radiation.* Cranbrook Institute of Science, Bloomfield Hills, MI, 1942.

Woodhouse, J. M., and Campbell, F. W. The role of the pupil light reflex in aiding adaptation to the dark. *Vision Res.* 15 (1975), 649–653.

Zusi, R. L., and Bridge, D. On the slit pupil of the black skimmer. *J. Field. Ornithol.* 52 (1981), 338–340.

2 Exploring the Image

Hans-Ortwin Nalbach, Friederike Wolf-Oberhollenzer, and Monika Remy

The image projected on the retina by the optics of the eye results in a pattern of differentially stimulated photoreceptor cells that must be analyzed by an array of neural networks from the retina to the brain. In this section we examine regional variations in the retinas of birds and their possible functional significance for visual information processing.

THE PHOTORECEPTOR LAYER

The background of the avian eye, the fundus oculi, is characterized by two prominent morphological features, the pecten, a comb-like structure protruding from the optic nerve head into the vitreous, and the granulation of the retina, which is caused by specular reflections from oil droplets within the cones.

The Pecten

This is a highly pigmented and manifoldly pleated structure whose shape varies widely among avian species. Although it has been hypothesized to play a role in visual perception (reviews in Martin, 1985; Meyer, 1986), it is primarily involved in the nutrition of the inner retinal layers. Evidence indicative of this function includes the absence of intraretinal blood vessels in birds, the considerable vascularization of the pecten, the presence of an oxygen gradient from the pecten to the retina, and the passing of nutrients from the pecten into the vitreous (Wingstrand and Munk, 1965; Bellhorn and Bellhorn 1975). Retinal perfusion is optimized by saccadic eye movements with the pecten acting as an agitator to propel nutrients and oxygen toward the central retina (Pettigrew et al., 1990).

The Photoreceptors

The avian photoreceptor complex, which may be arranged in a highly regular pattern ("retinal mosaic": Engstroem, 1958; Morris, 1970) comprises rods, double cones, and several types of single cones (Oehme 1961, 1962, 1964; Morris and Shorey 1967; Morris 1970; Mariani and Leure-DuPree, 1978). Cones may usually be distinguished from rods by the presence of an oil droplet (but see Sillman et al., 1981). Rods mediate vision at low light levels and cones in bright light (Blough, 1956). Not surprisingly, the retinas of diurnal birds are dominated by cones, which may constitute up to 80% of the visual cells (Bowmaker, 1980), while rods make up 30–40% of extrafoveal photoreceptors (Oehme, 1962, 1964; Meyer and May, 1973). Almost 90% of the receptors in some owl species are rods (Oehme, 1961; Fite, 1973), while they constitute only about 11% of the photoreceptor population in swifts (Oehme, 1962). Rod density may vary across the retina, as in the pigeon with rods making up to 30% of all photoreceptors in the yellow field (see below) and only 5% in the red field (Schultze, 1866; van Genderen Stort, 1887).

Double cones, which are present in all vertebrates except placentalia, consist of a principal member and an adjacent accessory member (review in Meyer, 1986), one or both of which may contain an oil droplet (Bowmaker, 1977; Mariani and Leure-DuPree, 1978; Cserhati et al., 1989). In some birds, double cones represent up to 50% of the total cone population (Oehme, 1962; Bowmaker and Knowles, 1977; Bowmaker, 1977; Jane and Bowmaker, 1988); in others they are rare (Oehme, 1962; Gallego et al., 1975) or even lacking (Oehme, 1961; Fite, 1973; Bowmaker and Martin, 1978, 1985; Sillman et al., 1981). The functional significance of this interspecific variation is not known.

The retina of birds contains a number of different photopigment types (Jane and Bowmaker, 1988; Varela et al., this volume). Rhodopsin, the rod pigment, has an absorption maximum between 500 and 506 nm (Bowmaker, 1977; Sillman et al., 1981). Iodopsin and related cone pigments have absorption maxima around 567, 514, 467, and 413 nm in chicken and pigeons (Bowmaker 1977; Govardovskij and Zueva 1977). Short wavelength-sensitive (near-ultraviolet) receptors have been reported in pigeon and several passerines (Chen et al., 1984; Chen and Goldsmith 1986).

The Oil Droplets

The presence of oil droplets is a common feature of the cones (but not the rods) of most vertebrate retinas (Muntz, 1972). Oil droplets consist of lipids in which carotenoid pigments, usually xantophylls, are dissolved (Goldsmith et al., 1984). Depending on the type and amount of carotenoids, the droplets appear transparent, clear, pale yellow to green, orange, or red (see Varela et al., this volume). Positioned at the distal end of the inner cone segment, they comprise the entire width of the receptor. Thus light has to traverse the oil droplet before entering the photosensitive outer segment. Microspectrophotometric measurements revealed that oil droplets act as cut-off filters, absorbing light below their characteristic wavelengths of transmission and conveying only longer wavelengths to their associated photopigments.

The various types of oil droplets are distributed in layers within the retina, with yellow droplets most sclerad, the pale and greenish most vitread, and the red and orange ones in between (Waelchli, 1883; van Genderen Stort, 1887; Mariani and Leure-DuPree, 1978; Cserhati et al., 1989). There are also differences in the distribution of oil droplets across the various retinal areas (Muntz, 1972; Goldsmith et al., 1984; Partridge, 1989). Pale droplets appear to dominate the ventral area; long wavelength transmitting droplets and colorless droplets dominate the dorsal retina. Furthermore, there are proportionally more red oil droplets in the area or fovea centralis than in its periphery (Waelchli, 1883; Galifret, 1968; Nalbach et al., 1990). The inhomogeneous distribution of oil droplets is most striking in the pigeon retina. Large numbers of red and orange droplets—in combination with microdroplets (Pedler and Boyle, 1969)—are found in the dorsotemporal (red) field, and yellow or yellow-greenish droplets dominate the remaining part of the retina, the yellow field (Waelchli, 1883). The wavelengths transmitted by oil droplets in the red field are in general 10 nm longer than those transmitted through the corresponding type of droplets in the yellow field (Bowmaker, 1977).

Function of Oil Droplets

The optic media of the avian eye transmit all wavelengths from red to ultraviolet (Emmerton et al., 1980). This transparency allows vision in the near–UV, possibly at the cost of considerable blur of the image due to chromatic aberration. By absorbing short wavelengths, colored oil droplets in birds, like the yellow lenses of mammals (Walls and Judd, 1933), would reduce the blur, and, additionally, might provide a selective shield against harmful effects of UV radiation (Lythgoe, 1979; Kirschfeld, 1982; Goldsmith, 1990). Oil droplets may also act as lenses focusing light onto the outer segment of the photoreceptors, thus enhancing the quantum catch of the visual pigments (Young and Martin, 1984). Finally, because the oil droplets modify the spectral composition of light incident on the photopigments, it has long been assumed that they play some role in color vision (see the chapter by Varela et al., this volume).

Spectral Sensitivity

The pigeon's spectral sensitivity comprises the range from ultraviolet to infrared (320–650 nm). Slight differences in the spectral sensitivity of the red and yellow fields over a range from 450 to 650 nm have been demonstrated using both electrophysiological and behavioral techniques (Muntz, 1972; Martin and Muntz, 1978; Wortel et al., 1984). However, the two methods yielded conflicting data for the UV portion of the range (figure 2.1); an electrophysiological study (using a 12° stimulus) finding no differences (Wortel et al., 1984), while a behavioral study in the head-fixed pigeon (using a 1° stimulus) found that UV sensitivity was high in the yellow field and low in the red field (Remy and Emmerton, 1989; Wortel et al., 1987). The discrepancy may be related to differences in stimulus size, since, in humans, large stimuli presented to the peripheral retina (where cones are sparse) produce the same color sensation as a small stimulus presented foveally (Gordon and Abramov, 1977).

Differences in the UV sensitivity of the red and yellow fields may reflect differences in the number of colorless oil droplets, since these droplets, in association with specific photoreceptor pigments, may mediate UV vision in birds. Since pigeons show excellent behavioral dis-

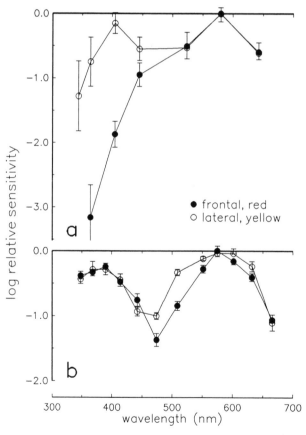

Figure 2.1 Relative spectral sensitivities of pigeons stimulated in their lateral yellow or their frontal red field. (a) After Remy and Emmerton (1989). (b) After Wortel et al. (1984).

crimination of patterns illuminated by UV light (Emmerton, 1983a) they may use the high UV sensitivity of the yellow field to detect and analyze objects that specifically reflect UV radiation (e.g., berries, plumage; Burkhardt, 1982, 1989). In chickens, UV sensitivity is controlled by a diurnal rhythm and is highest at dusk, enhancing orientation in twilight (Schaeffel et al., 1991). Thus endogenous activity as well as regional variations in receptor distribution may alter the spectral sensitivity of a retinal field.

NEURONAL WIRING OF THE AVIAN RETINA

Structural Organization of the Retinal Layers

In its gross anatomy and division into six layers the avian retina (figure 2.2) resembles that of other vertebrates (for review of older literature see Hayes, 1982; Martin, 1985). Its general structure is constant over the whole eye cup, but its thickness increases from the periphery to the parafoveal region because of corresponding increases in the inner plexiform and inner nuclear layers (IPL; INL). In pigeon, rods and principal members of the double cones terminate in the outer sublayer of the outer plexiform layer (OPL), the straight single cones in its middle sublayer while the oblique single cones end exclusively in the inner sublayer (Mariani and Leure-duPree, 1978; Mariani, 1987). In nocturnal

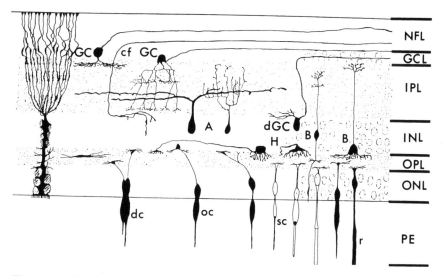

Figure 2.2 Sketch of the layering in the avian retina (after Franz, 1934). PE, pigment epithelium, containing the outer parts of the photoreceptors (r, rod; sc, single straight cone; oc, oblique cone; dc, double cone): ONL, outer nuclear layer; OPL, outer plexiform layer; INL, inner nuclear layer; IPL, inner plexiform layer; GCL, ganglion cell layer; NFL, nerve fiber layer; A, amacrine cell; B, bipolar cell; cf, centrifugal fiber; GC, ganglion cell; dGC, displaced ganglion cell; H, horizontal cell.

birds with a reduced set of cones a distinct layering is missing (Gallego et al., 1975).

Based on their locations and dendritic morphology, Mariani (1987) distinguished four types of horizontal cells (H1–H4) and eight types of bipolar cells (B1–B8). The axonal terminations of the bipolars extend into the IPL, which is differentiated into five sublayers (S1–S5) with each bipolar type showing a distinct pattern of arborization in the INL. Golgi studies in the pigeon revealed several types of amacrine cells of which only one type possesses an axon (Mariani, 1982). Among the axonless amacrines some have radially protruding dendrites (Mariani, 1982; Hayes, 1984) while the dendritic trees of others extend ventrodorsally over the retina (Mariani, 1983). In addition to "orthotopic" amacrines, i.e., cells with soma in the INL, there are "displaced amacrine" cells whose somata lie in the ganglion cell layer GCL (Hayes, 1984). In the chicken, "proprioretinal" amacrines provide long intraretinal connections with no axons joining the optic nerve (Catsicas et al., 1987a). Finally, there are cells with somata in the INL that send axons through the IPL to join the optic nerve. Because of their nonorthotopic somata these cells are called "displaced" ganglion cells and they all project to one central nucleus in the accessory optic system, the nucleus of the basal optic root (nBOR) (Karten et al., 1977; Fite et al., 1981). The orthotopic ganglion cells together with the displaced amacrines constitute the ganglion cell (GC) layer and its cells may be divided into several morphological and biochemical types (see review by Karten et al., 1990).

In all visual systems, convergence from photoreceptors via bipolars onto ganglion cells determines light sensitivity as well as spatial resolution. Accordingly, retinal locations that correspond to high acuity in the visual field (fovea, area centralis, or visual streak) are distinguished by a high density of photoreceptors as well as by an increased number of bipolars and ganglion cells per photoreceptor compared to peripheral parts of the retina. At such specialized locations, there is less convergence of signals from photoreceptors onto ganglion cells. Indeed, in the primate fovea the ratio of photoreceptor to bipolar to ganglion cells attains a value of 1:1:1, earning the name "midget system" (Boycott and Dowling, 1969).

Similarly, variation in photoreceptor density in the ONL of the pigeon is paralleled by a variation in the density of cells in the INL and in the GCL (Galifret, 1968). In these three layers the highest cell densities occur foveally and parafoveally, but nearly the same densities have been observed in the dorsotemporal quadrant of the retina (figure 2.3B), which corresponds to the red field (Hayes, 1982). However, regional variation in cell density does not necessarily correlate with synaptic complexity (Yazulla, 1974). In pigeons, for example, there are many more amacrine synapses in the red field than in parafoveal regions. The IPL is most complex in the red field followed by the temporal and the nasal yellow field. It is least complex in the area centralis, which is

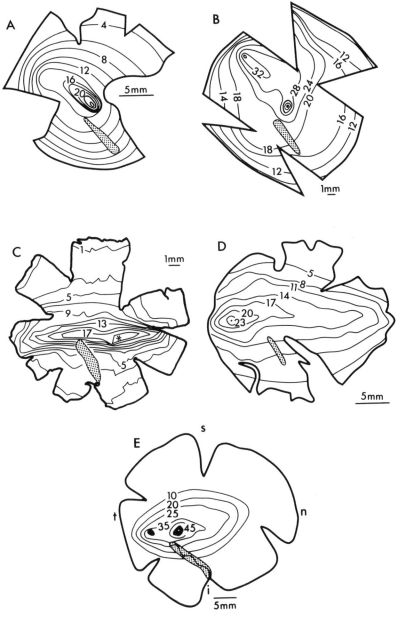

Figure 2.3 Radial distribution of retinal ganglion cell densities. (A) Chicken. Method: Nissl stain. After Ehrlich (1981). (B) Pigeon. Method: silver stain after Palmgren. After Bingelli and Paule (1969). (C) Manx shearwater. Method: Nissl stain. *Peak density of 21,500 cells/mm². After Hayes and Brooke (1990). (D) Burrowing owl. Method: Nissl stain. Dot: fovea. After Bravo and Pettigrew (1981). (E) Chilean eagle. Method: Nissl stain. Black areas: highest ganglion cell densities parafoveally. After Inzunza et al. (1991). (A)–(E) Orientation as shown in (E): i, inferior; n, nasal; s, superior; t, temporal. Stippled area, pecten. Numbers indicate 10³/mm².

thought to be specialized for precise point-to-point transmission by a "midget system" that does not require extensive processing by amacrine cells. Bipolar cells that have dendritic trees small enough to relay signals from only a single photoreceptor and could plausibly be components of a midget system have been described in several species (Cajal, 1933; Lockhart, 1979; Mariani, 1987; Quesada et al., 1988).

Comparative Considerations

The structural diversity of the avian retina may be viewed as a set of variations on a common groundplan. In species that live in a unique and clearly defined visual habitat, certain features of retinal structure appear to reflect ecological constraints (Meyer, 1977; Hughes, 1977; Martin, 1985). Birds living in open scenery typically possess a ribbon-like area centralis (figure 2.3C; Duijm, 1958), which is nearly aligned with the horizon and with the horizontal semicircular canals, when the head is in the "alert" head position (see below). In contrast, the streak of slightly increased ganglion cell density connecting the central and temporal retina in both granivorous (figure 2.3A,B) and predatory birds (figure 2.3D,E) may reflect a behavioral function in gaze shifts from lateral to frontal fixation rather than adaptation to a specific visual environment. In falconiformes, which possess both a temporal and a central fovea, the temporal fovea is pronounced only in those species that actually capture their prey from the air or perches but not in species that pick up carrion, insects, and fruit from the ground (Inzunza et al., 1991). On the other hand, a single (temporal) fovea characterizes nocturnal predators like owls (figure 2.3D; Oehme, 1961; Fite and Rosenfield-Wessels, 1975; Wathey and Pettigrew, 1989) and frogmouths (Wallman and Pettigrew, 1985). The need to summate information from both eyes under dim light conditions might have constrained frontal eye placement and a single, binocular fovea in these predominantly nocturnal birds. However, such constraints would not account for the existence of a single temporal fovea in diurnal swifts (Oehme, 1962), nor the presence of both a (deep) central and a (shallow) temporal fovea in swallows (Slonaker, 1897). The differences in the retinal structures of swifts and swallows may thus reflect their different evolutionary origins rather than differences in behaviour. Finally, both pigeon (figure 2.3B) and chicken (figure 2.3A) are granivorous, ground feeding birds, but only the pigeon possesses both a proper central fovea and a second area of high ganglion cell density in the dorsotemporal quadrant of the eye ("area dorsalis") (Galifret, 1968; Hayes, 1982; Meyer and May, 1973; Morris, 1987). Such observations suggest that interspecific retinal diversity reflects phylogenetic, ecological, and behavioral constraints.

Position and shape of the retinal pit characterizing a proper fovea vary widely among different species (for a review see Meyer, 1977). The emerging picture is that the pit helps to maintain accurate fixation of an object by three different properties. Because the neural retina has a higher refracting index than the vitreous, the bottom of the pit acts like a magnifying lens (Snyder and Miller, 1978). For this mechanism to improve resolution it is necessary that the angular width of the foveal pit is equal or broader than the cone of light converging onto its center (determined by the angular aperture of the eye) since the steep wall of the pit distorts the image (Pumphrey, 1948). Available data indicate that this condition is generally fulfilled (Donner, 1951; Oehme, 1964; Reymond, 1985, 1987). Rays of light will fall onto the wall when the image is out of focus so that the retinal pit may act as a focus indicator (Harkness and Bennet-Clark, 1978). Finally, when the image slips out of the pit its angular velocity is accelerated, transversing the circumference of the pit. Thus a fixed object seen at some distance is less likely to "creep" out of the fovea (Pumphrey, 1948). The three functions are more important in the lateral monocular visual field, which usually will look at distant objects, rather than in the frontal binocular visual field, which looks onto nearby objects. This may explain why the laterally pointing central fovea is generally deeper and has a higher ganglion cell density than the temporal fovea.

Central Distribution of Retinal Ganglion Cells

The avian visual system is composed of three parallel pathways: tectofugal, thalamofugal, and accessory optic (AOS) systems. In the first two, the retina projects, respectively, on the optic tectum (TO) and the principal optic nucleus of the thalamus (OPT). However, the organization of the retinal projection on the visual pathways differs for lateral-eyed (pigeon) and frontal-eyed (owl) birds. In pigeon, the whole retina is represented in TO, but retinal input to OPT originates, not from the frontal-facing red field, but from the yellow field (figure 2.4D). In owl, the OPT projection originates from the single temporal fovea and its surround (figure 2.4F), while TO seems to be the target of ganglion cells originating from an elongated stripe around the eye equator (figure 2.4E).

The retinal projection to AOS has two components, one of which originates in a distinct population of orthotopic ganglion cells located in a narrow strip around the eye equator (figure 2.4C) and projects topographically on the nucleus lentiformis mesencephali (LM) of the midbrain. The second, the nucleus of the basal optic root (nBOR) receives inputs from medium to large displaced retinal GCs (figure 2.4B), most of which, in contrast with orthotopic GCs (figure 2.3B), are located in peripheral retina (Karten et al., 1977; Fite et al., 1981; Reiner et al., 1979; Yang et al., 1989). The nBOR processes whole field motion (Morgan and Frost, 1981; Burns and Wallman, 1981), which, together with signals from LM and the semicircular canals, provides the animal with information about head and body movements (Gioanni et al., 1984).

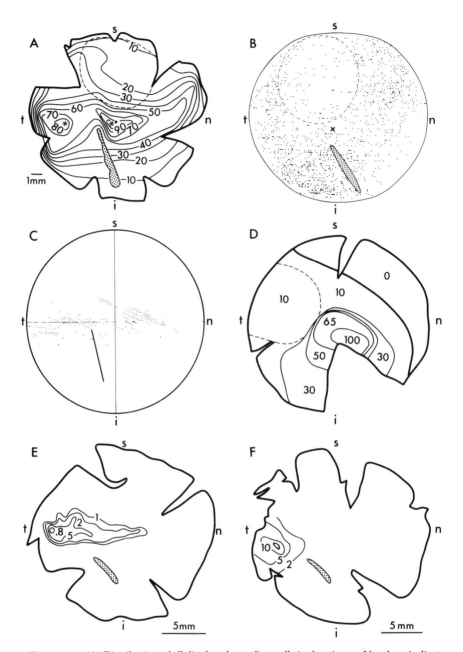

Figure 2.4 (A) Distribution of all displaced ganglion cells in the pigeon. Numbers indicate cells/mm². *Peak densities; dashed, red field. After Hayes and Holden (1983a). (B)–(F) Distribution of ganglion cells projecting to particular targets in the brain. (B) Large displaced ganglion cells that project to the nucleus of the basal optic root in the pigeon. x, fovea; dashed, red field. After Fite et al. (1981). (C) Orthotopic ganglion cells projecting to the nucleus lentiformis mesencephali in the chicken. Line indicates pecten. After Bodnarenko et al. (1988). (D) Distribution of ganglion cells projecting to the nucleus principalis thalami in the pigeon. After Remy and Güntürkün (1991); dashed, red field; numbers, cells/mm², (E) Density of ganglion cells projecting to the tectum opticum in the burrowing owl. (F) Distribution of ganglion cells projecting to the thalamus in the burrowing owl. (E) and (F) After Bravo and Pettigrew (1981). (A)–(F) i, inferior; n, nasal; s, superior; t, temporal; stippled area, pecten.

Physiology of the Retina

Avian retinal ganglion cells have little or no spontaneous activity, respond transiently to stimulation, and possess small receptive fields with diameters of 0.5°–2.5° (pigeon). They have been divided into ON, OFF, and ON/OFF classes and into various subclasses depending on their directional selectivity. A few pigeon ganglion cells respond to certain wavelengths or to large horizontal bars moving vertically through their receptive field. The concentrically organized receptive fields of the pigeon retina have an antagonistic surround such that stimulation of either center or surround excites the cell. They may also have a suppressive surround that inhibits the center response (for review see Holden, 1982).

A significant proportion (14–38%) of ganglion cells in pigeons is directionally selective, independent of background illumination, stimulus color, or background contrast. The directional tuning sharpens as the stimulated area grows larger and extends into the surround of the ganglion cell's receptive field. Thus an asymmetric inhibitory surround may play an important role in directional selectivity. The receptive field of such cells consists of partly overlapping excitatory and inhibitory patches. Since individual patches are not directionally selective, directional responses can be generated only when the target crosses the overlapping area (Holden, 1977). Theoretical accounts of directional selectivity must explain how correlated fluctuations in light intensity over neighboring photoreceptors ("local movement detectors") can be transformed into directionally selective output. Current neural models (e.g., Borst and Egelhaaf, 1989) assume that the response of a cell onto which many of these local movement detectors converge depends not only on the velocity of a moving pattern, but also on the distribution of contour lines (i.e., its spectrum of spatial wavelengths). That is, the response maximum of a cell should occur not at a particular stimulus velocity but at a particular temporal frequency (velocity/wavelength). Interestingly, neurons in the nBOR have their response maxima at one or two particular temporal frequencies, independent of the spatial wavelength of the test pattern (figure 2.5; Yang, 1989; Wolf-Oberhollenzer and Kirschfeld, 1990, 1991), suggesting the applicability of the model to birds.

Recently, it was found that the directional selectivity of rabbit retinal cells may be linked to characteristic excitatory (ACh) and inhibitory (GABA) neurotransmitters (Ariel and Daw, 1982), with a special role for the cholinergic amacrine cells (Masland and Tauchi, 1986). Three types of cholinergic amacrines have been found in the chick retina (Millar et al., 1987), of which the type I cells colaminate with "displaced" GCs possessing nicotinic acetylcholine receptors (Keyser et al., 1988). Selective destruction of these cells abolished directional responses in nBOR (Yang, 1989).

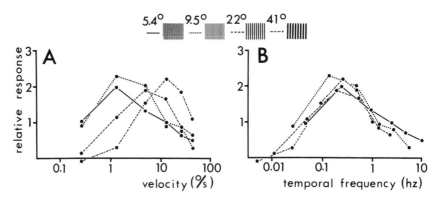

Figure 2.5 Responses of a directionally selective neuron in the nucleus of the basal optic root of the pigeon. Stimuli were sinewave gratings with different spatial wavelengths as shown in the inset. (A) Responses of the neuron calculated as the reaction in preferred direction minus reaction in antipreferred direction divided by the spontaneous activity and drawn as a function of the stimulus velocity. (B) Same responses as shown in (A) but calculated as a function of the temporal frequency of the stimulus. After Wolf-Oberhollenzer and Kirschfeld (1990).

Centrifugal Influences on the Retina

The possibility of central control of retinal processes is suggested by the presence of a pathway originating in the midbrain isthmo-optic nucleus (ION) and from a surrounding population of "ectopic" cells. ION receives topographically organized retinal input via the optic tectum and projects back in an orderly fashion on the retina, synapsing on amacrine and displaced ganglion cells (Maturana and Frenk, 1965; Hayes and Holden, 1983b; Hayes and Webster, 1981; Wolf-Oberhollenzer, 1987). In pigeons, centrifugal terminals are concentrated around the equator, barely penetrating the red field. Two types of terminal arborizations have been distinguished: "convergent" (restricted) and "divergent" (widespread) types, the former presumed to originate from ION neurons, the latter from the ectopic cells (Catsicas et al., 1987b; Fritzsch et al., 1990). Despite considerable speculation and a number of neurophysiological and neurobehavioral studies, the functional significance of centrifugal influences remains obscure (Uchiyama, 1989; Holden, 1990).

HEAD ORIENTATION, EYE MOVEMENTS, AND THE VISUAL FIELD

The projection of the visual field on the retina is often treated as a static phenomenon, but in fact the organization of that projection will vary continuously as the eye moves with respect to the head, and the head with respect to the body. Each such shift in position will project the visual field on a different set of retinal locations. Detailed analysis of such positional effects is critical to understanding the functional significance of the bird's retinal organization. A useful starting point for this analysis is the identification of standardized "resting" positions for the head and eyes. In pigeons (for which the most extensive data are available), the head is oriented such that the lateral semicircular canals are approximately horizontal (Duijm, 1951), so that a line projected from the center of the eye to the bill tip makes an angle of between 25° and 35° below the horizon. During walking or low flight the head moves downward (Erichsen et al., 1989); during fast flight it rotates up, reducing the angle to about 10° (Barlow and Ostwald, 1972). Similarly, in awake birds, there appears to be a "resting" position to which the eye returns after a saccade, and this position seems to approximate that measured ophthalmoscopically in anesthetized birds (figure 2.6; Bloch et al., 1984; Wallman and Pettigrew, 1985; Wallman and Velez, 1985). The position seems to be actively maintained, since curarizing the eye muscles results in unpredictable eye rotations (Nalbach et al., 1990).

Ophthalmoscopic observations indicate that in normal head orientation the optic axis of the eye of an anesthetized pigeon points 64° to 70° away from the midsagittal plane into the horizon, producing a small binocular overlap of the visual fields of about 22° in the horizontal plane

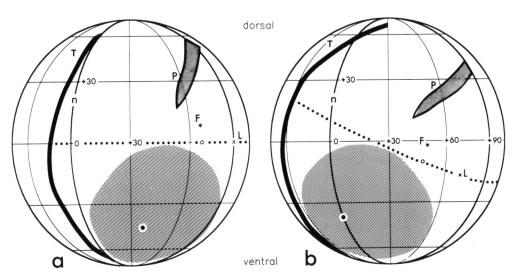

Figure 2.6 Retinal landmarks of the pigeon projected into external space of the left eye in its resting position during the anaesthetized state (a) and converged (yaw, −20°; pitch, 15°; roll, −20°) as might occur during pecking a grain (b). Azimuth (yaw) is defined as rotation of the eye away from the midsagittal plane, positive elevation (pitch) is the angular position of the optic axis above the horizon, and cyclotorsion (roll) is its clockwise rotation around the optic axis. The head is assumed to be held upright with the eye-to-beak axis pointing 30° below the horizon; n denotes the nasal meridian. The dotted line indicates the eye equator, which delimits the upper emmetropic or hyperopic half and the lower myopic half of the eye according to Fitzke et al. (1985). F, fovea centralis; L, lateral view onto the eye; o, optic axis; P, pecten; T, ora terminalis; hatched area, red field with area dorsalis (dot). After Nalbach et al. (1990).

(Barlow and Ostwald, 1972; Nalbach et al., 1990; Martin, this volume). However, the pigeon's red field is strictly monocular and directed onto the ground in the lower frontal visual field.

Hayes et al. (1987) suggested that the red field may serve to search for food on the ground, a hypothesis consistent with the observation that the dorsal retina, including the red field, is characterized by a gradient of myopia that enables the pigeon to obtain a sharp image of the groundplane simultaneously for any distance (Fitzke et al., 1985; see Martin, this volume). This function is assisted in walking pigeons and a vast number of mainly groundfeeding birds (Dunlap and Mowrer, 1930; Whiteside, 1967; Friedman, 1975; Dagg, 1977) by compensatory head movements ("head-bobbing") that reduce retinal image speed and thus prevent blurring of the ground seen close to the eyes where pieces of food may be hidden. However, these observations appear to conflict with the long-standing assumption that the pigeon's red field functions as a binocular "pecking field," controlling peck localization during feeding (Bloch and Martinoya, 1983; Goodale, 1983).

This conflict may be resolved by taking into account the role of eye movements, which, in birds, are often overlooked because of the extensive use of head movements. In pigeons, the range of eye movements may be considerable, covering at least 17° in yaw (convergence/divergence) and 24° in pitch (Bloch et al., 1984), and up to 30° in roll (cyclotorsion; Benjamins and Huizinga, 1927; Nalbach et al., 1990).

An object moving within a monocular visual field may be tracked in a sequence of saccades by the ipsilateral eye alone. When it enters the frontal visual field, the contralateral eye (even if occluded) also fixates the target (Bloch et al., 1987). Thus, eye movements are synchronized when an object enters the binocular visual field, and converging eye movements are prominent during the final head thrusts of a feeding peck (Jaeger et al., 1987). It seems that in pigeons two separate eye movement mechanisms are operative: one controlling independent motion of either eye, and the other mediating the coordinated use of the temporal retinas to examine binocular visual space (Bloch et al., 1987). In kestrel, these modes are mediated, respectively, by the lateral and temporal fovea (Pettigrew, 1978).

By taking into account eye movements around all three axes, we may describe the location in the visual field of the various retinal landmarks just prior to pecking at a grain (see figure 2.1b; cf. Bloch et al., 1987). A simulation of such a situation for the pigeon shows that convergent eye movements can produce a shift from a "monocular" to a "binocular" mode of vision, increasing the maximal binocular overlap from 30° in the resting position (figure 2.6a: elevation about 15° above the beak) to 80° in the converged eye position (figure 2.6b: elevation about 10° below the beak). In this position, the red fields of both eyes overlap up to 60° and their areae dorsales are directed into the midsagittal plane, 10° below the beak. Thus, the effect of the eye movements is to project the myopic optics into the binocular visual field, which is specifically adapted to view near-by objects (cf. Bloch and Martinoya, 1982; Uhlrich et al., 1982).

A relation between visual optics and eye mobility has been shown for a variety of species. In lateral-eyed birds, vergence movements, which make possible a shift from panoramic to binocular vision, have been shown to occur over a range from at least 19° (chicken; Benner, 1938) to 40° (sparrow: Slonaker, 1918). In contrast, such movements are minimal in the mallard duck (Martin 1986), which has the most complete panoramic visual field known, and in owls, birds with frontally placed eyes (Steinbach and Money, 1973; Pettigrew and Konishi 1976). Direct inspection of long billed birds, like pelicans or toucans, suggests that they may use eye movements to overcome the relatively high rotational momentum of their head. Furthermore, the easily overlooked eye roll is quite appropriate to converge the excentrical temporal region of acute vision (area or fovea) into the frontal visual field even without excessive eye-yaw (for further discussion see Wallman and Letelier, chapter 14).

CONCLUSIONS

In a natural situation, both eyes are constantly stimulated by a continuous flow of impressions from the visual environment. A variety of observations suggest that different retinal areas must be specialized to deal with certain aspects of that environment. Thus, the (lower) frontal retinal area seems to be used for searching for, pecking at, and grasping food, while the area centralis or fovea may be used to fixate novel, complex, or distant objects (Oehme, 1962; Blough, 1979; Friedman, 1975; Fox et al., 1976; Hirsch, 1982; Reymond, 1985, 1987; Bischof, 1988; Maldonado et al., 1988; Kirmse, 1990; Frost et al., 1990). Behavioral experiments with localized stimuli are an important tool to understand regional variation of properties of optics and retinal structure (for reviews see Bloch and Martinoya, 1983; Emmerton, 1983b; Hodos, this volume). However, to respond adequately, attention must be directed toward selected visual events such that their projection falls on the optically appropriate portion of the retinal field. Eye movements provide one mechanism for attentional shifts but inter- and intraocular transfer mechanisms and cerebral lateralization of certain functions must also be involved and these are discussed in detail elsewhere in this book (see Remy and Watanabe, and Rogers and Adret, this volume).

ACKNOWLEDGMENTS

We thank Susana Bloch, Sally McFadden, Onur Güntürkün, Graham Martin, Carlos Martinoya, and Phil Zeigler for their helpful and authoritative comments on the manuscript.

REFERENCES

Ariel, M., and Daw, N. W. Pharmacological analysis of directionally sensitive rabbit retina ganglion cells. *J. Physiol.* 324 (1982), 161–185.

Barlow, H. B., and Ostwald, T. J. Pecten of the pigeon's eye as an intra-ocular eye shade. *Nature (London)* 236 (1972), 88–90.

Bellhorn, R. W., and Bellhorn, M. S. The avian pecten. *Ophthalmic Res.* 7 (1975), 1–7.

Benjamins, C. E., and Huizinga, E. Untersuchungen über die Funktion des Vestibular-apparates von Tauben I. *Pflügers Arch.* 217 (1927), 105–123.

Benner, J. Untersuchungen über die Raumwahrnehmung der Hühner. *Z. wiss. Zool.* 151 (1938), 382–444.

Bingelli, R. L., and Paule, W. J. The pigeon retina quantitative aspects of the nerve and ganglion cell layer. *J. Comp. Neurol.* 137 (1969), 1–18.

Bischof, H.-J. The visual field and visually guided behavior in the zebra finch (*Taeniopygia guttata*). *J. Comp. Physiol.* 163 (1988), 329–337.

Bloch, S., and Martinoya, C. Comparing frontal and lateral viewing in the pigeon I. Tachistoscopic visual acuity as a function of distance. *Behav. Brain Res.* 5 (1982), 231–244.

Bloch, S., and Martinoya, C. Specialization of visual functions for different retinal areas in the pigeon, In J.-P. Ewert, R. R. Capranica, and D. J. Ingle (Eds.), *Advances in Vertebrate Neuroethology.* Plenum Press, New York, 1983, pp. 359–368.

Bloch, S., Rivaud, S., and Martinoya, C. Comparing frontal and lateral viewing in the pigeon III. Different patterns of eye movements for binocular and monocular fixation. *Behav. Brain Res.* 13 (1984), 173–182.

Bloch, S., Lemeignan, M., and Martinoya, C. Coordinated vergence for frontal fixation, but independent eye movements for lateral viewing, in the pigeon. In J. K. O'Regan and A. Levy-Schoen (Eds.), *Eye Movements: From Physiology to Cognition.* Elsevier, Amsterdam, 1987, pp. 47–56.

Blough, D. S. Dark adaptation in the pigeon. *J. Comp. Physiol. Psychol.* 49 (1956), 425–430.

Blough, P. M. Functional implications of the pigeon's peculiar retinal structure, In A. M. Granda and J. H. Maxwell (Eds.), *Neural mechanisms of Behavior in the Pigeon.* Plenum Press, New York, 1979, pp. 71–88.

Bodnarenko, S. R., Rojas, X., and McKenna, O. Spatial organization of the retinal projection to the avian lentiform nucleus of the mesencephalon. *J. Comp. Neurol.* 269 (1988), 431–447.

Borst, A., and Egelhaaf, E. Principles of visual motion detection. *TINS* 12 (1989), 297–306.

Bowmaker, J. K. The visual pigments, oil droplets and spectral sensitivity of the pigeon. *Vision Res.* 17 (1977), 1129–1138.

Bowmaker, J. K. Colour vision in birds and the role of oil droplets. *TINS* 8 (1980), 196–199.

Bowmaker, J. K, and Knowles, A. The visual pigments and oil droplets of the chicken retina. *Vision Res.* 17 (1977), 755–764.

Bowmaker, J. K., and Martin, G. R. Visual pigments and color vision in a nocturnal bird (*Strix aluco*), the tawny owl. *Vision Res.* 18 (1978), 1125–1130.

Bowmaker, J. K., and Martin, G. R. Visual pigments and oil droplets of the penguin, *Spheniscus humboldti*. *J. Comp. Physiol. A* 156 (1985), 71–77.

Boycott, B. B., and Dowling, J. E. Organization of the primate retina: Light microscopy. *Philos. Trans. R. Soc. London* 255 (1969), 109–184.

Bravo, H., and Pettigrew, J. D. The distribution of neurons projecting from the retina and visual cortex to the thalamus and tectum opticum of the barn owl, *Tyto alba*, and the burrowing owl, *Speotyto cunicularia*. *J. Comp. Neurol.* 199 (1981), 419–441.

Burkhardt, D. Birds, berries, and UV. *Naturwissenschaften* 69 (1982), 153–157.

Burkhardt, D. UV vision: A bird's eye view of feathers. *J. Comp. Physiol. A* 164 (1989), 787–796.

Burns, S., and Wallman, J. Relation of single unit properties to the oculomotor function of the nucleus of the basal optic root (accessory optic system) in chickens. *Exp. Brain Res.* 42 (1981), 171–180.

Cajal, S. R. La retine des vertebres. Trav. labor Rech. biol. L'Univ. Madrid, 28 (1933). As translated in S. A. Thorpe and M. Glickstein (Eds.), *The Structure of the Retina*. CC Thomas, Springfield, IL, 1972.

Catsicas, S., Catsicas, M., and Clarke, P. G. H. Long-distance intraretinal connections in birds. *Nature (London)* 326 (1987a), 186–187.

Catsicas, S., Thanos, S., and Clarke, P. G. H. Major role of neuronal death during brain development: Refinement of topographical connections. *Proc. Natl. Acad. Sci. U. S. A.* 84 (1987b), 8165–8168.

Chen, D., and Goldsmith, T. H. Four spectral classes of cone in the retinas of birds. *J. Comp. Physiol. A* 159 (1986), 473–479.

Chen, D., Collins, J. S., and Goldsmith, T. H. The ultraviolet receptors of the bird retinas. *Science* 225 (1984), 337–339.

Cserhati, P., Szel, A., and Rölich, P. Four cone types characterized by anti-visual pigment antibodies in the pigeon retina. *Inv. Ophthalmol. Visual Sci.* 30 (1989), 74–81.

Dagg, A. I. The walk of the silver gull (*Larus novohollendiae*) and of other birds. *J. Zool. (London)* 182 (1977), 529–540.

Donner, K. O. The visual acuity of some passerine birds. *Acta Zool. Fennica* 66 (1951), 1–40.

Duijm, M. On the head posture in birds and its relation to some anatomical features. *Proc. Kon. Ned. Akad. Wet. C* 54 (1951), 202–211, 260–271.

Duijm, M. On the position of a ribbon like central area in the eyes of some birds. *Arch. Neerl. Zool.* 13 (1958), 128–145.

Dunlap, K., and Mowrer, O. H. Head movements and eye functions of birds. *J. Comp. Psychol. Physiol.* 11 (1930), 99–113.

Ehrlich, D. Regional specialization of the chick retina as revealed by the size and density of neurons in the ganglion cell layer. *J. Comp. Neurol.* 195 (1981), 643–657.

Emmerton, J. Pattern discrimination in the near-ultraviolet by pigeons. *Perc. Psychophys.* 34 (1983a), 555–559.

Emmerton, J. Vision, In M. Abs (Ed.), *Physiology and Behaviour of the Pigeon*. Academic Press, London, 1983b, pp. 245–266.

Emmerton, J., Schwemer, J., and Muth, J. Spectral transmission of the ocular media of the pigeon (*Columba livia*). *Inv. Ophthalmol. Vis. Sci.* 19 (1980), 1382–1387.

Engstroem, K. On the cone mosaic in the retina of *Parus Major*. *Acta Zool.* 44 (1958), 65–69.

Erichsen, J. T., Hodos, W., Evinger, C., Bessette, B. B., and Phillips, S. J. Head orientation in pigeons—Postural, locomotor and visual determinants. *Brain Behav. Evol.* 33 (1989), 268–278.

Fite, K. V. Anatomical and behavioral correlates of visual acuity in the great horned owl. *Vision Res.* 13 (1973), 219–230.

Fite, K. V., and Rosenfield-Wessels, S. A comparative study of deep avian foveas. *Brain Behav. Evol.* 12 (1975), 97–115.

Fite, K. V., Brecha, N., Karten, H. J., and Hunt, S. P. Displaced ganglion cells and the accessory optic system of pigeon. *J. Comp. Neurol.* 195 (1981), 279–288.

Fitzke, F. W., Hayes, B. P., Hodos, W., Holden, A. L., and Low, J. C. Refractive sectors in the visual field of the pigeon eye. *J. Physiol. (London)* 369 (1985), 33–44.

Fox, R., Lehmkuhle, S. W., and Westendorf, D. H. Falcon visual acuity. *Science* 192 (1976), 263–265.

Franz, V. Höhere Sinnesorgane: Vergleichende Anatomie des Wirbeltierauges. In L. Bolk, E. Göppert, E. Kallius, and W. Lubosch (Eds.), Handbuch der vergleichenden Anatomie der Wirbeltiere. Urban und Schwarzenberg, Berlin, 1934, p. 1157.

Friedman, M. B. How birds use their eyes. In P. Wright, P. Caryl, and D. M. Vowles (Eds.), Neural and Endocrine Aspects of Behavior in Birds, Elsevier, Amsterdam, 1975, pp. 182–204.

Fritzsch, B. Crapon de Crapona, M.-D. and Clarke, P. G. H., Development of two morphological types of retinal fibers in chick embryos, as shown by the diffusion along axons of a carbocyane dye in fixed retina. *J. Comp. Neurol.* 300 (1990), 405–421.

Frost, B. J., Wise, L. Z., Morgan, B., and Bird, D. Retinotopic representation of the bifoveate eye of the kestrel (*Falco sparverius*) on the optic tectum. *Visual Neurosci.* 5 (1990), 231–239.

Galifret, Y. Les diverses aires fonctionelles de la retine du Pigeon. *Z. Zellforsch* 86 (1968), 535–545.

Gallego, A., Baron, M., and Gayoso, M. Organization of the outer plexiform layer of the diurnal and nocturnal bird retinae. *Vision Res.* 15 (1975), 1027–1028.

Gioanni, H., Rey, J., Villabos, J., and Dalbera, A. Single unit activity in the nucleus of the basal optic root (nBOR) during optokinetic vestibular and visual-vestibular stimulations in the alert pigeon (*Columba livia*). *Exp. Brain Res.* 57 (1984), 49–60.

Goldsmith, T. H. Optimization, constraint, and history in the evolution of eyes. *Q. Rev. Biol.* 65 (1990), 281–322.

Goldsmith, T. S., Collins, J. S., and Licht, S. The cone oil droplets of avian retinas. *Vision Res.* 24 (1984), 1661–1671.

Goodale, M. A. Visually guided pecking in the pigeon (*Columba livia*). *Behav. Brain Evol.* 22 (1983), 22–41.

Gordon, J., and Abramov, I. Color vision in the peripheral retina. II. Hue and saturation. *J. Opt. Soc. Am.* 67 (1977), 202–207.

Govardovskij, V. I., and Zueva, L. V. Visual pigments of chicken and pigeon. *Vision Res.* 17 (1977), 537–543.

Harkness, L., and Bennet-Clark, H. C. The deep fovea as a focus indicator. *Nature (London)* 272 (1978), 814–816.

Hayes, B. P. The structural organization of the pigeon retina. In N. N. Osborne, and G. J. Chader (Eds.), *Retinal Research*, Vol. 1. Pergamon Press, Oxford, 1982, pp. 197–226.

Hayes, B. P. Cell populations of the ganglion cell layer: Displaced amacrine and matching amacrine cells in the pigeon retina. *Exp. Brain Res.* 56 (1984), 565–575.

Hayes, B. P., and Brooke, M. de L. Retinal ganglion cell distribution and behavior in procellariiform seabirds. *Vision Res.* 30 (1990), 1277–1289.

Hayes, B. P., and Holden, A. L. The distribution of displaced ganglion cells in the retina of the pigeon. *Exp. Brain Res.* 49 (1983a), 181–188.

Hayes, B. P., and Holden, A. L. The distribution of centrifugal terminals in the pigeon retina. *Exp. Brain Res.* 49 (1983b), 189–197.

Hayes, B. P., and Webster, K. E. Neurons situated outside the isthmo-optic nucleus and projecting to the eye in adult birds. *Neurosci. Lett.* 26 (1981), 107–112.

Hayes, B. P., Hodos, W., Holden, A. L., and Low, J. C. The projection of the visual field upon the retina of the pigeon. *Vision Res.* 27 (1987), 31–40.

Hirsch, J. Falcon visual sensitivity to grating contrasts. *Nature (London)* 300 (1982), 57–58.

Holden, A. L. Responses of directional ganglion cells in the pigeon retina. *J. Physiol. (London)* 270 (1977), 253–269.

Holden, A. L. Electrophysiology of the avian retina. In N. N. Osborne and G. J. Chader (Eds.), *Retinal Research*, Vol. 1. Pergamon Press, Oxford, 1982, pp. 179–196.

Holden, A. L. Centrifugal pathways to the retina: Which way does the "searchlight" point? *Visual Neurosci.* 4 (1990), 493–495.

Hughes, A. The topography of vision in mammals. In F. Crescitelli (Ed.), The Visual System of Vertebrates, Handbook of Sensory Physiology, Vol. VII/5. Springer Verlag, Berlin, 1977, pp. 613–756.

Inzunza, O., Bravo, H., Smith, R. L., and Angel, M. Topography and morphology of retinal ganglion cells in falconiforms: A study on predatory and carrion eating birds. *Anat. Rec.* 229 (1991), 271–277.

Jäger, R., Martinoya, C., Lemeignan, M., and Bloch, S. Oculomotor behavior during walking in the pigeon. In G. Lüer and U. Lass (Eds.), Proc. Fourth European Conf. Eye Movements Vol. 1. C. J. Hogrefe, Toronto, 1987, pp. 112–114.

Jane, S. D., and Bowmaker, J. K., Tetrachromatic color-vision in the duck (*Anas platyrhynchos* L.)—Microspectrophotometry of visual pigments and oil droplets. *J. Comp. Physiol. A* 162 (1988), 225–235.

Karten, H. J., Fite, K. V., and Brecha, N. Specific projection of displaced retinal ganglion cells upon the accessory optic system in the pigeon (*Columba livia*). *Proc. Natl. Acad. Sci. U. S. A.* 74 (1977), 1753–1756.

Karten, H. J., Keyser, K. T., and Brecha, N. C. Biochemical and morphological heterogeneity of retinal ganglion cells. In B. Cohen and I. Bodis-Wollner (Eds.), Vision and the Brain. Raven Press, New York, 1990, pp. 19–33.

Keyser, K. T., Hughes, T. E., Whiting, P. J., Lindstrom, J. M., and Karten H. J. Cholinoceptive neurons in the retina of the chick: An immunohistochemical study of the nicotinic acetylcholine receptors. *Visual Neurosci.* 1 (1988), 349–366.

Kirmse, W. Kritische Übersicht zur selektiven Sensomotorik des Blickens und multifoveales Spähen bei Vögeln. *Zool. Jb. Physiol.* 94 (1990), 217–228.

Kirschfeld, K. Carotenoid pigments: their possible role in protecting against photooxidation in eyes and photoreceptor cells. *Proc. R. Soc. London B* 216 (1982), 71–85.

Lockhart, M. Quantitative morphological investigations of retinal cells in the pigeon: a golgi, light microscopic study. In A. M. Granda and J. H. Maxwell (Eds.), *Neural Mechanisms of Behavior in the Pigeon*. Plenum Press, New York, 1979, pp. 371–394.

Lythgoe, J. N. *The Ecology of Vision*. Oxford University Press, Oxford, 1979.

Maldonado, P. E., Maturana, H., and Varela, F. J. Frontal and lateral visual system in birds. Frontal and lateral gaze. *Brain Behav. Evol.* 32 (1988), 57–62.

Mariani, A. P. Association amacrine cells could mediate directional selectivity in the pigeon retina. *Nature (London)* 298 (1982), 654–655.

Mariani, A. P. A morphological basis for verticality detectors in the pigeon retina: Asymmetric amacrine cells. *Naturwissenschaften* 70 (1983), 368–369.

Mariani, A. P. Neuronal and synaptic organization of the outer plexiform layer of the pigeon retina. *Am. J. Anat.* 179 (1987), 25–39.

Mariani, A. P., and Leure-du Pree, A. E. Photoreceptors and oildroplet colors in the red area of the pigeon retina. *J. Comp. Neurol.* 182 (1978), 821–838.

Martin, G. R. Eye. In A. S. King and J. McLelland (Eds.), *Form and Function in Birds*, Vol. 3. Academic Press, London, 1985, pp. 311–373.

Martin, G. R. Total panoramic vision in the mallard duck, *Anas platyrynchos*. *Vision Res.* 26 (1986), 1303–1305.

Martin, G. R., and Muntz, W. R. A. Spectral sensitivity of the red and yellow oil droplet fields of the pigeon (*Columba livia*). *Nature (London)* 274 (1978), 620–621.

Masland, R. H., and Tauchi, M. The cholinergic amacrine cell. *TINS* 9 (1986), 218–223.

Maturana, H. R., and Frenk, S. Synaptic connections of the centrifugal fibers in the pigeon retina. *Science* 150 (1965), 359–361.

Meyer, D. B. The avian eye and its adaptations. In F. Crescitelli (Ed.), The Visual System of Vertebrates, Handbook of Sensory Physiology, Vol. VII/5. Springer-Verlag, Berlin, 1977, pp. 549–611.

Meyer, D. B. The avian eye and vision. In P. D. Sturkie (Ed.), Avian Physiology, 4th ed. Springer-Verlag, Berlin, 1986, pp. 38–48.

Meyer, D. B., and May, H. C., Jr. The topographical distribution of rods and cones in the adult chicken retina. *Exp. Eye Res.* 17 (1973), 347–355.

Millar, T. J., Ishimoto, I., Chubb, I. W., Epstein, M. L., Johnson, C. D., and Morgan, I. G. Cholinergic amacrine cells of the chicken retina: a light and electron microscope immunocytochemical study. *Neuroscience* 21 (1987), 725–743.

Morgan, B., and Frost, B. J. Visual response characteristic of neurons in nucleus of basal optic root of pigeons. *Exp. Brain Res.* 42 (1981), 181–188.

Morris, V. B. Symmetry in a receptor mosaic demonstrated in the chick from the frequency, spacing and arrangement of the types of retinal receptors. *J. Comp. Neurol.* 140 (1970), 359–398.

Morris, V. B. An afoveate area centralis in the chick retina. *J. Comp. Neurol.* 210 (1987), 198–203.

Morris, V. B., and Shorey, C. D. An electromicroscope study of types of receptor in the chick retina. *J. Comp. Neurol.* 129 (1967), 313–340.

Muntz, W. R. A. Inert absorbing and reflecting pigments. In H. J. A. Dartnell (Ed.),

Photochemistry of Vision, Handbook of Sensory Physiology, Vol. VII/1. Springer-Verlag, Berlin, 1972, pp. 529–565.

Nalbach, H.-O. Wolf-Oberhollenzer, F., and Kirschfeld, K., The pigeon's eye viewed through an ophthalmoscopic microscope: Orientation of retinal landmarks and significance of eye movements. *Vision Res.* 30 (1990), 529–540.

Oehme, H. Vergleichend-histologische Untersuchungen an der Retina von Eulen. *Zool. Jb. Anat. Ontol.* 79 (1961), 439–478.

Oehme, H. Das Auge von Mauersegler. *Star und Amsel J. Ornithol.* 103 (1962), 189–212.

Oehme, H. Vergleichende Untersuchungen an Greifvogelaugen. *Z. Morph. Ökol. Tiere* 53 (1964), 618–635.

Partridge, J. C. The visual ecology of avian cone oil droplets. *J. Comp. Physiol. A* 165 (1989), 415–426.

Pedler, C., and Boyle, M. Multiple oil droplets in the photoreceptors of the pigeon. *Vision Res.* 9 (1969), 525–528.

Pettigrew, J. D. Comparison of the retinotopic organization of the visual wulst in nocturnal and diurnal raptors, with a note on the evolution of frontal vision. In S. J. Cool and E. L. Smith (Eds.), Frontiers in Visual Science. Springer-Verlag, Berlin, 1978, pp. 328–335.

Pettigrew, J. D., and Konishi, M. Binocular neurones selective for orientation and disparity in the visual wulst of the barn owl (*Tyto alba*). *Science* 193 (1976), 675–678.

Pettigrew, J. D., Wallman, J., and Wildsoet, C. F. Saccadic oscillations facilitate ocular perfusion from the avian pecten. *Nature (London)* 343 (1990), 362–363.

Pumphrey, R. J. The theory of the fovea. *J. Exp. Biol.* 25 (1948), 299–312.

Quesada, A., Prada, F. A., and Genis-Galvez, J. M. Bipolar cells in the chicken retina. *J. Morphol.* 197 (1988), 337–351.

Reiner, A., Brecha, N., and Karten, H. J. A specific projection of retinal displaced ganglion cells to the nucleus of the basal optic root in the chicken. *Neuroscience* 4 (1979), 1679–1688.

Remy, M., and Emmerton, J. Behavioural spectral sensitivities of different retinal areas in pigeons. *Behav. Neurosci.* 103 (1989), 170–177.

Remy, M., and Güntürkün, O. Retinal afferents to the tectum opticum and the nucleus opticus principalis thalami in the pigeon. *J. Comp. Neurol.* 304 (1991), 1–14.

Reymond, L. Spatial visual acuity of the eagle *Aquila audax:* A behavioural, optical and anatomical investigation. *Vision Res.* 25 (1985), 1477–1491.

Reymond, L. Spatial visual acuity of the falcon, *Falco berigora:* A behavioural, optical and anatomical investigation. *Vision Res.* 27 (1987), 1859–1874.

Schaeffel, F., Rohrer, B., Lemmer, T., and Zrenner, E. Diurnal control of rod function in the chicken. *Visual Neurosci.* 6 (1991), 641–653.

Schultze, M. Zur Anatomie und Physiologie der Retina. *Arch. Mikrosk. Anat.* 2 (1866), 175–286.

Sillman, A. J., Bolnick, D. A., Haynes, L. W., Walter, A. E., and Loew, E. R. Microspectrophotometry of the photoreceptors of palaeognathos birds—the emu and tinamu. *J. Comp. Physiol.* 144 (1981), 271–276.

Slonaker, J. R. A comparative study of the area of acute vision in vertebrates. *J. Morphol.* 13 (1897), 445–493.

Slonaker, J. R. A physiological study of the anatomy of the eye and its accessory parts of the English sparrow. *J. Morphol.* 31 (1918), 351–450.

Snyder, A. W., and Miller, W. H. Telephoto lens system in falconiform eyes. *Nature (London)* 275 (1978), 127–129.

Steinbach, M. J., and Money, K. E. Eye movements of the owl. *Vision Res.* 13 (1973), 889–891.

Uchiyama, H. Centrifugal pathways to the retina—Influence of the optic tectum. *Visual Neurosci.* 3 (1989), 183–206.

Uhlrich, D. J., Blough, P. M., and Blough, D. S. The pigeon's distant visual acuity as a function of viewing angle. *Vision Res.* 22 (1982), 429–431.

van Genderen Stort, A. G. H. Über Form- und Ortsveränderungen der Netzhautelemente unter Einfluß von Licht und Dunkel. *von Graefes Arch. Ophthal.* 33 (1887), 229–247.

Waelchli, G. Zur Topographie der gefärbten Kugeln der Vogelnetzhaut. *v. Graefe's Arch Ophthalm.* 29 (1883), 205–223.

Wallman, J., and Pettigrew, J. D. Conjugate and disjunctive saccades in two avian species with contrasting oculomotor strategies. *J. Neurosci.* 5 (1985), 1418–1428.

Wallman, J., and Velez, J. Directional asymmetries of optokinetic nystagmus: Developmental changes and relation to the accessory optic system and to the vestibular system. *J. Neurosci.* 5 (1985), 317–329.

Walls, G. L., and Judd, H. D. The intraocular colour filters of vertebrates. *Br. J. Ophthalm.* 19 (1933), 705–725.

Wathey, J. C., and Pettigrew, J. D. Quantitative analysis of the retinal ganglion cell layer and optic nerve of the barn owl *Tyto alba. Brain Behav. Evol.* 33 (1989), 279–292.

Whiteside, T. C. D. The head movements of walking birds. *J. Physiol. (London)* 188 (1967), 31P–32P.

Wingstrand, K. G., and Munk, O. The pecten oculi of the pigeon with particular regard to its function. *Biol. Skr. Danske Vid. Selsk.* 14 (1965), 1–64.

Wolf-Oberhollenzer, F. A study of the centrifugal projections to the pigeon retina using two fluorescent markers. *Neurosci. Lett.* 73 (1987), 16–20.

Wolf-Oberhollenzer, F., and Kirschfeld, K. Temporal frequency dependence in motion sensitive neurons of the accessory optic system of the pigeon. *Naturwissenschaften* 77 (1990), 296–298.

Wolf-Oberhollenzer, F., and Kirschfeld, K. Processing of spatially and temporally modulated stimuli in the nucleus of the basal optic root of the pigeon. *Proc. Göttingen Neurobiol. Conf.* 19 (1991), 218.

Wortel, J. F., Wubbels, R. J., and Nuboer, J. F. W. Photopic spectral sensitivities of the red and yellow field of the pigeon retina. *Vision Res.* 24 (1984), 1107–1113.

Wortel, J. F., Rugenbrink, H., and Nuboer, J. F. W. The photopic spectral sensitivity of the dorsal and ventral retinae of the chicken. *J. Comp. Physiol.* A 160 (1987), 151–154.

Yang, G. Neural circuitry and information processing in the inner retina of the chicken. Ph. D. Thesis, Australian National University, Canberra, 1989.

Yang, G., Millar, T. J., and Morgan, I. G. Co-lamination of cholinergic amacrine cell and displaced ganglion cell dendrites in the chicken retina. *Neurosci. Lett.* 103 (1989), 151–156.

Yazulla, S. Intraretinal differentiation in the synaptic organization of the inner plexiform layer of the pigeon retina. *J. Comp. Neurol.* 153 (1974), 309–324.

Young, S. R., and Martin, G. R. Optics of retinal oil droplets: a model of light collection and polarization detection in the avian retina. *Vision Res.* 24 (1984), 129–137.

3 Constructing the Three-Dimensional Image

Sally A. McFadden

Birds, like most animals, must operate within a three-dimensional (3D) visual environment using stimuli presented on two-dimensional (2D) retinal surfaces. The apparent missing third dimension can be obtained from the perceptual integration of these 2D retinal representations of space. Reconstruction of the third dimension facilitates the perception of two fundamental spatial attributes. First, it permits estimation of the relative position of points, features, or surfaces with respect to some reference position (usually the fixation plane). This "relative depth perception" need only be of a qualitative nature (whether an object is nearer or further than the fixation point) for the 3D perception of unambiguous surfaces relative to their background. The grouping of unambiguous surfaces into figure and ground facilitates object detection. In situations at the limits of depth resolution, (such as flight maneuvers in a cluttered environment or for breaking camouflage of a detailed textured local surface) and possibly for veridical space perception, quantitative estimates of position relative to a fixation point are required.

Second, a three-dimensional frame of reference can allow the estimation of the absolute distance of a point, object, or local surface relative to the observer. Because it is generally used to guide reaching movements, such absolute distance ("egocentric") perception requires quantitative computations.

Traditionally (see review in Graham, 1965), the perception of three-dimensional space has been thought to involve three mechanisms: (1) multiple sampling of the visual image either from different positions in space (stereopsis) or time (motion parallax), (2) oculomotor adjustment of the optical system of each eye (accommodation) or both eyes (convergence) to maintain a sharp image on the photoreceptors, and (3) cognitive interpretation of the image of an object that had previously been actively explored. Despite species differences in optical and neural constraints, most visual systems have adapted these three mechanisms to their particular niche characteristics. The three methods are interdependent. Thus accurately sampling the same image with each eye (in stereopsis) depends on binocular convergence for fusion of that image and, in the case of extremely ambiguous images, can be enhanced by prior knowledge for expected image matching. Which mechanisms are emphasized in a particular species will depend on the behavioral requirements of different visuomotor tasks. However, any behavior will utilize multiple linked visual strategies at different stages of the movement pattern.

The contribution of monocular cues to space perception is likely to be quite important, but has only begun to be explored (see Martinoya et al., 1988; Davies and Green, 1990; Martinoya and Delius, 1990). In contrast, because of the salience of binocular vision for the relatively automatic appreciation of depth, the almost universal presence of a binocular field (Walls, 1942), its strong association with stereoscopic capacity (see Fox, 1978; Hughes, 1977), and its applicability to human perception, the role of binocular vision has dominated the literature on space perception. This chapter reviews evidence for the existence, utilization, and possible mechanisms of binocular vision in mediating 3D space perception in birds. (For comparative studies see reviews by Walls, 1942, Fox, 1981: general; Hughes, 1977: mammals; House, 1989: frogs and toads; Rossel, 1992: insects).

BINOCULAR SAMPLING OF THE VISUAL IMAGE

Retinal Disparity and Stereopsis

The presence of two separate eyes allows each point in space to be simultaneously sampled from two different vantage positions. Integration of these two disparate retinal images allows an automatic appreciation of the third dimension known as stereopsis. Stereopsis is based on the associated horizontal (but not vertical) retinal disparity and allows a direct angular measure of depth with respect to a fixation point (F in figure 3.1). Geometrically defined, horizontal retinal disparity directly measures the difference between the visual (θ) or convergence angles (γ) such that

$$\theta_R - \theta_L = \gamma_F - \gamma_P \tag{3.1}$$

The horizontal retinal disparity (δ) can be calculated as

$$\delta^\circ = 2 \left[\tan^{-1} \frac{I/2}{D} - \tan^{-1} \frac{I/2}{D + \Delta d} \right] \tag{3.2}$$

Equation (3.2) relates to symmetric convergence conditions in which $\phi \approx 0$, that is, for objects close to a central line of sight. For asymmetric conditions, the visual direction ϕ has to be taken into account (see figure 3.1 for variable definitions). The horizontal retinal disparity predicts the relative distance between F and P dependent on the interocular separation (I) and the absolute distance of the fixation point (D).

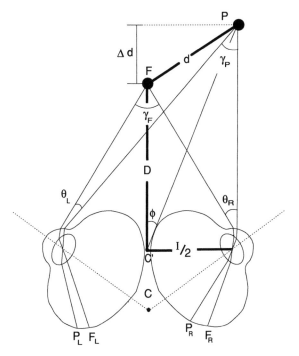

Figure 3.1 Diagrammatic representation of retinal disparity. Variables are defined as follows: F, fixation point; P, arbitrary point; d, depth; D, absolute distance of F; ϕ, visual direction of point P; γ_F and γ_P, convergence angles of F and P, respectively; θ_L and θ_R, visual angles of P with respect to the fixation point for the left and right eyes, respectively; $I/2$, half the interocular separation; C and C', cyclopean centers, C $\approx$ C' when I is small relative to D; P_L and P_R, corresponding retinal points for point P on the left and right retinas, respectively; F_L and F_R, corresponding retinal points for the fixation point F on the left and right retinas, respectively; dotted lines represent the projection of the optic visual axes; $\Delta d \approx d$ for symmetrical convergence, i.e., when the visual direction $\phi = 0$.

Levels of Stereopsis

Stereopsis is based on horizontal retinal disparity and requires that corresponding points on each retina (see [F_L,F_R] and [P_L,P_R] in figure 3.1) be binocularly combined. This combination involves two levels of processing called local and global stereopsis. In humans, these levels are dissociable since global stereopsis can be impaired (from temporal lobe excision) while local stereopsis remains intact (Ptito et al., 1991).

Local stereopsis refers to the assignment of a retinal disparity value to unambiguous matched corresponding points (Julesz, 1978). The retinal disparity values can be one of three classes: crossed, uncrossed, or zero disparity, depending on the position of the target with respect to the fixation plane (Richards, 1970). For local stereopsis in all classes, some characteristic local micropattern provides sufficient information so that there is no ambiguity in which two receptive fields correspond.

However, with more complex images, there may be ambiguity in determining which pair of points or features in each eye's image correspond. Solving this ambiguity requires global stereopsis. This ambiguity is exemplified in random dot stereograms (RDS) (Julesz, 1960). In a RDS, each eye is separately presented with an apparently identical random dot pattern, except for a small subpopulation of dots that is slightly shifted in one eye's image. The shift creates a small disparity when the two arrays are binocularly fused and the disparate dots will be seen in a different depth plane to the background dots. However, since the shifted dots cannot be seen in the monocular image and all the dots are the same, there is ambiguity in determining which dot pairs actually correspond.

Computationally, this "correspondence problem" (see Julesz, 1971; Poggio and Poggio, 1984) can be resolved by selecting the most probable set of matched pairs based on comparison of the disparity values assigned to neighboring pairs from the local stereoscopic process. Determining the most probable set requires a global solution and can be based on assumptions about the image (such as surface continuity) (Blake and Wilson, 1991). Alternatively, it may be that global stereopsis operates by first reducing the false matches either by using vertical disparities (Mayhew and Longuet-Higgins, 1982) in addition to horizontal disparity or possibly by sequential spatial filtering of the image (Poggio and Poggio, 1984, Blake and Wilson, 1991). This latter suggestion is based on the knowledge that the required degree of similarity between the two corresponding images is dependent on the spatial frequency of the disparity detector (Bishop and Henry, 1971). Thus fine stereopsis (disparity $< 0.5°$) requires a high degree of similarity between the two images otherwise retinal rivalry and suppression occurs, while coarse stereopsis can operate with quite dissimilar images. Fine and coarse stereopsis are independent channels at the level of local stereopsis but may be coupled at the level of global stereopsis (Poggio and Poggio, 1984).

Local and Global Stereopsis in Birds

Local coarse stereopsis has been demonstrated behaviorally in pigeons (McFadden and Wild, 1986). Subjects were trained to discriminate two-dimensional (2D), flat stimuli from three-dimensional (3D) depth stimuli. These stimuli were made by separating in space two nonoverlapping arrays of random sized triangles so that when viewed binocularly, a central circle appeared behind the foreground array (figure 3.2a). In these stimuli local features (such as orientation of an edge or corner of a triangle, particularly near the edges of the stereoscopic circle) could be matched in each eye's image. When the density of the triangle pattern was reduced so that cues for local matching were more sparse, the discrimination took longer to learn (McFadden, 1984). Discrimination was also sensitive to the sign of the disparity, so that no

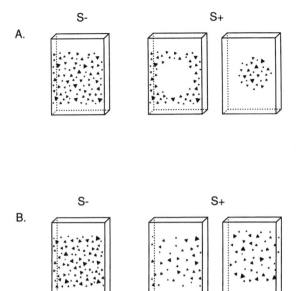

Figure 3.2 Stimuli used for testing stereopsis in the pigeon. (A) A displaced circle was presented behind the background; (B) no coherent displaced form was present, half the triangles were in the foreground and half were in the background.

immediate generalization was seen when, after training with the opposite arrangement, the circle was presented in front of the surrounding plane. In addition, discrimination between crossed and uncrossed disparity, a relative depth task, was easily obtained. Discrimination of depth was possible only under binocular viewing conditions, and consistently fell to chance when the binocular field was reversibly blocked. Interestingly, adult birds that have had monocular visual deprivation from day 1–30 of life are unable to learn even the easiest of our depth discriminations and fail on the visual cliff (McFadden, unpublished observations). Thus it would appear that the pigeon has at least a local stereoscopic capacity which may require balanced binocular input during development.

A behavioral demonstration of global stereopsis has been attempted in the kestrel using random dot stereograms (Fox et al, 1977). The bird was rewarded for flying to a display containing a stereoscopic vertical rectangle displaced in depth (8–12° uncrossed disparity). The stimuli were produced with dynamic RDS using red/green filters placed before the eyes. In dynamic RDS's different static RDS are presented in fast temporal succession. However, replacing the pattern of red and green random dots every 16 msec on a color television monitor brings additional problems, since the flicker fusion frequency of the kestrel is unknown but in the pigeon has been measured up to 150 cps (Powell and Smith, 1968). Thus, although perhaps unlikely, it is possible that the discrimination was based on the onset delay in which the pattern was generated rather than on global stereopsis. The reported decline in performance at disparities about the training disparity could be ascribed to a generalization gradient, particularly given inequalities in training at the different data points. The discrimination of the stereoscopic form was found to be orientation sensitive, which is interesting since in monkeys the complex cells that respond to RDS have been found to be orientation insensitive (Poggio and Poggio, 1984).

Using pigeons, McFadden (1984) presented stimuli similar to those described in figure 3.2a, except that no particular form was present, and the stimuli appeared as two lacy transparent planes of random sized triangles separated in depth (figure 3.2b). This pattern contains a small number of ambiguities in determining the corresponding points for each eye's image. (Note that a global solution for eliminating false matches is unlikely to rely on assumptions about surface continuity.) Pigeons can discriminate the presence of depth in these lacy stimuli and performance consistently fell to chance under monocular conditions, but they took twice as long to learn the task (> 2000 trials) as when the stimuli contain a displaced form in depth. Pigeons proved impossible to train when a large number of ambiguities are presented (as in an RDS) (Blough, personal communication). This suggests that in the pigeon, global processes may operate on a very simple level and as shown below, at a fairly coarse resolution.

RESOLUTION LIMITS

Stereoacuity in Birds

Within the constraints of the optical apparatus, the limits of visual resolution are normally set by the spacing of the photoreceptor array. Thus spatial grating acuity in birds appears matched to the anatomical resolving power of the eye (wedge tailed eagle—Reymond, 1985; American kestrel—Hirsch, 1982). However, neural summation of the signal in each eye can improve acuity limits, much as occurs for the superiority of binocular compared to monocular visual acuity (Campbell and Green, 1965). For example, binocular grating acuity in the pigeon is better than monocular acuity by the expected $\sqrt{2}$ factor (McFadden, unpublished data). Some visual acuity tasks permit hyperacuity (Westheimer, 1975) in which the visual acuity supersedes that predicted on the basis of physiological optics. In humans, local stereoacuity is one such hyperacuity, with the best estimates being 2–4 sec of arc (compared with a minimum angle of resolution of 25 min of arc). This capacity for fine stereoacuity is more than one order of magnitude smaller than the width of tuning of disparity sensitive cells found in monkeys. Westheimer (1979) has suggested that such fine stereopsis can be generated cooperatively from much larger local disparities (thus requiring only a relatively coarse disparity input) by detecting a difference (Δ) between the disparity (δ) of two simultaneously seen targets, such that

$$\Delta = \delta_P^F - \delta_i^F \tag{3.3}$$

Only limited data are available on the stereoacuity of birds. In the RDS study with the kestrel (Fox et al., 1977) thresholds were not measured, but best performance was at 8–12 min of arc, 60 times the minimum angle of resolution (grating acuity of 160 cycles/degree, see Fox et al., 1976), well outside the hyperacuity range. In the pigeon, stereoacuity for local stereopsis is 1 min of arc (figure 3.3a). This value matches the minimum receptor spacing and possibly approaches the hyperacuity range (McFadden, 1987). Such a capacity may conceivably arise through a differencing mechanism of the kind suggested by Westheimer (1979) working at the borders of the displaced circle shown in figure 3.2a. This is not the case for the global stereoscopic process (see figure 3.3b) where threshold stereoacuity is only 9.5 min of arc. The implication of these data is that in birds, the neural solution for global stereopsis may occur at the expense of disparity resolution.

Limits of Stereoscopic Vision

The limiting far point of stereopsis is defined as the greatest distance at which an object can be just detected as nearer than an object at infinity (Ogle, 1962). In figure 3.1, this would be equivalent to the detection of point F as nearer than point P, with P at infinity. Since the just detectable distance should be equivalent to the threshold for stereopsis ($\delta_t = \gamma_F - \gamma_P$), and since for P at infinity $\gamma_P \approx 0$, then $\delta_t = \gamma_F$. Thus, theoretically the limiting distance (D) is

$$D = \frac{I/2}{\tan(\delta_t^0/2)} \tag{3.4}$$

In man, the limiting range of stereopsis is often calculated based on such theoretical considerations (Graham, 1965: 453 m for a threshold of 30 sec of arc; Reading, 1983: 1.3 km for a threshold of 10 sec of arc). In the pigeon, with a threshold of approximately 9.5 min of arc (for global stereopsis) and an interocular separation of 22 mm, Eq. (3.4) predicts that the limiting far point for stereopsis should be 8 m, but in practice is only 190 mm (figure 3.4). This discrepancy possibly arises because the Eq. (3.4) does not take into account the far and resting points of convergence, the latter being in man at an intermediate distance (approximately 70 cm) rather than at infinity (Owens, 1984).

The restricted range of stereoscopic vision found in the pigeon may reflect a limiting range of convergence or accommodation. The former is possibly more important, since the near point of stereopsis (90 mm, figure 3.4) is not equivalent to the near point of accommodation predicted from pecking fixation distance to be 50 mm (Hodos et al., 1976).

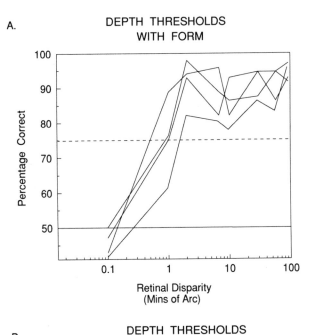

A.

DEPTH THRESHOLDS
WITH FORM

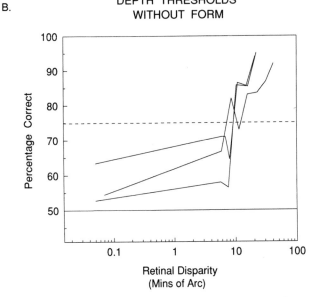

B.

DEPTH THRESHOLDS
WITHOUT FORM

Figure 3.3 Psychometric threshold curves for measuring stereoacuity for two different types of stimuli: (A) stimuli contained a central circle displaced in depth as shown in figure 3.2A; and (B) stimuli contained no actual displaced form but appeared with binocular vision as two lacy transparent planes separated in depth as shown in figure 3.2B In both cases the discrimination was between zero depth difference between the background and foreground (negative stimulus) and a descending range of small depth differences (positive stimulus). Each curve represents the psychometric function generated by different pigeons with each point being the mean of 3–5 threshold estimates measured with a descending series of depth differences. The stimuli were presented behind adjacent pecking keys as described in McFadden (1986). Viewing distance was approximately 8 cm from the eye to the front surface of the stimuli. Thresholds were taken where the psychometric function crossed the 75% line (dotted).

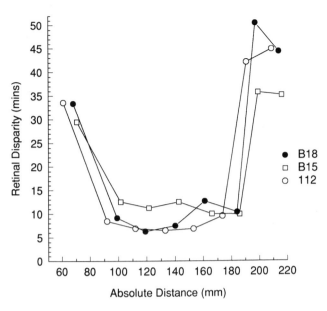

Figure 3.4 Threshold stereoacuity as a function of viewing distance in the frontal field of the 3 pigeons. Stimuli were back illuminated and presented down two white tunnels placed behind two adjacent pecking keys. Luminance was held constant and as measured through the response key was 500 cd/m^2. The discrimination was between depth versus no depth. The depth stimuli were as described in figure 3.2b.

In addition, the accommodative resting state is about 500 cm based on the myopic refractive error we have found in the frontal binocular field (anesthetized, $-2D$, SE = 0.4D). Whatever the source, the limitations suggest that the use of stereopsis in the pigeon is restricted to between 9 and 19 cm, thus encompassing relatively near range activities.

COORDINATION OF THE TWO IMAGES

Binocular fixation without active fusion of the two monocular images can be used to estimate the absolute position (and indeed the relative qualitative position) of objects. For example, species that lack a vergence system and thus have a fixed horopter (defined as the locus of points stimulating hypothetical corresponding retinal points) can use binocular cues to guide prey reaching movements (Collett, 1977: toads; Ingle, 1976: frogs; Rossel, 1983: mantids). However, for a qualitative estimate of the relative position of objects, in which depth and disparity covary, active fusion is necessary.

Binocular Fixation and the Role of the Fovea

Binocular fusion depends on a capacity for coordinated binocular fixation. Birds have a range of eye movements including vergence (Bloch et al., 1987) and conjugate saccades (Wallman and Pettigrew, 1985). In birds with a temporal fovea, binocular fixation might be expected to utilize this structure. However, the finding of stereoscopic capabilities in lateral-eyed birds lacking a temporal fovea (McFadden and Wild, 1986) but with a specialization known as the "area dorsalis" (Galifret, 1968) suggests that a fovea as such is not a requirement. The vulture has no temporal binocular fovea, but exhibits the usual pattern of over-representation of this part of the retina in the visual Wulst (Pettigrew, 1979a).

In pigeons, the high estimates of stereoacuity indicate that if binocular fixation occurs, it may be through the entrainment of the center of the area dorsalis on the object of regard. During key-pecking, the mean eye position at the next to the last fixation point would place the center of the stimulus image 8.6° below the eye beak axis. This is functionally consistent with the observation that with the eyes in a rest position, the "area dorsalis" projects the image into the lower binocular visual field (McFadden and Reymond, 1985; Nalbach et al., 1990; McFadden, 1990). The increased ganglion cell density, increased synaptic density of the inner plexiform layer, and reduced rod content of the area dorsalis (Yazulla, 1974), while often not as great as that surrounding the mon-ocular fovea, would still allow enhancement of spatial acuity (pigeon: 15 cycles/degree, McFadden and Rounsley, unpublished data; kooka-burra, up to 15 cycles/degree, Moroney and Pettigrew 1987). However, it is not clear how binocular fixation may be mediated by such a struc-ture. Perhaps fine stereopsis requires a binocular fovea which could detect small movements, while an area dorsalis may only support coarse stereopsis. It is also possible that the limited stereoscopic range may be related to limitations in fixation capacity in a species without a binocular fovea.

VERIDICAL SPACE PERCEPTION

Horizontal retinal disparity measures depth intervals relative to a fixa-tion plane, but because it is an angular measure, cannot alone predict the absolute value of these depth intervals. For a constant physical depth, retinal disparity increases in proportion to the square of the absolute physical distance (Graham, 1965) according to the following approximation:

$$\Delta d \approx \frac{(D^2 \cdot \gamma)}{I} \tag{3.5}$$

where the variables are defined as in Eq. (3.1). For example, a depth of 10 mm at a distance of 1 m has an associated horizontal retinal disparity in the pigeon of 2 min of arc, while the same 10-mm depth at 200 cm from the bird will have an associated disparity of 50 min of arc. Unless absolute distance is specified, depth perception from horizontal retinal disparity is nonveridical. The visual system in man can rescale horizontal retinal disparity with respect to absolute distance up to a distance of 200 cm (Ono and Comerford, 1977), a capacity referred to as depth constancy.

Depth Constancy in the Pigeon

The pigeon also has a capacity for depth constancy measured for distances less than 20 cm in the frontal binocular field (McFadden, 1991). Depth constancy was measured using a task involving discrimination between 10 and 3 mm depth stimuli (similar to those shown in figure 3.2b). Pigeons took 6000 trials to learn the task under binocular conditions and could not learn it under monocular conditions. Subsequent tests examined the effects of confounding retinal disparity with physical depth information. (For all tests, retinal image size was held constant at 12.5°.) Despite different absolute distances, the pigeon always used the physical depth difference to guide operant behavior, showing that retinal disparity was calibrated in terms of the absolute distance of the stimuli.

SPECIES DIFFERENCES IN BINOCULAR SPATIAL PERCEPTION

Binocular spatial perception arises from a number of processes, some of which are interdependent, and some of which are dissociable. The initial process involves the detection of horizontal retinal disparity called local stereopsis, probably on a fairly coarse scale. The orientation sensitive local disparity neurons in the visual Wulst of the Barn Owl and American kestrel (preferred disparity 3–5°) (Pettigrew and Konishi, 1976a; Pettigrew, 1979b) provide a neural basis for coarse local stereopsis and such a capacity is supported by the behavioral studies in the pigeon and the kestrel. Such local coarse stereopsis would allow the discrimination of whether an object is further or nearer than a fixation point, and could be suitable for object localization. However, for a finer local stereoscopic capacity, greater control of vergence eye movements is required to enable more accurate fixation, and it is possible that these finer eye movements may be driven by the retinal disparity output of the coarse local detectors. (Thus we might expect to see output from the visual Wulst to the eye movement centers.) It is also possible that fine local stereopsis may require a binocular fovea for fixation control. It can be speculated that in birds that have such a fine control system, a neural difference mechanism could also allow the discrimination of hyperacute depth differences.

A separate form of binocular depth perception is global stereopsis. In birds, behavioral evidence suggests that coarse global stereopsis may be present in both granivorous birds and raptors. Neurophysiological evidence for global stereopsis has been shown in the rhesus monkey (Poggio and Poggio, 1984) and requires input from local stereoscopic detectors. Thus, if such detectors were to be found in birds, they could be in the efferent connections of the superficial layers of the visual Wulst. Global stereopsis is dependent on inbuilt assumptions of the visual world such as surface continuity and probably involves comparison of neighboring parts of an image to allow the ambiguity inherent in complex textures to be resolved. Global stereopsis is likely to allow breaking an image into its background and foreground components (such as in decoding camouflage) and may be one spatial cue used in object identification.

The discrimination of figure from ground from a great height such as can occur in predatory raptors may not be aided by global stereopsis, as it usually operates within a limited range. It would also depend on hyperacute local stereopsis and fine oculomotor control. However, in birds that use their talons to catch prey, local stereopsis would be very useful in estimating the relative position of its limbs in relation to the prey object during the final phase of the movement. This behavior involves reaching movements with greater than one degree of freedom for prey localization. As the limbs move, the binocular field would also need to be large enough to encompass activity within a binocular field without recourse to head and/or excessive eye movement.

Birds that use a fixed frame of reference (e.g., the beak) to grasp stationary objects also have a need for spatial localization. Local stereopsis would aid in the detection of the position of the seed relative to its background. Global stereopsis would be required only under conditions in which the background pattern is similar to the seed being pecked. The advantage of a fixed frame of reference is that the size of the binocular field does not need to be very great. However, the fixed frame of reference also means that absolute distance information can guide the initial pecking movement. Experiments with prisms and lenses indicate that accommodation appears to be an effective cue in the owl (Wagner and Schaeffel, 1991) and the pigeon, which also relies on binocular convergence (Bloch et al., 1987; McFadden, 1990).

Absolute distance is also required to recalibrate retinal disparity so that depth perception is veridical. We have shown that veridical depth perception occurs at least in a granivorous bird, and it is probable that other birds may also have this capacity, particularly during flight when absolute distance is constantly changing. In figure 3.1, either γ_F is directly calculated from an extraretinal signal related to the convergence state of the eyes or is neurally transformed from the local disparity signal. Veridical depth can then be obtained as a function of the perceived absolute distance and the retinal disparity signal. It should be noted that perceived absolute distance is dependent on the visual direction (ϕ, figure 3.1). It is possible that the visual direction is determined by saccade amplitude, but would require a conjugate eye movement system. Since conjugate saccades in the little eagle and the frogmouth are limited to less than 6° (Wallman and Pettigrew, 1985), it is possible that veridical depth fails for objects laterally separated by greater than 6°. If this is true, then veridical depth perception may be restricted to objects close to the line of the beak. This would not present a problem for locating an object with a fixed frame of reference. However, in raptors, it may be expected that location of an object with moving limbs would be best when the talons are bought into a central line of regard.

The old notion that frontal vision, large binocular fields, a prominent visual Wulst, and predatory life-styles should go hand in hand with binocular vision and stereopsis has difficulty explaining exceptions, such as the South American oilbird, and does not take into account the fact that binocular depth perception and stereopsis are not unitary phenomenon, nor a high level capacity bestowed only on some subset of "elite" species (see Fox, 1978), but may occur in various forms, and vary with both a bird's ecological niche and its behavioral needs.

REFERENCES

Bishop, P. O., and Henry, G. H. Spatial vision. *Annu. Rev. Physiol.* 22 (1971), 119–160.

Blake, R., and Wilson, H. R. Neural models of stereoscopic vision. *TINS* 14 (1991), 445–452.

Bloch, S., Lemeignan, M., and Martinoya, C. Coordinated vergence for frontal fixation, but independent eye movements for lateral viewing, in the pigeon. In J. K. O'Regan and A. Levy-Schoen (Eds.), *Eye Movements: From Physiology to Cognition*. Elsevier, Amsterdam, 1987, pp. 47–56.

Campbell, F. W., and Green, D. G. Monocular versus binocular visual acuity. *Nature (London)* 208 (1965), 191–192.

Collet, T. Stereopsis in toads. *Nature (London)* 267 (1977), 349–351.

Davies, M. N. O., and Green, P. *Naturwissenschaften* 77 (1990), 142–144.

Fox, R. Binocularity and stereopsis in the evolution of vertebrate vision. In S. J. Cool and E. L. Smith (Eds.), *Frontiers in Visual Science*, Vol. 3, Springer-Verlag, Berlin, 1978, pp. 316–327.

Fox, R. Stereopsis in animals and human infants: A review of behavioral investigations. In R. N. Aslin, J. R. Albert, and M. R. Petersens (Eds.), *Development of Perception: Psychobiological Perspectives*, Vol. 2. Academic Press, New York, 1981, Ch. 12, pp. 335–381.

Fox, R., Lehmkuhle, S. W., and Westendorf, D. H. Falcon visual acuity. *Science* 192 (1976), 263–265.

Fox, R., Lehmkuhle, S. W., and Bush, R. C. Stereopsis in the falcon. *Science* 197 (1977), 79–81.

Galifret, Y. Les diverses aires fonctionelles de la retine du pigeon. *Z. Zellforsch.* 86 (1968), 535–545.

Graham, C. H. Visual space perception. In C. H. Graham (Ed.), *Vision and Visual Perception*. Wiley, New York, 1965, pp. 504–547.

Hirsch, J. Falcon visual sensitivity to grating contrasts. *Nature (London)* 300 (1982), 57–58.

Hodos, W., Leibowitz, R. W., and Bonbright, J. C. Jr. Near-field visual acuity of pigeons: Effects of head location and stimulus luminance. *J. Exp. Anal. Behav.* 25 (1976), 129–141.

House, D. Depth perception in frogs and toads: A study in neural Computing. In S. Levin (Ed.), *Lecture Notes in Biomathematics*, Vol. 80, Springer-Verlag, Berlin, 1989, pp. 1–135.

Hughes, A. The topography of vision in mammals of contrasting lifestyle: Comparative optics and retinal organisation. In F. Cresticelli (Ed.), *Handbook of Sensory Physiology, The Visual System in Vertebrates*, Vol VII/5. Springer, Berlin, 1977, Ch. 11, pp. 614–642.

Ingle, D. Spatial vision in anurans. In K. Kite (Ed.), *The Amphibian Visual System: A Multidisciplinary Approach*. Academic Press, New York, 1976, pp. 119–140.

Julesz, B. Binocular depth perception of computer generated patterns. *Bell System Tech. J.* 39 (1960), 1125.

Julesz, B. *Foundations of Cyclopean Perception*. University of Chicago Press, Chicago, 1971.

Julesz, B. Global stereopsis: Cooperative phenomena in stereoscopic depth perception. In R. Held, H. W. Leibowitz, and H.-L. Teuber (Eds.), *Handbook of Sensory Physiology, Perception*, Vol 8. Berlin, Springer, 1978, Ch. 7, pp. 215–256.

Martinoya, C., and Delius, J. D. Perception of rotating spiral patterns by pigeons. *Biol. Cybern.* 63 (1990), 127–134.

Martinoya, C., Le Houezec, J., and Bloch, S. Depth resolution in the pigeon. *J. Comp. Physiol. A* 163 (1988), 33–42.

Mayhew, J. E. W., and Longuet-Higgins, C. A computational model of binocular depth perception. *Nature (London)* 297 (1982), 376–378.

McFadden, S. A. Depth perception in the pigeon. Ph.D. Thesis, The Australian National University, 1984.

McFadden, S. A. The binocular stereoacuity of the pigeon and its relation to the anatomical resolving power of the eye. *Vision Res.* 27 (1987), 1741–1746.

McFadden, S. A. Eye design for depth and distance perception in birds: An observer orientated perspective. *Comp. Psychol.: Comp. Studies on Perception Cognition* 3 (1990), 1–31.

McFadden, S. A. Depth Constancy in the pigeon. *Proc. Soc. Comp. Psychol.* (1991), Brussels.

McFadden, S. A., and Reymond, L. A further look at the binocular visual field of the pigeon Columba Livia). *Vision Res.* 25 (1985), 1741–1746.

McFadden, S. A., and Wild, J. M. Binocular depth perception in the pigeon (Columba Livia). *J. Exp. Anal. Behav.* 45 (1986), 149–160.

Moroney, M. K., and Pettigrew, J. D. Some observations on the visual optics of kingfishers (Alves, Coraciformes, Alcedinidae). *J. Comp. Physiol. A* 160 (1987), 137–149.

Nalbach, H.-O., Wolf-Oberhollenzer, F., and Kirschfeld, K. The pigeon's eye viewed through an ophthalmoscopic microscopic: Orientation of retinal landmarks and significance of eye movements. *Vision Res.* 30 (1990), 525–540.

Ogle, K. N. *Spatial Localisation through Binocular Vision, The Eye*, Vol 4. Academic, New York, 1962, pp. 271–320.

Ono, H., and Comerford, T. Stereoscopic depth constancy. In W. Epstein (Ed.), *Stability and Constancy in Visual Perception: Mechanisms and Processes*. New York, Wiley, 1977, pp. 91–128.

Owens, D. A. The resting state of the eyes. *Am. Scient.* 72 (1984), 378–387.

Pettigrew, J. D. Comparison of the retinotopic organisation of the visual Wulst in nocturnal and diurnal raptors, with a note on the evolution of frontal vision. In S. J. Cool and E. L. Smith (Eds.), *Frontiers of Visual Science*, Vol. III. Springer-Verlag, New York, 1979a, pp. 328–335.

Pettigrew, J. D. Binocular visual processing in the owl's telencephalon. *Proc. R. Soc. London Ser. B.* 204 (1979b), 435–454.

Pettigrew, J. D., and Konishi, M. Neurones selective for orientation and binocular disparity in the visual Wulst of the barn owl (Tyto alba). *Science* 193 (1976a), 675–678.

Poggio, G. F., and Poggio, T. The analysis of stereopsis. *Annu. Rev. Neurosci.* 7 (1984), 379–412.

Powell, R. W., and Smith, J. C. Critical flicker-fusion thresholds as a function of very small pulse-to-cycle fractions. *Psychol. Rec.* 18 (1968), 35–40.

Ptito, A., Zatorre, R. J., Larson, W. L., and Tosoni, C. Stereopsis after unilateral anterior temporal lobectomy. *Brain* 114 (1991), 1323–1333.

Reading, R. W. *Binocular vision—foundations and Applications.* Butterworth's, London, 1983, p. 124.

Reymond, E. Spatial visual acuity of the eagle Aquila audax: A behavioural, optical and anatomical investigation. *Vision Res.* 25 (1985), 1477–1491.

Richards, W. Stereopsis and stereoblindness. *Exp. Brain Res.* 10 (1970), 380–388.

Rossel, S. Binocular stereopsis in an insect. *Nature (London)* 302 (1983), 821–822.

Rossel, S. Vertical disparity and binocular vision in the praying mantis. *Visual Neurosci.* 8 (1992), 165–170.

Wagner, H., and Schaeffel, F. Barn owls (Tyto alba) use accommodation as a distance cue. *J. Comp. Physiol. A.* 169 (1991), 515–521.

Wallman, J., and Pettigrew, J. D. Conjugate and disjunctive saccades in two avian species with contrasting oculomotor strategies. *J. Neurosci.* 5 (1985), 1418–1428.

Walls, G. L. *The Vertebrate Eye and Its Adaptive Radiation.* Hafner, New York, 1942.

Westheimer, G. Visual acuity and hyperacuity. *Invest. Ophthal. Visual Sci.* 14 (1975), 570.

Westheimer, G. Cooperative neural processes involved in stereoscopic acuity. *Exp. Brain. Res.* 36 (1979), 585–597.

Yazulla, S. Intraretinal differentiation in the synaptic organisation of the inner plexiform layer of the pigeon retina. *J. Comp. Neurol.* 153 (1974), 309–324.

4 The Visual Capabilities of Birds

William Hodos

Of all the vertebrate classes, birds are the most visual dependent. Many aspects of their adaptation to their environment and their survival depend on precise and sometimes quite subtle visual discrimination. Such behaviors as foraging for food, defense of territory and the nest, selection of mates, orientation, homing, and navigation depend on a well developed and highly sensitive visual system. We have already seen in the preceding chapters how exquisitely designed is the avian eye as an optical device; in the next chapter (Varela et al.) we will see how finely tuned it is to detect the most subtle differences in color. In this chapter we shall explore the abilities of the avian visual system (eye and visual brain) for the detection and discrimination of small differences in the spatial distribution and intensity of achromatic light.

PSYCHOPHYSICS

Psychophysics is that branch of psychology that deals with the measurement of sensory events. It attempts to answer such questions as What is the dimmest light that can be detected? or What is the smallest gap between two bars that can be visualized? Although psychophysics is one of the oldest branches of human psychology, its use in the realm of animal psychology is a much more recent development that was largely made possible by the marriage of human psychophysical methodology with the sophisticated and highly automated techniques for training animals developed by B. F. Skinner. One of the pioneers of this approach was Donald Blough, who used these methods to determine the course of dark adaptation (Blough, 1956) and spectral sensitivity (Blough, 1957) in pigeons.

Psychophysicists who study humans often measure absolute thresholds and difference thresholds. The basic principle of animal psychophysics is to train the animal to respond differently in the presence of a stimulus than in its absence for the determination of an absolute threshold. To measure difference thresholds, the animals are trained to respond differently in the presence of one stimulus than in the presence of a quantitatively different stimulus. In either case, this usually is accomplished by rewarding the animal in one stimulus condition and not rewarding it in the other. The difference between the amount of behavior in the presence of the rewarded stimulus condition and the nonrewarded stimulus condition becomes a measure of the animal's ability to differentiate between the two stimuli. The threshold usually is considered to be that value of the stimulus that results in performance that is halfway between perfect detection and performance that is based on chance or random guessing. Another variant is to require the animal to select one response option (such as pecking on the right) in the presence of one stimulus and another response option (such as pecking on the left) for the other stimulus.

Once the animal has learned the "rules of the game," the experimenter begins to manipulate the intensity or some other property of the stimulus (or the difference between two stimuli) until it can no longer be detected. The stimulus may be varied according to some predetermined or random sequence or it may be adjusted according to the animal's performance. In the latter approach, known as "tracking," if the animal does well, the stimulus is weakened or the difference is made smaller; if the animal does poorly, the stimulus is strengthened or the difference increased.

BRIGHTNESS

Brightness is the psychological response to the intensity of a visual stimulus. We have investigated the abilities of pigeons to detect small differences in the intensity or luminance or visual targets (Hodos and Bonbright, 1972). Two types of targets are presented to the birds: a standard luminance of 300 cd/m^2 and variable stimuli that are dimmer by a specified amount. The pigeon views each target and must decide if it is seeing the standard or one of the dimmer, variable stimuli. It registers its choice by pecking to the right or to the left. If it is correct in its selection it is rewarded with grain; if it has made an error, it gets no grain for its efforts and must start again.

A plot, known as a psychometric function, is made of the percentage of correct responses as a function of the difference between the standard and the variable stimuli. The difference threshold is determined from that difference between the standard and the variable that corresponds to 75% correct, which is halfway between chance responding (50%) and perfect detection (100%). This intensity difference is known as the point of subjective equality (PSE). The difference between the PSE and the standard is the difference threshold. We determined from a large group of pigeons that were studied over the years in a number of experiments that the mean threshold for intensity differences in pigeons is 0.11 log unit ($\pm$ 0.003 SEM), which corresponds to the amount of light attenuation that would be produced by two microscope cover glasses interposed in the beam path (Hodos et al., 1985). The most sensitive pigeons had difference thresholds of approximately 0.05 log unit, which corresponds to a difference of about 10% in luminance.

The reader should note that these data were collected in a successive viewing of the stimuli, i.e., the pigeon must compare each stimulus to its memory of the standard and then decide if it is looking at the standard or one of the variable stimuli. When the stimuli were viewed simultaneously, we were unable to produce (by means of optical density) differences that were small enough to be undetectable by the pigeons. By extrapolation, however, we estimated that the simultaneous discrimination difference threshold for pigeons is about 0.01 log unit.

BRIGHTNESS SCALING

Psychophysics is a process that measures sensory events in physical units such as cd/m^2, decibels, g/cm^2, nanometers, etc. In contrast, psychophysical scaling attempts to measure sensory events in psychological units. A detailed discussion of psychophysical scaling is beyond the scope of this review, but some examples from our laboratory may indicate how this approach can be used.

If we consider the size of the difference threshold as a unit of discriminability, then we can construct a psychological scale by successively adding these discriminability units together. This is feasible as Sommers (1972) showed and the result is a scale that is a linear function of the logarithm of intensity. This outcome is consistent with the psychophysical law of G. T. Fechner (1966) that relates the perceived psychological magnitude of a stimulus to the logarithm of the intensity of the physical stimulus. Thus, in the situation in which the standard (brightest) stimulus is 300 cd/m^2 and the dimmest variable stimulus is 50 cd/m^2, the PSE is 240 cd/m^2 and the difference threshold would be 60 cd/m^2. By using this Fechnerian scaling technique we could state that the animal would be able to fractionate the physical continuum from 50 to 300 cd/m^2 into approximately seven discriminable, psychological units of brightness (Hodos and Bonbright, 1974; Hodos, 1976). The implication of such a scaling analysis is that if an animal is very sensitive (i.e., has a low difference threshold), very small changes in the size of the difference threshold translate into very large changes in the number of discriminable units. On the other hand, if the animal has low sensitivity, even fairly large changes in the difference threshold have only minor effects on the number of discriminable steps between the brightest and dimmest stimuli.

BRIGHTNESS CONTRAST

We should not lose sight of the fact that stimuli rarely exist in the absence of a background or surround condition. Moreover, the interaction between the surround and the target can have by important consequences for the subjects psychological response to the target. These effects are well known in human visual perception where the nature of the surround can have dramatic effects on the apparent brightness color or size of the target. We have demonstrated (Hodos and Leibowitz, 1978) that such effects also occur in the avian visual system. Pigeons were trained to discriminate the difference in brightness between two self-luminous disks. Each disk was surrounded by a self-luminous annulus. When the annuli were of equal luminance, the pigeons were rewarded for pecking the disc with the higher intensity, which presumably appeared brighter to them. When this discrimination was well established, the birds intermittently were presented with a situation in which the disks were equally luminous, but the annuli differed. To human observers the effect was very obvious; the disk within the less luminous (dimmer) annulus appeared brighter than the disk within the more luminous annulus. This is the well-known phenomenon of brightness contrast. In the case of the avian observers, the overwhelming majority consistently responded as did the humans and chose the disc that was within the less luminous of the two annuli.

SIZE

A second property of visual stimuli that is important to animals is the spatial extent or size of a stimulus. Just as we measured the pigeons' ability to detect small differences in luminance, we were able to use the same methodology to measure their ability to detect small differences in the size of a target (Hodos et al., 1985). The standard target was an annulus with a diameter of 3.0 mm. The birds initially were trained to discriminate this annulus from one that had a diameter of 15.0 mm. Once the large vs. small discrimination was established, we systematically varied the size of the variable annulus. The mean difference threshold was 0.94 mm ($\pm$ 0.08). In other words, the typical pigeon could just barely differentiate a 3.00-mm annulus from a 3.94-mm annulus. The most sensitive pigeons could detect a 3.0-mm annulus from a 3.3-mm annulus; like brightness differences, the limit of size difference discrimination also is about 10%.

SIZE SCALING

The same psychophysical scaling approach as we used for brightness was applied to stimulus size (Kertzman and Hodos, 1988). The analysis revealed that the average pigeon could fractionate the size range from 3 to 15 mm into about six or seven discriminable units.

TILT

Another important property of visual stimuli is its orientation in space. To determine how well pigeons can detect differences in orientation, we trained pigeons to discriminate a self-luminous bar that was tilted 45° to the right from one that was tilted 45° to the left. When this discrimination was established, we presented the birds with stimuli that were less tilted and plotted their percentages of correct detection of the degree of tilt on a psychometric function. The results indicated that the pigeons were quite readily able to detect all but the smallest differences in tilt to the right or left; indeed the actual mean difference threshold for tilt was 11.3° (± 0.42). For comparison purposes, consider that when the hour hand of a clock moves from 1:00 to 1:05 it changes its tilt by 30°. To detect a tilt of 11.3° we would have to notice something that was slightly less than the difference between 1:00 and 1:02 on a clock with no numbers and no indication of the positions of any of the minutes.

ACUITY

In addition to their ability to detect small differences in the sizes of stimuli, birds also are excellent at the detection of the fine details of stimuli. Such an ability is known as visual acuity. We have tested the visual acuity of pigeons (Hodos et al., 1976) using our psychophysical procedure but with stimuli that consisted of fine, square-wave optical gratings that ranged in frequency from 1 to 20 lines/mm. The gratings were presented immediately behind an optically neutral, glass window by means of a motorized wheel. The pigeons were required to discriminate the grating from a neutral-density filter that transmitted the same intensity of light, but which was completely blank. The percentage of correct responses was plotted as a function of the spatial frequencies of the gratings to form a typical psychometric function. The threshold of detectability in lines/mm was determined from this function by observing which grating frequency corresponded to 75% correct.

The threshold of detectability in lines/mm unfortunately is of little use by itself as an indicator of the resolving power of the visual system because the size of the retinal image of a target depends on the distance of that target from the eye; the closer to the eye, the larger the image on the retina. To estimate the size of the image, we performed a photographic analysis of the pigeons as they were observing the stimulus. From this analysis we could determine the viewing distance (Hodos et al., 1991a; Macko and Hodos, 1984, 1985) from which we were able to calculate the size of the retinal image in terms of the number of cycles (line/space pairs) of the grating that subtended one degree of visual angle. The average pigeon had a visual acuity of 12.7 cycles/deg (± 0.43), which would correspond to human acuity on the familiar

Snellen eye chart of approximately 20/50 or 6/14 in metric units. This corresponds well with the values reported by Fite et al. (1975) for blue jays and Blough (1971) for the acuity of pigeons that were viewing distant targets. In practical terms this means that in good illumination the typical pigeon could just barely detect a seed with a width of 0.3 mm at a distance of 50 cm. The best of our pigeons, however, had acuities of approximately 18 cycles/deg, which corresponds to 20/33 (6/10) and is not far from normal human acuity of 20/20 (6/6). Excellent as the pigeon's acuity is, however, it does not rival that of predatory birds such as hawks and eagles, which are better than that of pigeons by at least an order of magnitude (Fox et al., 1976; Reymond, 1985, 1987). Among the factors that affect visual acuity are the luminance and wavelength of the target illuminant and the adaptation level of the subject. The influence of these factors in turn is affected by the relative proportions of photoreceptor types that are present in the retina. Thus we would expect pigeons, which are diurnal birds and have a rod-poor retina, to perform less well under conditions of dark adaptation than would owls, which are nocturnal and have a rod-rich retina. Such indeed is the case; under conditions of photopic illumination pigeons have higher acuity (Hodos and Leibowitz, 1977) than do owls (Fite, 1973; Martin and Gordon, 1974), but under scotopic adaptation, the reverse is true. Likewise, when the spectral composition of the grating illuminant changes, the visual acuity of the subject changes in accordance with the spectral sensitivities of its various cone types. Hodos and Leibowitz (1977) reported that pigeons, like humans, are in the range of 525–575 nm. Longer and shorter wavelengths result in losses of acuity; the most severe losses occur at the short wavelength end of the spectrum, which suggests a paucity of blue sensitive cones.

The luminance of the acuity stimulus also has a great affect on its detectability as we all have discovered when we noticed how the finer details of an object were better visible in stronger illumination. As in humans and other mammals, such also is the case in pigeons (Hodos et al., 1976) for which optimal acuity occurs when the stimulus luminance is in the range of 300–1000 cd/m^2.

VELOCITY

In the visual world, stimuli do not always remain in a fixed position. Movement, absolute or relative, thus is a fundamental property of visual stimuli. Hodos et al. (1975) investigated the movement-detection thresholds of stimuli that exhibited either linear or radial movement. The psychophysical techniques were virtually identical to those described above for intensity and spatial vision. In particular, the pigeons were required to respond differentially in the presence of a moving or a stationary target. The results of our studies indicated that the velocity-detection thresholds of pigeons ranged from 4.4 to 6.5 mm/sec which correspond to retinal velocities of 4.1–6.01 deg/sec. Similar data were reported by Mulvanny (1978). In contrast, human observers can detect retinal velocities of 3 min/sec (Graham, 1968).

Maldonado et al. (1988) report that pigeons use frontal viewing for slow or static stimuli, but adopt a lateral viewing orientation to fast moving stimuli. Since the velocity thresholds reported here were determined in frontal viewing, one must consider the possibility that the retinal regions that view the frontal and lateral visual fields may be specialized for different aspects of viewing, such as static versus dynamic acuity.

Studies that base their findings on the minimal stimulus velocity necessary to activate the optokinetic reflex may not be dealing with the same phenomenon as that in which an animal must decide whether to peck left or right depending on whether the target is moving or stationary. In other words, we do not know whether an animal "sees" the movement of the visual world that causes these reflex movements of its eyes just as we have no awareness of the reflex changes in our pupil diameter in response to changes in the level of illumination in the environment.

VISUAL SEARCH

One of the most common visual tasks for animals or humans is to find an object somewhere in the visual environment. Tasks that are designed to investigate this are known as visual-search tasks. In the commonly used procedure, the subject is presented with an array of objects that are similar, except for one. The subject's task is to locate the dissimilar object. We have devised a variant of this task for pigeons (Hodos et al., 1993a). The pigeon is confronted by a video monitor that produces a retinal image that subtended 34° × 40° on the retina. On this screen either a + or an = (2.7° × 2.7°) could appear in any one of 16 locations on the screen. The pigeon first makes an "observing response" that indicates to the experimenters that it is ready to begin a trial. The observing response causes the stimulus to appear somewhere on the monitor screen where it remains for a duration that may be as short as 150 msec or as long as 1500 msec. The pigeon's task is to detect the stimulus during the observation interval and then to indicate by pecking right or left whether the stimulus was the + or the =. By plotting a psychometric function of the percentage of correct responses as a function of the duration of the observation interval, we have determined that the mean search time for pigeons under these experimental conditions is 373.8 msec (± 20). This value compares favorably with the data of Blough (1977, 1979), who reported similar search times for pigeons but with different psychophysical methods and different stimuli.

EFFECTS OF AGING ON VISION

As animals age, various changes occur in their vision. Some of these changes are due to changes in the optical media of the eye, some due to degenerative changes in the retina, and some due to changes in the central visual system (Bagnoli and Hodos, 1991). Among the causes of the changes in the eye are such factors as the intensity, duration, and spectral composition of the animal or human's light-exposure history (Fite et al., 1991; Werner, 1991).

In both pigeons and quail, visual acuity shows a progressive decline with age from young adulthood to senescence (Hodos et al., 1991a,b; Porciatti et al., 1991. This decline has been correlated with losses of certain classes of photoreceptors (Hodos, et al., 1991a). In addition to the acuity losses, pigeons also suffer from senile miosis, a progressive diminution in maximum pupil diameter with age that also occurs in human visual aging (Hodos et al., 1991a). These age-dependent changes should be taken into account by investigators who use the less expensive retired breeders as their subjects or who keep well-trained, experienced pigeons as subjects in their laboratories for many years. Those who use feral pigeons as their subjects should consider that animals reared in the wild age more rapidly than those reared in captivity and may not be comparable to domesticated animals of the same chronological age (Hodos, 1991).

Kurkjian and Hodos (1992) reported little change in intensity difference thresholds over the same age span in which acuity showed a serious decline. Likewise, visual search, a sensitive indicator of human visual aging (Plude and Hoyer, 1981), showed no age-related change in pigeons over the same age span that resulted in visual acuity losses. These findings are of particular interest because they indicate plainly that the acuity losses in pigeons (and probably quail as well) are specific to spatial vision and are not indicative of global age-dependent changes that could affect cognitive functions such as memory or attention.

CONTRAST SENSITIVITY

Visual acuity tells us about a bird's or a person's ability to resolve small differences between objects that have high contrast. But this does not tell the complete story of an eye's or an optical system's ability to form useful images. An image, such as a square, consists of low spatial-frequency components, that give us information about global properties of the stimulus such as its size. The square also contains high spatial-frequency components that tell us about the small details, such as the sharpness of the corners. High-frequency filtering of the optical image of the square would thus round the corners of the square and make its edges blurry. Visual acuity only tell us how the visual or optical system handles the fine details; high contrast is required to see these fine details. Contrast is the difference in luminance between the darkest and lightest parts of an image expressed as a percentage of the total luminance; in the case of a grating, contrast is the difference in the luminances of the dark and light bars as a percentage of their combined luminances.

Visual and optical systems also can form useful images of objects at low contrast, even though the fine details may be lost. Visual acuity tells only about the ability to resolve high-contrast, high spatial-frequency objects; it tells us nothing about ability to detect the low-frequency properties of stimuli, which can be accomplished quite well at relatively low levels of contrast.

A contrast-sensitivity function is an assessment of a visual system's ability to form useful images in over a wide range of spatial-frequency ranges and over a wide range of contrasts. The procedure involves determining the lowest contrast at which a grating of a given spatial frequency can be detected. A contrast-sensitivity curve thus is a plot of the reciprocal of the contrast threshold (i.e., sensitivity) as a function of the spatial frequencies of the gratings in cycles per degree of visual angle. Contrast-sensitivity functions typically have the form of an inverted U. By extrapolating the high-frequency limb of the curve to the baseline (i.e., to the highest contrast) and noting the spatial frequency at the intercept (the so-called "high-frequency cutoff"), an estimate of visual acuity can be made since visual acuity is the ability to detect high-frequency, high-contrast gratings.

Figure 4.1 shows contrast-sensitivity curves for pigeons (Nye, 1968; Hodos et al., 1993b), an eagle (Reymond and Wolfe, 1981), and a falcon (Hirsch, 1982). The data of Nye (1968) are unusual because he used a binomial probability measure of threshold that is roughly equivalent to 66% correct on a psychometric function rather than the conventional 75% correct. This may account for the unusually broad range of spatial frequencies and the very high estimate of visual acuity for pigeons. The high-frequency-cutoff data of Hodos et al. (1993b) are consistent with the visual acuity data of Hodos et al. (1976) for stimuli of this luminance. Jassik-Gerschenfeld and Hardy (1979), who recorded contrast sensitivity curves of single cells in the pigeon optic tectum using virtually the same target luminance as Hodos et al. (1993b), reported that they were unable to record high-frequency cutoffs above 7 cycles/deg, which is consistent with the observations of Hodos et al. (1993b), but not those of Nye (1968). Hodos et al. (1991a) were able to obtain visual acuities as high as the high-frequency cutoff of Nye (1968), but only with much higher target luminance. The high-frequency cutoff of the falcon is approximately 35 cycles/deg and that of the eagle is in the vicinity of 100 cycles/deg.

Figure 4.2 shows the effects of age on contrast sensitivity. Data are shown for two human subjects and four pigeons. All six subjects were tested with the same apparatus (Hodos et al., 1993b). For both species,

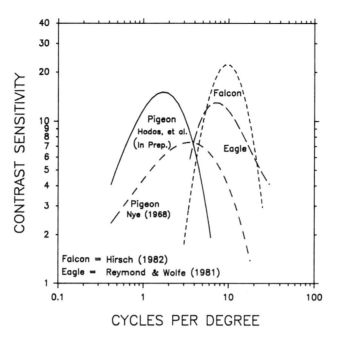

Figure 4.1 Contrast-sensitivity curves for pigeons (Nye, 1968; Hodos, et al., 1993b), an eagle (Reymond and Wolfe, 1981), and a falcon (Hirsch, 1982).

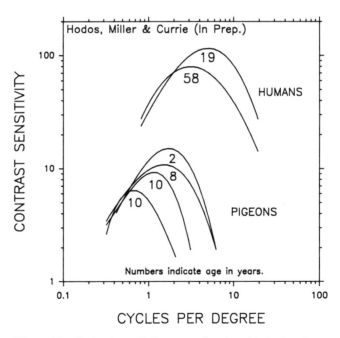

Figure 4.2 Contrast-sensitivity curves for six subjects: two humans and four pigeons (Hodos et al., 1993b). All subjects were tested using the same apparatus. The numbers in the figure indicate the ages of the subjects in years.

the typical effects of age (Owsley et al., 1983) can be seen, i.e., a progressive loss of high spatial frequencies with increasing age, but little change in the low frequencies. Increasing age also results in a progressive decrease in the maximum sensitivity to contrast and in a shift of the location of this maximum to progressively lower frequencies. In other words, the elderly lose the ability to resolve high and intermediate spatial-frequency components of stimuli, but the low-frequency components are little affected.

A major difference between the contrast sensitivities of birds and humans is the maximum sensitivity. The peak pigeon contrast sensitivity was approximately 14, which corresponds to about 7% contrast. The falcon's peak sensitivity was 28, which corresponds to 3.6% contrast. The humans, on the other hand, peaked at about 150, which equals 0.7% contrast. Peak sensitivities of humans, and mammals in general typically are in the contrast-sensitivity range of 100–200. Why birds, which have visual systems so highly adapted for virtually every aspect of the visual world, should be so relatively poor at detecting low contrast targets is not clear. Without doubt birds are well adapted to the high-contrast properties of the visual world. This weaker ability to detect the low-contrast properties of the visual environment may reflect a trade-off in the optical design of the eye to permit high acuity with relatively small eyes and relatively small pupils.

EFFECTS OF VISUAL SYSTEM LESIONS

A full survey of the effects of visual system lesions on psychophysical indicators is beyond the scope of this review. But a few general observations should be mentioned. We have compared the effects of lesions of the tectofugal and thalamofugal pathways (see chapter by Shimizu and Karten (this volume) using visual acuity, brightness difference threshold, size difference threshold, and visual search. In general we have found that lesions of the tectofugal pathway (nucleus rotundus or ectostriatum) result in elevations of intensity difference threshold, size threshold, and search time as well as losses in visual acuity (Hodos and Bonbright, 1974; Hodos et al., 1984, 1986, 1988; Kertzman and Hodos, 1988; Macko and Hodos, 1984). In contrast, lesions of the thalamofugal pathway (OPT complex or visual wulst) result in little or no change in intensity difference threshold or visual acuity (Hodos et al., 1984; Macko and Hodos, 1984; Pasternak and Hodos, 1977). A tempting explanation has been that only the tectofugal pathway processes visual information and that the thalamofugal pathway is involved in processing "something else." No convincing explanations of what that something else might be have been offered. Recently, Remy and Güntürkün (1991) have reported that the OPT complex receives very few ganglion cell axons from the retinal red field, which is the part of the retina used for viewing close objects such as the stimuli in visual-discrimination experiments. A similar result was reported by Britten (1987). Thus we must consider the possibility that our lack of effects from thalamofugal lesions may be the result of the fact that our apparatus has put the stimuli on the wrong part of the retina. Further research will be necessary to see if this is a reasonable conclusion. We should add, however, that we cannot state that OPT is totally uninvolved with the processing of information coming from the retinal red field because when lesions of the thalamofugal pathway are combined with lesions of the tectofugal pathway, the effects are much larger than those of tectofugal pathway lesions alone. Indeed they often are larger than the sum of the tectofugal and thalamofugal effects combined. Moreover, the sequence of the combined lesions can be an important factor (Riley et al., 1988). These effects suggest that we still have some way to go before we can feel that we have a complete understanding of the function of these two visual pathways in the processing of visual information.

ACKNOWLEDGMENTS

I am grateful to Mrs. Ellen Carta for assistance in manuscript preparation and to the National Eye Institute, which supported much of the research reported here through Grant EY-00735.

REFERENCES

Bagnoli, P., and Hodos, W. (Eds.). *The Changing Visual System: Maturation and Aging in the Central Nervous System*. Plenum, New York, 1991.

Blough, D. S. Dark adaptation in the pigeon. *J. Comp. Physiol. Psychol.* 49 (1956), 425–430.

Blough, D. S. Spectral sensitivity in the pigeon. *J. Opt. Soc. Am.* 47 (1957), 827–833.

Blough, D. S. Visual search in pigeons: Hunt and peck method. *Science* 196 (1977), 1013–1014.

Blough, D. S. Effect of number and form of stimuli in visual search in the pigeon. *J. Exp. Psychol., Animal Behav. Proc.* 5 (1979), 211–223.

Blough, P. M. The visual acuity of the pigeon for distant targets. *J. Exp. Anal. Behav.* 15 (1971), 57–68.

Britten, K. H. Receptive fields of neurons of the principal optic nucleus of the pigeon (*Columba livia*). Ph. D. Dissertation, State University of New York at Stony Brook, 1987.

Fechner, G. T. *Elements of Psychophysics*. Holt, Rinehart & Winston, New York, 1966. Translation of 1860 German edition.

Fite, K. V. Anatomical and behavioral correlates of visual acuity in the great horned owl. *Vis. Res.* 13 (1973), 219–230.

Fite, K. V., Stone, R. J., and Conley, M. Visual acuity in the northern blue jay: Behavioral and anatomical correlates. *Neurosci. Abstr.* 1 (1975), 82.

Fite, K. V., Bengston, L., and Donaghy, B. Age, sex and light damage in the avian retina. In P. Bagnoli and W. Hodos (Eds.), *The Changing Visual System: Maturation and Aging in the Central Nervous System*. Plenum, New York, 1991, pp. 283–294.

Fox, R., Lemkuhle, S. W., and Westendorf, D. H. Falcon visual acuity. *Science* 192 (1976), 263–265.

Graham, C. H. Depth and movement. *Am. Psychol.* 23 (1968), 18–26.

Hirsch, J. Falcon visual sensitivity to grating contrast. *Nature (London)* 300 (1982), 57–58.

Hodos, W. Vision and the visual system: a bird's eye-view. In J. M. Sprague and A. N. Epstein (Eds.) *Progress in Psychobiology and Physiological Psychology*, Vol. 6 Academic Press, New York, 1976, pp. 29–62.

Hodos, W. Animal models of life-span development. In P. Bagnoli and W. Hodos (Eds.), *The Changing Visual System: Maturation and Aging in the Central Nervous System*. Plenum, New York, 1991, pp. 21–32.

Hodos, W., and Bonbright, J. C., Jr. The detection of visual intensity differences in pigeons. *J. Exp. Anal. Behav.* 18 (1972), 471–479.

Hodos, W., and Bonbright, J. C., Jr. Intensity difference thresholds in pigeons after lesions of the tectofugal and thalamofugal visual pathways to the telencephalon. *J. Comp. Physiol. Psychol.* 87 (1974), 1013–1031.

Hodos, W., and Leibowitz, R. W. Near-field visual acuity of pigeons: Effects of scotopic adaptation and wavelength. *Vis. Res.* 17 (1977), 463–467.

Hodos, W., and Leibowitz, R. W. Simultaneous brightness contrast induction in pigeons. *Vis. Res.* 18 (1978), 179–181.

Hodos, W., Smith, L., and Bonbright, J. C., Jr. Detection of the velocity of movement of visual stimuli by pigeons. *J. Exp. Anal. Behav.* 25 (1975), 143–156.

Hodos, W., Leibowitz, R. W., and Bonbright, J. C., Jr. Near-field visual acuity of pigeons: Effects of head position and stimulus luminance. *J. Exp. Anal. Behav.* 25 (1976), 129–141.

Hodos, W., Macko, K. A., and Bessette, B. B. Near-field acuity changes after visual system lesions in pigeons, II. Telencephalon. *Behav. Brain Res.* 13 (1984), 15–30.

Hodos, W., Bessette, B. B., Macko, K. A., and Weiss, S. R. B. Normative data for pigeon vision. *Vis. Res.* 25 (1985), 1525–1527.

Hodos, W., Weiss, S. R. B., and Bessette, B. B. Size-threshold changes after lesions of the visual telencephalon in pigeons. *Behav. Brain Res.* 28 (1986), 203–214.

Hodos, W., Weiss, S. R. B., and Bessette, B. B. Intensity difference thresholds after lesions of ectostriatum in pigeons. *Behav. Brain Res.* 30 (1988), 43–53.

Hodos, W., Miller, R. F., and Fite, K. V. Age-dependent changes in visual acuity and retinal morphology in pigeons. *Vis. Res.* 31 (1991a), 669–677.

Hodos, W., Miller, R. F., Fite, K. V., Porciatti, V., Holden, A. L., Lee, J.-Y., and Djamgoz, M. B. A. Life-span changes in the visual acuity and retina in birds. In P. Bagnoli and W. Hodos (Eds.), *The Changing Visual System: Maturation and Aging in the Central Nervous System*. Plenum, New York, 1991b, pp. 137–148.

Hodos, W., Miller, R. F., and Shimizu, T. (1993a). In preparation.

Hodos, W., Miller, R. F., and Currie, D. G. (1993b). In preparation.

Jassik-Gerschenfeld, D., and Hardy, O. Single-neuron responses to moving sine-wave gratings in the pigeon optic tectum. *Vis. Res.* 19 (1979), 993–999.

Kertzman, C., and Hodos, W. Size difference thresholds after lesions of thalamic visual nuclei in pigeons. *Vis. Neurosci.* 1 (1988), 83–92.

Kurkjian, M. L., and Hodos, W. Age-dependent intensity-difference thresholds in pigeons. *Vis. Res.* 32 (1992), 1249–1252.

Macko, K. A., and Hodos, W. Near-field acuity after visual system lesions in pigeons. I. Thalamus. *Behav. Brain Res.* 13 (1984), 1–14.

Macko, K. A. and Hodos, W. Near point of accommodation in pigeons. *Vis. Res.* 25 (1985), 1529–1530.

Maldonado, P. E., Maturana, H., and Varela, F. J. Frontal and lateral visual system in birds. *Brain Behav. Evol.* 32 (1988), 57–62.

Martin, G. R., and Gordon, I. E. Visual acuity in the tawny owl *(Strix aluco)*. *Vis. Res.* 14 (1975), 1393–1397.

Mulvanny, P. Velocity discrimination by pigeons. *Vis. Res.* 27 (1978), 531–536.

Nye, P. The binocular acuity of the pigeon measured in terms of the modulation transfer function. *Vis. Res.* 8 (1968), 1041–1053.

Owsley, C., Sekuler, R., and Siemsen, D. Contrast sensitivity throughout adulthood. *Vis. Res.* 23 (1983), 689–699.

Pasternak, T., and Hodos, W. Intensity difference thresholds after lesions of the visual wulst in pigeons. *J. Comp. Physiol. Psychol.* 91 (1977), 485–497.

Plude, D. J., and Hoyer, W. J. Adult age differences in visual search as a function of stimulus mapping and information load. *J. Gerontol.* 36 (1981), 598–604.

Porciatti, V., Hodos, W., Signorini, G., and Bramanti, F. Electroretinographic changes in aged pigeons. *Vis. Res.* 31 (1991), 661–668.

Remy, M., and Güntürkün, O. Retinal afferents to the tectum opticum and the nucleus opticus principalis thalami in the pigeon. *J. Comp. Neurol.* 305 (1991), 57–70.

Reymond, L. Spatial visual acuity of the eagle, *Aquila audax:* A behavioural, optical and anatomical investigation. *Vis. Res.* 25 (1985), 1477–1491.

Reymond, L. Spatial visual acuity of the falcon, *Falco berigora.* A behavioural, optical and anatomical investigation. *Vis. Res.* 27 (1987), 1859–1874.

Reymond L., and Wolfe, J. Behavioural determination of the contrast sensitivity function of the eagle. *Aquila audax, Vis. Res.* 27 (1981), 263–271.

Riley N., Hodos, W., and Pasternak, T. Effects of serial lesions of telencephalic components of the visual system in pigeons. *Vis. Neurosci.* 1 (1988), 387–394.

Sommers, D. I. The scaling of visual intensity differences by pigeons. M.A. Thesis. University of Maryland, College Park, 1972.

Werner, J. S. The damaging effects of light on the eye and implications for understanding changes in vision across the life span. In P. Bagnoli and W. Hodos (Eds.), *The Changing Visual System: Maturation and Aging in the Central Nervous System.* Plenum, New York, 1991, pp. 295–310.

5 Color Vision of Birds

Francisco J. Varela, Adrian G. Palacios, and
Timothy H. Goldsmith

The role of color vision in an animal's perception, behavior, and ecological setting, and its underlying retina and neuronal mechanisms vary
enormously in different groups of animals. Amidst this diversity, birds
have arguably the most elaborate and interesting color vision. The
evidence for this assertion comes from various sources. (1) Foremost
are existing knowledge about different types of cells and pigments in
the retina and (2) behavioral experiments demonstrating various chromatic abilities. Less extensive evidence can be drawn from (3) physiological analyses of neural mechanisms and (4) occasional ecological
observations. A potential sources of evidence, only now becoming available for birds, is (5) identification and analysis of genes for the proteins
(opsins) of visual pigments (Okano et al., 1992). Information from all
these levels needs to be brought together for a detailed understanding
of the color vision in any animal group. This chapter summarizes for
birds the existing knowledge in the first four of these categories of
evidence. Supplementary information of a broader comparative nature
can be found elsewhere (Goldsmith, 1990; Neumeyer, 1991; Thompson
et al., 1992).

RETINAL BASES

The cones of birds (see Nalbach et al., chapter 2) present more morphological complexity and diversity than those of mammals. First, the
inner segment characteristically contains a colored oil droplet adjacent
to the base of the outer segment, forming a filter through which light
must pass before reaching the visual pigment. The oil droplets are of
several colors, due to the presence of different carotenoids. Second, in
addition to single cones, there are also double cones, consisting of two
closely contiguous cells known as the principal and accessory members
of the pair.

Cone Oil Droplets

Knowledge of cone spectral sensitivity is critical to understanding how any color vision functions. The spectral sensitivity of a bird cone, however, is determined jointly by the product of the spectral transmittance of the oil droplet and the spectral absorptance (i.e., l-transmittance) of the visual pigment. The most direct method of determining the transmittance spectrum of individual oil droplets would appear to be microspectrophotometry, but this measurement involves a serious technical problem. The concentrations of carotenoids, particularly in the deeper-colored droplets, are very high, with peak absorbances (i.e., optical densities) greater than 10 or even 20. In other words, only a minute fraction of the incident light is transmitted by the droplet. The signal from the detector used to measure transmittance therefore becomes dominated by stray light, and an accurate measurement of the droplet's absorption spectrum is not possible. The seriousness of this problem is evident in published records of oil droplet spectra in which the apparent peak absorbance of the dense red and yellow droplets is only 0.7 (Bowmaker and Martin, 1985; Jane and Bowmaker, 1988). In some early work this problem was not recognized; in more recent work on birds it has been dealt with in two different ways.

The simplest approach is to assume that the droplets function as long-pass cut-off filters and to characterize them by the wavelength at 50% transmission and the slope of the transmittance curve in the cut-off region, which the experimenter tries to determine at wavelengths where the transmittance is still high enough to be measured accurately. From this information it is possible to calculate the effect of the droplet on the absorptance of the underlying visual pigment. This approach gives no information on the chemical identity of the absorber, a point of interest because differences in the spectral region of cut off can be due either to different carotenoids or to differences in concentration of the same carotenoid.

A more elaborate approach, first introduced by Liebman and Granda (1975) in a study of turtle oil droplets, is to expand individual cone oil droplets by fusing them with larger droplets of mineral oil. The resulting droplet is not only larger, it has a lower concentration of carotenoid, permitting a sufficiently accurate measurement of spectral absorbance to be useful in chemical identification (Goldsmith et al., 1984). In principle, no information is lost, because with knowledge of the diameters of the original and final droplets it is possible to calculate the transmittance as it was in vivo. An important finding from this approach is that one class of droplets commonly present in many orders of birds contains a mixture of two carotenoids whose proportions frequently vary in different cells in the same retina (table 5.1, P droplets). What appears superficially to be a homogeneous class of droplets is therefore actually

Table 5.1. Classification of Avian Cone Oil Droplets Based on Carotenoid Content (Goldsmith et al., 1984) and Its Possible Relation to Other Schemes Based on Cut-off Wavelengths[a]

Type	Appearance	Identified carotenoids	λ_{max} (nm)	Termi-nology of Bowmaker[b]	Termi-nology of Partridge[c]
R	Red	Astaxanthin	477	red	R
O	Orange	Uncertain	425–477	C(?)	
Y	Yellow	Zeaxanthin	435–455	C	Y_2
P	Pale	Galloxanthin (405 nm) or X (375 nm) plus e-carotene	375–455	B_1	P_1(?)P_2,Y_1
C	Colorless or (pale yellow)	Galloxanthin or X (375 nm)	375–405	A(?)	P_1(?)
T	Transparent	No carotenoid	None	Clear	

[a]X (375 nm) is an apocarotenoid known only from its absorption spectrum in MSP measurements. P droplets contain variable mixtures of e-carotene and an apocarotenoid. Except for e-carotene, all the identified carotenoids in oil droplets are xanthophylls and occur as esters of fatty acids.
[b]Bowmaker (1977) and Bowmaker and Knowles (1977).
[c]Partridge (1989).

heterogeneous. The implications for the spectral properties of afferent chromatic channels are not yet known.

Unfortunately no common agreement has yet emerged on a terminology to characterize avian oil droplets, due mainly to variation (for example, in the aforementioned P droplets), to uncertainties in relating results obtained by the two methods in different laboratories, and to uncertainties whether new measurements from sparsely studied species fit an existing scheme of classification. Table 5.1 tries to relate the measurements and classification of Goldsmith et al. (1984), who reduced the concentration of carotenoids by expanding individual droplets (first column), to the results of Bowmaker (1977), Bowmaker and Knowles (1977), and Partridge (1989), who measured the cut-off properties of undiluted droplets (last columns). As suggested by the interrogation marks (?) in the last two columns, there is considerable uncertainty in bringing these systems into agreement. Confusion abounds, for recently Jane and Bowmaker (1988) have also loosely employed the terminology in column 1, with the result that in early papers this research group used "C" to refer to bright yellow droplets containing high concentrations of C40 xanthophyll, and later to the virtually colorless, galloxanthin-containing droplets.

There are a number of additional issues that require clarification. First, orange droplets are not yet adequately defined; some may contain carotenoids not listed in table 5.1; others may simply hold a higher concentration of zeaxanthin (or lutein) or a lower concentration of astaxanthin. Second, microspectrophotometry in the near UV suggests subclasses of C and P droplets containing an apocarotenoid with λ_{max} at 375 nm (and thus with fewer double bonds than galloxanthin). As has now been noted by several workers, some sauropsid oil droplets fluoresce weakly (e.g., Kolb and Jones, 1987). In bird retinas the fluorescence is associated with droplets containing the apocarotenoid galloxanthin or the unknown carotenoid absorbing maximally about 375 nm (Goldsmith et al., 1984), but the source of the fluorescence has not been identified.

The functions of oil droplets remain a subject for speculation. Suggested functions, would are not mutually exclusive, include narrowing of the spectral sensitivity functions of the cones, with implications for avian color space (Lythgoe, 1979; Barlow, 1982; Govardovskii, 1983; Goldsmith, 1990), protecting the outer segment from short wavelength photo damage (Kirschfeld, 1982), improvement of contrast or relief from chromatic aberration (Muntz, 1972; Miller, 1979), and concentration of light on the outer segment (Baylor and Fettiplace, 1975; Ives et al., 1983; Young and Martin, 1984).

The distributions and proportions of the different colors of oil droplets show variations between species in ways that correlate with diet or other aspects of the ecology (Peiponen, 1964; Partridge, 1989). The dorsal retina tends to have more of the deeply colored red and yellow droplets, particularly in birds that look through an air–water interface (Muntz, 1972). (In pigeons the red and orange droplets are associated with a quadrant of the retina directed forward and down [the "red field"], but this is not characteristic of most other orders of birds.) Of the droplets containing galloxanthin (droplets P and C in the first column of table 5.1), those supplemented with an additional carotenoid (P) are frequently more abundant in the ventral retina, the ones with less color (C), the dorsal retina (Goldsmith et al., 1984). In general, birds with nocturnal or crepuscular habits have many fewer deeply pigmented droplets. See also Nalbach et al., this volume.

Visual Pigments of Cones

Light is trapped in the cones of the eye by pigments consisting of a protein (opsin) conjugated to a fat-soluble molecule called retinal, which is the aldehyde of vitamin A. Cone cells sensitive in different regions of the spectrum owe their different spectral absorption to the presence of different opsins. The retinas of birds characteristically express the genes for three or more cone opsins, each located in a distinct subset of cones. A major source of information about the spectral properties of these pigments has been the microspectrophotometric measurements of Bowmaker and his colleagues. Figure 5.1 summarizes what is known from direct measurements of pigments (filled symbols); in a number of instances the properties of the associated oil droplets have also been determined, and figure 5.1 also indicates the amount of spectral shift

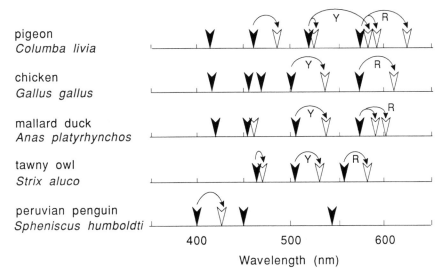

pigeon
Columba livia

chicken
Gallus gallus

mallard duck
Anas platyrhynchos

tawny owl
Strix aluco

peruvian penguin
Spheniscus humboldti

400   500   600

Wavelength (nm)

Figure 5.1 Cone pigments in several species of birds in which there is evidence for three or more opsins. Filled symbols: spectral positions of the wavelengths of maximal absorption of known cone pigments. Most of the data are based on microspectrophotometry. Small curved arrows and open symbols: calculated spectral shifts produced by red (R) and yellow (Y) oil droplets. The absence of an indicator for the droplet means that an unambiguous designation of the droplet type (usually as one of the less deeply colored types in column 1 of table 5.1) is not possible from the published data. Note, however, that the deeply colored (red and yellow) droplets are necessarily found only with the visual pigments that absorb at long wavelengths. Furthermore, some filtering by oil droplets attenuates the short wavelength limb and thus narrows the absorption spectrum of the visual pigment without shifting the wavelength of maximal absorption; such effects are not shown in this diagram. References: Pigeon microspectrophotometry (MSP) of 460, 497, and 569 nm pigments (Bowmaker, 1977); fast photovoltage ("early receptor potential"), 413 nm pigment (Govardovskii and Zueva, 1977). Chicken MSP of 497 and 569 nm pigments (Bowmaker and Knowles, 1977); fast photovoltage, 413 and 449 nm pigments (Govardovskii and Zueva, 1977); extraction of 417 and 467 nm pigments (Fager and Fager, 1981). Mallard duck (including two domestic strains) MSP (Jane and Bowmaker, 1988). Tawny owl, MSP (Bowmaker and Martin, 1978). Penguin MSP (Bowmaker and Martin, 1985).

that these filters can impose on the effective absorption by the accompanying cone pigments (curved arrows and open symbols).

A wide selection of birds have at least three or four cone pigments, and as one pigment may be associated with more than one type of oil droplet (in different cells), the possible number of chromatic channels could, in principle, be larger than the number of cone pigments. In every species examined so far, the pigment absorbing at longest wavelengths (near 570 nm, roughly the spectral region that is occupied by the "red"- and "green"-sensitive pigments in the primate retina) is by far the most abundant. This is iodopsin, first extracted from chickens by Wald et al. (1955), and it appears to be the visual pigment that dominates the photopic spectral sensitivity of birds (Wright, 1979; Wortel et al., 1984; Remy and Emmerton, 1989). The measurements on penguins suggest that in this species the pigment has responded to natural selection for vision in a blue aquatic environment by shifting its absorption spectrum to shorter wavelengths, to an λ_{max} at 543 nm (Bowmaker and Martin, 1985). Birds characteristically have more than one cone pigment absorbing at short wavelengths, but in general those pigments absorbing in the blue and violet are known from small samples of cones, in some cases as few as a single cell (but see also Fager and Fager, 1981).

Physiological Measurements of Spectral Sensitivity in the Retina

By recording light-elicited, transretinal voltages (electroretinogram) in opened eyecups of a variety of birds, mostly passerines, Chen and Goldsmith (1986) were able to measure spectral sensitivity functions under different states of adaptation to colored lights. The conditions were photopic, and the presence of aspartate (used to block the synapses between receptors and retinal neurons) indicated that the spectral responses reflected the properties of receptors. As the light was incident from the vitreal side, the receptors were filtered by oil droplets as they would in vivo. In all species the dark-adapted retinas were maximally sensitive over a broad wavelength band around 580 nm, indicating the presence of the 570-nm cone pigment referred to above. When the retinas were adapted with increasing intensities of orange and yellow lights, the spectral sensitivity functions shifted to shorter wavelengths, finally leaving a distinct maximum in the near UV at 370 nm. Of the 15 species studied (ruby-throated hummingbird [*Archilochus colubris*], pigeon [*Columba livia*], and 13 passerines), all had sensitivity maxima at 370 and 570–580 nm. In the chickadee (*Parus atricapillus*), house sparrow (*Passer domesticus*), house finch (*Carpodacus mexicanus*), northern cardinal (*Cardinalis cardinalis*), and song sparrow (*Melospiza melodia*) (upper line) it was possible to isolate additional maxima at 450 and 480 nm by using adapting lights generated by mixing near UV with orange or yellow light. Other species (lower line) (American robin [*Turdus migratorius*], brown thrasher [*Hylocichla mustelina*], and barn swallow [*Hirundo rustica*] had a cone with λ_{max} at 510 nm. In still other species there was only a single bird with which to work and not all the sensitivity maxima shown in Figure 5.2 were detected before the experiment ended. For the pattern shown in the lower row, there is probably a fourth cone operating in the blue-violet region of the spectrum.

BEHAVIORAL EVIDENCE

Although physiological data may indicate that an animal has color vision, the final judgment about its presence and use must be based on behavioral experiments and ecological observations. A particularly im-

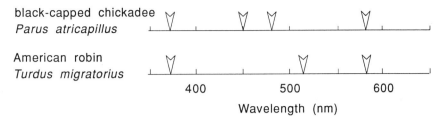

Figure 5.2 Spectral positions of the maxima of spectral sensitivity functions revealed by selective chromatic adaptation of isolated bird retinas. These spectral sensitivity data are believed to reflect the properties of cones, as filtered by oil droplets. The examples shown (chickadee and robin) are representative of a number of species of passerines. Data from Chen and Goldsmith (1986).

portant question that can be settled only by behavioral experiments is whether the animal is able to distinguish between wavelength (color) and intensity (brightness) cues. Only if this question can be answered in the affirmative is it possible to conclude that the animal has color vision. Behavioral experiments can also be used to quantify the capacity for color vision. For example, in which spectral regions is the capacity to discriminate between monochromatic lights of similar wavelengths the keenest? What mixtures of colors are indistinguishable to an animal? Knowledge of these and similar behavioral capacities is critical in understanding how information about color is being handled by the nervous system.

Wavelength Discrimination

Knowing how the animal's ability to discriminate one wavelength from another varies in different spectral regions can be very informative. The results of such measurements are plotted as $\Delta\lambda$ (the minimal separation between two wavelengths that can just be detected as different) vs. l. The animal's ability to discriminate is measured by increasing $\Delta\lambda$ from l until a criterion of (say) 70% correct responses is attained. Since for each wavelength one can obtain two values of $\Delta\lambda$ (one to either side of l), the final curve is usually plotted as the mean of the two. It is essential that wavelengths to be compared be adjusted for the animal's subjective brightness, which means that the experimenter must obtain the animal's spectral sensitivity function. As a consequence, these experiments are very time consuming, and only a handful of results are available.

Table 5.2 shows some results from the pigeon (*Columba livia*) (Hamilton and Coleman, 1933; Wright and Cumming, 1971; Blough, 1961; Riggs et al., 1972; Schneider, 1972; Wright, 1972; Jitsumori, 1978; Nuboer and Wortel, 1987; Palacios et al., 1990a). Each value of wavelength in table 5.2 corresponds to a minimum in the curve of $\Delta\lambda$ vs. λ and identifies a local spectral region of good wavelength discrimination. Figure 5.3a shows two wavelength discrimination functions (Emmerton

Table 5.2. Minima in Wavelength Discrimination Functions Measured in the Pigeon

Wavelength minima (nm)					Reference
		500		580	Hamilton and Coleman (1933)
			540	595	Wright and Cumming (1971)
	460		540	600	Blough (1961)
			530	585	Riggs et al. (1972)
		500	540	600	Schneider (1972)
		500	540	600	Wright (1972)
		510	530	600	Jitsumori (1978)
365–385	460		530	595	Emmerton and Delius (1980)
	470		540[a]	600[a]	Nuboer and Wortel (1987)
			560[b]	610[b]	
	450		530	600	Palacios et al. (1990b)

[a]Yellow field.
[b]Red field.

and Delius, 1980; Palacios et al., 1990a), one of which extends into the near UV. Best discrimination was observed at 370, 460, 530, and 595 nm. Whether the appearance of minima at 500 nm (and at shorter wavelengths) is due to differences in experimental design (caused, for example, by the birds imaging the target on different parts of the retina) or differences between individual birds remains to be determined. Results for the hummingbird (*Archilochus alexandri*) do not reveal a deterioration in wavelength discrimination at short wavelengths, indicating the need to base general conclusions on more than one species (Goldsmith et al., 1981) (figure 5.3b).

Wavelength discrimination curves are interesting because they are an indication, however partial and incomplete, of the different chromatic processes that are actually operating in color vision. Antagonistic interactions between neural signals (opponent mechanisms) are responsible for minima in the wavelength discrimination curve. The inputs to these neural mechanisms, however, need not correspond to single types of cone. There are more minima in the wavelength discrimination functions of pigeons than of Old World primates, suggesting that avian color vision may be more elaborate than the trichromacy of humans.

Color Mixing

In the color vision of Old World primates, three independent chromatic stimuli must be available in color mixtures to produce a visual match with any arbitrarily selected colored light. Our color vision is thus said to be trichromatic, and this is related to the fact that we have three different spectral classes of cone cells. Determining the dimensionality

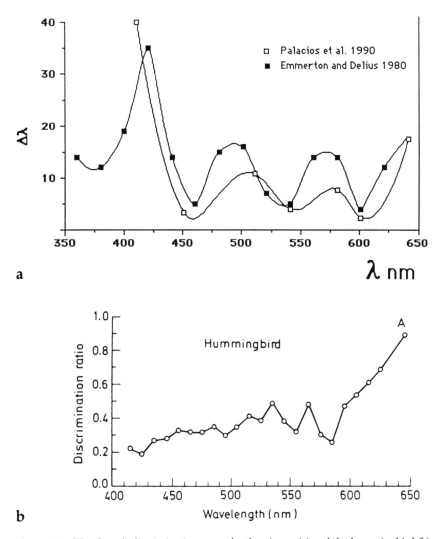

Figure 5.3 Wavelength discrimination curve for the pigeon (a) and the hummingbird (b) showing three minima. Data on pigeons from Emmerton and Delius (1980) and Palacios et al. (1990a); on hummingbird, from Goldsmith et al. (1981). The hummingbird data are a plot of fraction incorrect:fraction correct when test and training lights were a fixed 10 nm apart, and are therefore not a Δλ vs. λ function. They indicate, however, that these birds have optimal wavelength discrimination at the short wavelength region of the spectrum.

of color vision of other species is a major behavioral task and can be achieved only by color mixing and color matching experiments. Operationally, dimensionality refers to the minimum number of independent variables (i.e., colored lights, characterized by wavelength and intensity) required to generate all color matches of which the animal is capable. Data on color matching are frequently presented in graphic form, in which a color dimension is represented as an independent axis in a vector space (Wyszecki and Stiles, 1981). An example of such a plot appears in figure 5.5, and further explanation is provided below.

Until recently, color mixing data for birds were conspicuously absent. An early successful color match was reported in the qualitative observations of Delius et al. (1972). These authors tested young herring and lesser black-backed gulls (*Larus argentatus, L. fuscus*), which indicate a desire to be fed by pecking spontaneously at a bright orange spot on the parent's beak. When the experimenter replaced this target with two pure spectral lights (536 and 620 nm) or a mixture of both, the young bird pecked preferentially at the mixture.

A quantitative study on pigeons has recently been reported (Palacios et al., 1990b; Palacios and Varela, 1992). The principal method was a modified autoshaping procedure, which takes advantage of the animal's spontaneous tendency to peck. After a short period of training, the birds pecked continuously whenever a positive stimulus was present (Palacios et al., 1990a). When the animal compared a monochromatic reference stimulus (S−) with an appropriate mixture of two spectral sources, a decrease from 90% correct responses to 50% (chance) indicated that the animal was unable to distinguish the mixture from the reference wavelength. These experiments establish that pigeons can make a variety of color matches throughout their visible spectrum. Examples of dichromatic matches made by four pigeons at the long

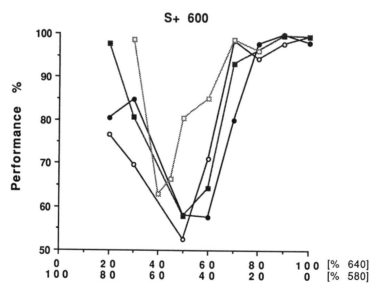

Figure 5.4 Color matches of a monochromatic light of 600 nm (S+) with mixtures of two spectral lights (580 and 640 nm) presented in varying proportions (indicated as percentage on the x-axis). Curves are for four individual pigeons. A fall to chance performance (50% correct) indicates that the animal confuses the two stimuli and thus establishes the match. Data from Palacios et al. (1990b). Like humans, the pigeon is dichromatic in this long wavelength region of the spectrum.

wavelength end of the spectrum are shown in figure 5.4, where the abscissa shows the proportion of 640 and 580 nm light required for confusion with S+ = 600 nm.

The fundamental principle that is involved in color matches is that two physically different lights (i.e., 600 nm monochromatic light [orange] and an appropriate mixture of 640 and 580 nm lights [red and yellow] in the example of figure 5.4) are able to excite the population of retinal cones in an identical manner. It therefore becomes appropriate to compare the results with predictions derived from knowledge of the spectral properties of those cones that are likely to have been activated during the color matching experiments (Palacios et al., 1990b; Palacios and Varela, 1992). These predictions can be made quantitative by calculating the fraction of the incident light that is trapped by each spectral type of cone, where the properties of each spectral type are determined by the absorption spectrum of the visual pigment and the effect of the overlying oil droplet.

As in our own eye, the color vision of the pigeon is dichromatic in a spectral region limited to long wavelengths, and the experimental data on pigeons are consistent with the presence of cone systems in the red field having maxima and 575 and 619 nm. For the middle-wavelength region, primary mechanisms with maxima at 485–nm for the red field and 525 nm for the yellow field appear to be present, along with two additional mechanisms in the violet at 415 nm and in the near UV at 350 or 360 nm. These experiments thus provide strong evidence for a pentachromatic nature to the pigeon's color space, but three- and four-way color mixtures are still needed to establish this point more fully.

The Maxwell color triangle is one of the graphic conventions that can be used to convey information about color matches. In this convention, the proportions in which the three receptors in a trichromatic system are activated are plotted on a triangular coordinate system in which points at the three vertices of the triangle correspond to exclusive activation of each of three cone systems (Rushton, 1972). Figure 5.5 shows how this graphic convention can be expanded to a color tetrahedron to accommodate a tetrachromatic color space.

Color Constancy and Color Contrast

In addition to several independent cone systems, neural interactions are also important participants in color vision. The well-known and related phenomena of color constancy (the relative invariance of perceived hue with changes in illumination) and color contrast (the appearance of complementary colors adjacent to or following the presentation of a colored stimulus) are manifestations of lateral neural interactions and play important roles in color vision theory (Hurvich, 1981; Jameson and Hurvich, 1989; Hurlbert, 1986). In fact, the integra-

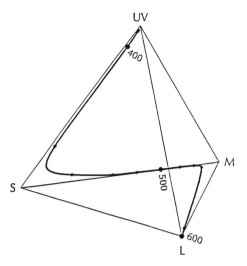

Figure 5.5 A calculated color tetrahedron for a passerine bird possessing the cone system shown in the upper part of figure 5.2. The calculated spectral locus is indicated by the heavy line. If only three receptors are present, the color space projects onto one of the faces of the tetrahedron, forming the more familiar color triangle. With a fourth (UV) receptor present, the spectral locus rises out of the floor of the tetrahedron at short wavelengths. From Goldsmith (1990).

tive processes underlying these psychophysical phenomena are universal participants in all color vision systems.

Color constancy has been shown quantitatively in the bee and qualitatively in the goldfish, and some preliminary evidence is available on color induction in pigeons (Budnik, 1985). In these experiments pigeons were trained to respond to a positive stimulus generated using broad band filters (Kodak Wratten) so that the animal effectively responded to a chromatic class. After the training phase, the animal was tested by replacing the positive stimulus with a neutral field surrounded by a ring of the complementary color. In many cases the animal responded to the test field as though it were colored like the original field. This effect was dependent on the area of the annular surround and the distance between surround and the spectrally neutral center, as is to be expected from a lateral integrative effect in which the center took on a hue complementary to the surround. In fact, these geometrical parameters seem quite comparable in humans, the pigeon and the honeybee, as shown in figure 5.6. Needless to say, quantitative data on color contrast and color constancy are sorely needed for birds.

NEUROPHYSIOLOGY

Surprisingly, a survey of the literature reveals very few experimental studies on the neural substrate of avian color vision. Birds and mammals use homologous structures in the brain in importantly different ways.

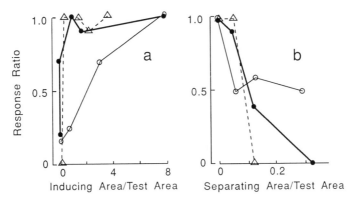

Figure 5.6 Induction of the training color in a neural test field by the presence of a surround of the complementary color, as indicated by behavioral responses to the test field. (a) The behavioral response (ordinate) is stronger the larger the ratio of inducing to test areas. (b) The presence of a ring separating the inducing and test areas diminishes the response as the area of the ring increases. Filled circles: pigeons; open circles: humans (Budnik, 1985); triangles, honeybees (Neumeyer, 1980). Data have been normalized for comparison.

For example, in birds the optic tectum, rather than the lateral geniculate nucleus of the thalamus, is the major relay center for ascending visual information. It is therefore not possible to transfer knowledge about areas of the mammalian brain that are involved in color vision to an understanding of the color vision of birds, and, conversely, other regions of the avian brain are involved in color vision than those that play a role in mammals. In view of the different evolutionary histories of avian and mammalian brains, comparative data should be very rewarding. The visual pathways are discussed in more detail in part II of this volume.

Optic Nerve

Donner (1953) was the first to study the responses of optic nerve fibers in the pigeon. More recently Marin (1983; see Varela et al., 1983) recorded from more than 200 fibers in the optic tract of the quail. Of these, 18% were tonic fibers exhibiting sustained responses that were readily modulated by changing the wavelength (adjusted for equal brightness) of the stimulus. The spectral preferences of these ganglion cells were clearly at short wavelengths; 42% responded best between 410 and 450 nm. (No UV stimuli were used in this study.) All of these cells showed an "off" response to lights of complementary color, which, if presented in color mixtures, could also inhibit the tonic response. The receptive fields of both chromatic actions were spatially coextensive; these cells are therefore color-opponent units without a center/surround organization.

Optic Tectum

A careful study on pigeons using substitution of chromatic stimuli of the same brightness demonstrated a small number of tectal units that responded when one color was changed to another (Jassik-Gerschenfeld et al., 1977). Instead of using static stimuli, Letelier (1983) studied the responses of 82 tectal cells to a moving bar of monochromatic light projected on a dark background. Using such stimuli, 30% of the cells responded; the spectral sensitivity functions were narrow, and most cells were maximally sensitive toward short wavelengths. When a monochromatic slit or edge was moved against its complementary wavelength of equal luminosity, the activity of the cell did not change, suggesting that these units do not have antagonist chromatic inputs. This inference may be wrong, however, since for many tectal cells the responses to leading and trailing edges varied differently with wavelength, even though the total spike count would have led one to classify these cells as broad-band luminosity units. When studied on a finer time scale, a moving bar against a chromatic background does modulate these responses, since the ratio of the size of the leading edge/trailing edge response varies with hue. We have tentatively named this behavior temporal-opponency (Varela et al., 1983). Whether this is a significant and novel feature of the neural basis of avian color vision remains to be confirmed by future experiments. On the other hand, it supports the view that the tectum is an important locus of information processing in avian color vision.

Diencephalon

In the avian homologue of the lateral geniculate nucleus of mammals, the complex designated as the nucleus opticus principalis thalami, color responses have not been detected yet (Maxwell and Granda, 1979). A few units sensitive to color have been reported in the nucleus rotundus, the thalamic relay nucleus between the optic tectum and the ectostriatum of the cortex (tectofugal pathway) (Yazulla and Granda, 1973).

Most thalamic color-sensitive units have been found in the ventral lateral geniculate nucleus (GLv). This structure is virtually nonexistent in mammals; in birds it projects reciprocally and topographically to the optic tectum as well as receiving ascending input from the retina and descending input from the Wúlst, the homologue of the mammalian visual cortex (Crossland and Uchwat, 1979; Guiloff et al., 1987). Many neurons (48% of 156 units studied) in the GLv are color opponent (Maturana and Varela, 1982). Like units in the optic tract, these cells respond tonically, their antagonistic receptive fields are similar, and sensitivity to blue and violet predominates. These cells are insensitive to luminance changes over 2 log units.

The anatomical location of the ventral thalamic nucleus (bridging the tecto- and thalamofugal pathways) and its small size make it hard to interpret its role in color vision. In a recent study pigeons were trained to make color discriminations before and after bilateral chemical lesions of the GLv (Palacios et al., 1991). After a transient phase, the discrimination thresholds were not altered, so at least for this task, the GLv does not seem to be essential. In contrast, even a small amount of damage to the nucleus rotundus immediately above the GLv induces a deficit in discrimination (Hodos, 1969; Palacios et al., 1991).

ECOLOGICAL CONSIDERATIONS

Although we still lack extensive knowledge of the ecological role of color vision in most animal species, the available evidence demonstrates that speculations about color vision should not be driven by simplified, top-down computational models that are based on the evolutionarily unique features of Old World primates, specifically humans. Instead, as the following examples will illustrate, color vision must be understood within the context of the behavioral repertoires of diverse animals.

The colors and distributions of retinal oil droplets of birds vary considerably among species (Martin, 1977, 1986; Jane and Bowmaker, 1988; Martin and Lett, 1985; Budnik et al., 1984). For example, the common tern, a fish-eating predator, has a large number of red and yellow droplets in the dorsal retina, while the barn swallow, which catches insects, has few deeply colored droplets (Peiponen, 1964; Goldsmith et al., 1984). Partridge (1989) has shown by means of cluster analysis that the ecological niche (herbivore, fishing, etc.) is more important in predicting the kinds and distribution of oil droplets than phylogenetic relationships. The evidence suggests that oil droplets respond to natural selection faster than opsins.

The presence of ultraviolet pigments in birds may also provide an example of variation with ecological niche, but too little is yet known of the distribution of UV receptors to draw firm conclusions. For example, the presence of UV visual pigments has been linked to bird-fruit coevolution, including the dissemination of seeds (Snow, 1971; Burkhardt, 1982), and to ethological factors involving animal recognition (Weedon, 1963; Durrer, 1986), but these hypotheses are propelled by the tradition in comparative physiology of seeking particular adaptive explanations for all phenomena. The reflectances of bird plumages have been shown to have shorter wavelength content than reflectances of natural objects of interest to humans and other primates (Burkhardt, 1989; Hudon and Brush, 1989; Brush, 1990), and this suggests the possibility of a perceptual color space of higher dimensionality than three (Barlow, 1982; Bonnardel and Varela, 1991). Evolutionary arguments supported by both comparative physiology and molecular genetics indicate the trichromacy of primate color vision is recently derived, and it is only in avian vision that it is possible to find the quintessence of diurnal capability, evolutionarily uncompromised by a long history of nocturnality as encountered in the mammalian line (Goldsmith, 1990). Seen this way, the question is not "Why do many birds see UV?" but rather "Why is it that most mammals do not?"

The question of how UV sensitivity is utilized by birds is not resolved. UV sensitivity is exploited, for if it were not, natural selection would have abandoned it, as almost certainly occurred in most of the evolutionary line that led to mammals. But in discussing birds, we remain in the realm of speculation. For example, Nuboer's (1986, pp. 370–371) words call attention to the possible use of UV sensitivity in aerial navigation as well as also illustrating the traditional appeal to special adaptation: "the excellent spectral discrimination within this range . . . represents an adaptation to the coloration of an unclouded sky. This property enables the pigeon to evaluate short-wave gradients in the sky, ranging from white at the sun's locus to highly saturated (ultra) violet at angles of 90° to the axis between observer and sun." Furthermore, since pigeon navigation is based on orientation with respect to the sun's azimuth, "the perception of colour gradients in the sky may control navigation indirectly when the sun is hidden by clouds." All of this may be true, but one could also generate adaptationist hypotheses having to do with feather or fruit reflectance, no one of which is likely to have sufficient generality to account for the wide distribution of UV sensitivity in birds.

A different but perhaps more important perspective on the ecological role of color vision is that the process yields a set of perceptual categories that have functional significance, even "cognitive significance" (Jacobs, 1981, pp. 170–171) for animals that must deal with a variety of behavioral interactions and ecological circumstances. A color category can guide behavior in various ways depending on the things that exemplify it: in the case of fruits, it guides feeding; in the case of animal coloration, it may guide various social interactions, such as mating; and these roles are not necessarily mutually exclusive. Pigeons have been shown to group spectral stimuli into categories of hue, and the brightly colored feathers of birds, particularly those exhibiting sexual dimorphism, must have cognitive significance for behavior, especially behavior involving sexual recognition. Finally, although discrimination of objects is obviously important for these kinds of behaviors, the cognitive significance of color may have an affective dimension (perhaps related to the overall hormonal/motivational level of the animal) that cannot be explained simply in terms of discrimination of objects.

CONCLUSIONS

Much research remains to be done on the relations among color vision, perceptual color categories, and animal behavior (Hailman, 1977; Burtt,

1979). Although color as a perceptual category with cognitive significance obviously plays a great role in human life, there is, with the exception of hymenopterous insects (Menzel and Backhaus, 1991), still little evidence about the roles of color perception in nonhuman animals, especially nonprimates. In the case of birds, however, it seems safe to conclude that the experience of color does exist. Moreover, the evidence that we have presented serves to demonstrate our point that the operation of color vision must ultimately be understood at all the levels of analysis to which we referred in the introduction, from molecular events in cells to the behavioral repertoires of animals seen in the ecological conditions in which their kind evolved.

In no species of bird is there a clear understanding of the number and properties of the pigment–oil droplet combinations and their distributions in the retina, providing a detailed description of the receptor basis for that animal's color vision. Multiple foveae and other specialized regions that are suggested by nonuniform distributions of oil droplets (such as the red quadrant of the pigeon's retina) indicate a degree of complexity that is not present in the human eye and for which our own sensory experience provides little intuitive understanding. Birds may have a generalized system of color vision, but individual species may also have features of their eyes adapted to specific visual tasks or conditions, and attention to this ecological dimension in formulating hypotheses about visual function is likely to be critical.

As in primates, pigments absorbing at relatively long wavelengths are the major contributors to photopic sensitivity, but at least some birds probably discriminate short wavelengths in the violet region of the spectrum rather better than primates. The presence of a receptor process in the near UV, long thought to be the exclusive province of insects and foreign to our own visual experience, now seems to be commonly present in many nonmammalian vertebrates (e.g., Kreithen and Eisner, 1978; Goldsmith, 1980; Avery et al., 1983; Harosi and Hashimoto, 1983; Arnold and Neumeyer, 1987) and has recently also been found in rodents (Jacobs et al., 1991). Birds can detect near UV, and it may have a chromatic quality of its own; the possible role of UV in avian color vision needs to be explored.

The information that is available on the receptor substate and on color abilities such as discrimination and color matches shows that at least four chromatic channels are likely to be very commonly present in the retinas of birds. This makes birds true tetrachromats, and perhaps the only pentachromats in the animal kingdom.

The evolutionary history and radiation of vertebrate color vision present us with enormous diversity, and the mammalian or even primate perspective is a narrow pedestal from which to view and understand this evolutionary scene. The tetra- or pentachromatic color space of birds appears to be the most complex in nature and is likely involved in virtually all areas of the animals' lives, from the discrimination and recognition of objects to more complex behavioral tasks such as navigation, the classification of objects, and social and sexual behavior. The next years should see considerable progress in understanding these various evolutionary, physiological, behavioral, and ecological factors and in solving the mysteries of this appealing facet of natural history.

ACKNOWLEDGMENTS

F.V. acknowledges with gratitude the support of the Prince Trust Fund, and C.N.R.S. (Unité Associée 1199); A.P., the Simone & Cino del Duca and Philippe Foundations; and T.H.G., National Eye Institute (NIH) Grants EY-00222 and EY-00785.

REFERENCES

Arnold, K., and Neumeyer, C. Wavelength discrimination in the turtle. *Pseudemys scripta elegans. Vision Res.* 27 (1987), 1501–1511.

Avery, J. A., Bowmaker, J. K., Djamgoz, M. B. A., and Downing, J. E. G. Ultraviolet sensitive receptors in a freshwater fish. *J. Physiol.* 334 (1983), 23–24.

Barlow, H. B. What causes trichromacy? A theoretical analysis using comb-filtered spectra. *Vision Res.* 22 (1982), 635–643.

Baylor, D. A., and Fettiplace, R. Light path and photon capture in turtle photoreceptors. *J. Physiol.* 248 (1975), 433–464.

Blough, D. S. The shape of some wavelength generalization gradients. *Percept. Psychophys.* 4 (1961), 31–40.

Bonnardel, V., and Varela, J. F. A frequency view of colour: Measuring the human sensitivity to square-wave spectral power distributions. *Proc. Roy. Soc. Ser. B* 245 (1991), 165–171.

Bowmaker, J. K. The visual pigments oil droplets and spectral sensitivity of the pigeon. *Vision Res.* 17 (1977), 1129–1138.

Bowmaker, J. K., and Knowles, A. The visual pigments and oil droplets of the chicken retina. *Vision Res.* 17 (1977), 755–764.

Bowmaker, J. K., and Martin, G. R. Visual pigments and colour vision in a nocturnal bird, strix aluco (*tawn owl*). *Vision Res.* 18 (1978), 1125–1130.

Bowmaker, J. K., and Martin, G. R. Visual pigments and oil droplets in the penguin, *Spheniscus humboldti. J. Comp. Physiol. A* 156 (1985), 71–77.

Brush, A. H. Metabolism of carotenoid pigments in birds. *FASEB* 4 (1990), 2969–2977.

Budnik, V. "Un estudio comparativo de la induccion cromatica." Tesis de Licenciatura, Facultad de Ciencias, Universidad de Chile, Santiago, Chile, 1985.

Budnik, V., Mpodozis, J., Varela, J., and Maturana, H. R. Regional specialization of the quail retina: Ganglion cell density and oil droplet distribution. *Neurosci. Lett.* 51 (1984), 145–150.

Burkhardt, D. Birds, berries and UV: A note on some consequences of UV vision in birds. *Naturwissenschaften* 69 (1982), 153–157.

Burkhardt, D. UV vision: a bird's eye view of feathers. *J. Comp. Physiol. A* 164 (1989), 787–796.

Burtt, E. H. The Behavioral Significance of Color. New York, Garland STPM Press, 1979.

Chen, D. M., and Goldsmith, T. H. Four spectral classes of cone in the retinas of birds. *J. Comp. Physiol. A* 159 (1986), 473–479.

Crossland, W. J., and Uchwat, C. J. Topographic projections of the retina and optic tectum upon the ventral lateral geniculate nucleus in the chick. *J. Comp. Neurol.* 185 (1979), 87–106.

Delius, J. D., Thompson, G., Allen, K. L., and Emmerton, J. Colour mixing and preferences in neonate gulls. *Experientia* 28 (1972), 1244–1246.

Donner, K. O. The spectral sensitivity of the pigeon's retinal elements. *J. Phisiol.* 122 (1953), 524–537.

Durrer, H. Colouration. In J. Bereiter-Hahn, A. G. Matoltsy, and K. S. Richards (Eds.), Biology of the Integument, the Skin of Birds. Springer, Berlin, 1986, Vol. 2, pp. 239–247.

Emmerton, J., and Delius, J. D. Wavelength discrimination in the 'visible' and ultraviolet spectrum by pigeons. *J. Comp. Physiol. A* 141 (1980), 47–52.

Fager, L. Y., and Fager, R. S. Chicken blue and chicken violet, short wavelength sensitive visual pigments. *Vision Res.* 21 (1981), 581–586.

Goldsmith, T. H. Hummingbirds near ultraviolet light. *Science* 207 (1980), 786–788.

Goldsmith, T. H. Optimization, constraint, and history in the evolution of eyes. *Q. Rev. Biol.* 65 (1990), 281–322.

Goldsmith, T. H., Collins, J. S., and Perlman, D. L. A wavelength discrimination function for the hummingbird *Archilochus alexandri*. *J. Comp Physiol. A* 143 (1981), 103–110.

Goldsmith, T. H., Collins, J. S., and Licht, S. The cone oil droplets of avian retinas. *Vision Res.* (1984), 1661–1671.

Govardovskii, V. I. On the role of oil drops in colour vision. *Vision Res.* 23 (1983), 1739–1740.

Govardovskii, V. I., and Zueva, L. V. Visual pigments of chicken and pigeon. *Vision Res.* 17 (1977), 537–543.

Guiloff, G. D., Maturana, R. H., and Varela, F. J. Cytoarchiteture of the avian ventral lateral geniculate nucleus. *J. Comp Neurol.* 264 (1987), 509–526.

Hailman, J. P. Optical Signals: Animal Communication and Light. Bloomington and London, Indiana University Press, 1977.

Hamilton, W. F., and Coleman, T. B. Trichromatic vision in the pigeon as illustrated by the spectral hue discrimination curve. *J. Comp. Psychol.* 15 (1933), 183–191.

Harosi, F. I., and Hashimoto, Y. Ultraviolet visual pigment in a vertebrate: A tetrachromatic cone system in the dace. *Science* 223, (1983) 1021–1023.

Hodos, W. Color discrimination deficits after lesions of the nucleus rotundus in pigeons. *Brain Behav. Evol.* 2 (1969), 185–200.

Hudon, J., and Brush, A. H. Probable dietary basis of a color variant of the cedar waxing. *J. Field Ornithol.* 60 (1989), 361–368.

Hurlbert, A. Formal connections between lightness algorithms. *J. Opt. Soc. Am. A* 3 (1986), 1684–1693.

Hurvich, L. M. Color Vision. Sinauer Associates, Sunderland, MA, 1981.

Ives, J. T., Normann, R. A., and Barber, P. W. Light intensification by cone oil droplets: electromagnetic considerations. *J. Opt. Soc. Am. A* 73 (1983), 1725–1731.

Jacobs, G. H. Comparative Color Vision. Academic Press, New York, 1981.

Jacobs, G. H., Neitz, J., and Deegan, II J. F. Retinal receptors in rodents maximally sensitive to ultraviolet light. *Nature (London)* 253 (1991), 655–656.

Jameson, D., and Hurvich, L. Essay concerning color constancy. *Annu. Rev. Psychol.* 40 (1989), 1–22.

Jane, S. D., and Bowmaker, J. K. Tetrachromatic colour vision in the duck (*Anas platyr-hynchos L.*): Microspectrophotometry of visual pigments and oil droplets. *J. Comp. Physiol. A* 62 (1988), 225–235.

Jassik-Gerschenfeld, D., Lange, R. L., and Ropert, N. Response of movement detecting cells in the optic tectum of pigeons to change of wavelength. *Vision Res.* 17 (1977), 1139–1146.

Jitsumori, M. Wavelength discrimination function derived from post-discrimination gradients in the pigeon. *Jpn. Psychol. Res.* 20 (1978), 18–28.

Kirschfeld, K. Carotenoid pigments: their possible role in protecting against photo-oxidation in eyes and photoreceptor cells. *Proc. Roy. Soc. London B* 216 (1982), 71–85.

Kolb, H., and Jones, J. The distinction by light and electron microscopy of two types of cone containing colorless oil droplets in the retina of the turtle. *Vision Res.* 27 (1987), 1445–1458.

Kreithen, M., and Eisner, T. Ultraviolet light detection by the homing pigeon. *Nature (London)* 272 (1978), 347–348.

Letelier, J. "Respuestas cromáticas en el tectum óptico de la paloma." Tesis de Licenciatura, Facultad de Ciencias, Universidad de Chile, Santiago, Chile, 1983.

Liebman, P. A., and Granda, A. M. Super dense carotenoid spectra resolved in single oil droplets. *Nature (London)* 253 (1975), 370–372.

Lythgoe, J. N. The Ecology of Vision. Clarendon Press, Oxford, 1979.

Marin, G. "Respuestas cromáticas en el tracto óptico de la codorniz." Tesis de Licenciatura, Facultad de Ciencias, Universidad de Chile, Santiago, Chile, 1983.

Martin, G. R. Absolute visual threshold and scotopic spectral sensitivity in the tawny owl, *Strix aluc. Nature (London)* 268 (1977), 636–638.

Martin, G. R. The eye of a passerifrom bird, the european starling (*Sturnus vulgaris*): Eye movement amplitude, visual fields and schematic optics. *J. Comp. Physiol. A* 159 (1986), 545–557.

Martin, G. R., and Lett, B. T. Formation of associations of coloured and flavoured food with induced sickness in five avian species. *Behav. Neural. Biol.* 43 (1985), 223–237.

Maturana, H. R., and Varela, F. J. Color-opponent responses in the avian lateral geniculate: a study in the quail (*Coturnix coturnix japonica*). *Brain Res.* 247 (1982), 227–241.

Maxwell, J. H., and Granda, A. M. Receptive fields of movement-sensitive cells in the pigeon thalamus. In A. M. Granda and J. H. Maxwell (Eds.), Neural Mechanism of Behavior in the Pigeon. Plenum Press, New York, 1979.

Menzel, R., and Backhaus, W. Colour vision in insects. In J. Cronly-Dillon (Ed.), Vision and Visual Dysfunction. Macmillan Press, London, 1991, Vol. 6, P. Gouras (Ed.), pp. 262–293.

Miller, W. H. Ocular optical filtering. In H. Autrum (Ed.), Handbook of Sensory Physiology, VII, Part 6A, Vision in Invertebrates. Springer-Verlag, Berlin, 1979, pp. 69–143.

Muntz, W. R. Inert absorbing and reflecting pigments. In H. J. A. Dartnall (Ed.), Handbook of Sensory Physiology, VII/1: Photochemistry of Vision. Springer-Verlag, Berlin, 1972, pp. 530–565.

Neumeyer, C. Simultaneous color contrast in the honeybee. *J. Comp. Physiol. A* 139 (1980), 163–176.

Neumeyer, C. Evolution of colour vision. In J. Cronly-Dillon (Ed.), Vision and Visual Dysfunction. Macmillan, London, 1991, Vol. 2, J. R. Cronly-Dillon and R. L. Gregory (Eds.), pp. 284–305.

Nuboer, J. F. A comparative view on color vision. *Netherlands J. Zool.* 36 (1986), 344–380.

Nuboer, J. K., and Wortel, J. F. Colour vision via the pigeon's red and yellow retinal fields. In J. Kulikowski, C. M. Dickinson, and I. J. Murray (Eds.), Seeing Contour and Colour. Pergamon Press, Oxford, 1987.

Okano, T., Kojima, D., Fukada, Y., Shichida, Y., and Yoshizawa, T. Primary structures of chicken cone visual pigments: vertebrate rhodopsins have evolved out of cone visual pigments. *Proc. Natl. Acad. Sci. U. S. A.* 89 (1992), 5932–5936.

Palacios, A. G., and Varela, F. J. Color mixing in the pigeon (*Columba livia*) II. A psychophysical determination in the middle, short and near-UV wavelength range. *Vision Res.* 32 (1992), 1947–1953.

Palacios, A., Bonnardel, V., and Varela, F. An autoshaping method for wavelength discrimination on birds. *C. R. Acad. Sci. Paris* 311(III) (1990a), 213–218.

Palacios, A., Martinoya, C., Bloch, S., and Varela, F. Color mixing in the pigeon. A psychophysical determination in the longwave spectral range. *Vision Res.* 30 (1990b), 587–596.

Palacios, A., Gioanni, H., and Varela, F. Chromatic discrimination in pigeons after thalamic lesions of nuclei Rotundus (Rt) and Geniculatus Lateralis ventralis (GLv): A psychophysical study. *C. R. Acad. Sci. Paris* 312(III) (1991), 113–116.

Partridge, J. C. The visual ecology of avian cone oil droplets. *J. Comp. Physiol. A* 165 (1989), 415–426.

Peiponen, V. A. Zur Bedeutung der Ölkugeln im Farbensehen der Sauropsiden. *Ann. Zool. Fenn.* 1 (1964), 281–302.

Remy, M., and Emmerton, J. Behavioral spectral sensitivities of different retinal areas in pigeons. *Behav. Neurosci.* 103 (1989), 170–177.

Riggs, L. A., Blough, P. M., and Schafer, K. L. Electrical responses of the pigeon eye to changes in wavelength of the stimulating light. *Vision Res.* 12 (1972), 981–991.

Rushton, W. A. H. Pigments and signals in colour vision. *J. Physiol.* 220 (1972), 1–31.

Schneider, B. Multidimensional scaling of colour differences in the pigeon. *Percept. Psychophys.* 12 (1972), 373–378.

Snow, D. W. Evolutionary aspects of fruit eating by birds. *Ibis* 113 (1971), 194–202.

Thompson, E., Palacios, A. G., and Varela, F. J. Ways of coloring: Comparative color vision as a case study for cognitive science. *Behav. Brain Sci.* 15 (1992), 1–75.

Varela, F. J., Letelier, J. C., Marin, G., and Maturana, H. R. The neuphysiology of avian color vision. *Arch. Biol. Med. Exp.* 16 (1983), 291–303.

Wald, G., Brown, P. K., and Smith, P. H. Iodopsin. *J. Gen. Physiol.* 38 (1955), 623–681.

Weedon, B. C. Occurence. In O. Isler (Ed.), Caretenoids. Birkhauser Verlag, Basel, 1963, pp. 29–59.

Wortel, J. F., Wubbels, R. J., and Nuboer, J. F. Photopic spectral sensitivity of the red and the yellow field of the pigeon retina. *Vision Res.* 24 (1984), 1107–1113.

Wright, A. A. Psychometric and psychophysical hue discrimination functions for the pigeon. *Vision Res.* 12 (1972), 1447–1464.

Wright, A. A. Color-vision psychophysics: A comparison of pigeon and human. In A. M. Granda and J. H. Maxwell (Eds.), Neural Mechanisms of Behavior in the Pigeon. Plenum Press, New York, 1979, pp. 89–127.

Wright, A. A., and Cumming, W. W. Color-naming functions for the pigeon. *J. Exp. Anal. Behav.* 15 (1971), 7–17.

Wyszecki, G., and Stiles, W. S. Color Science, 2nd ed. John Wiley, New York, 1981.

Yazulla, S., and Granda, A. M. Opponent-color units in the thalamus of the pigeon (*Columba livia*). *Vision Res.* 13 (1973), 1555–1563.

Young, S. R., and Martin, G. R. Optics of retinal oil droplets: a model of light collection and polarization detection in the avian retina. *Vision Res.* 24 (1984), 129–137.

II Functional Anatomy of the Avian Visual System

Introduction

Onur Güntürkün

Luigi Rolando, the distinguished late eighteenth-century Italian anatomist, was probably the first to study the functional anatomy of the avian brain. In his laboratory at the university of Sassari he studied hemispherectomized hens, ravens, falcons, and ducks and observed that they were able to walk, fly, drink, and feed, although often missing the food while pecking. Rolando therefore suspected that the avian telencephalon was of minor importance for most of these visually guided actions. Instead the forebrain seemed to furnish the birds with some sort of will and intelligence, since they behaved like drunkards when hemisphrectomized. Although Rolando's monograph provides a large number of completely new insights into brain functions, his conclusion remains rather pessimistic: "Despite countless experiments I rarely obtained consistent results; but this is not surprising, if one considers the mess of fibers which meet in this region" (Rolando, 1809, p. 188).

In the 200 years since Rolando's expression of frustration, many of this "mess of fibers" have been labeled, traced, and classified according to their biochemical content and their functional importance. The emerging pattern reveals that the *bauplan* of the avian visual system is consistent with that of many, perhaps all, vertebrates. For amniotes (i.e., reptiles, birds, and mammals) even the details of the connectivity and a good part of the chemoarchitecture of the two major ascending visual pathways to the forebrain are closely comparable. But these hodological similarities seem to be contradicted by the fact that, in birds, these projections terminate in structures that are organized differently from their putative mammalian counterparts. Target areas that, in mammals, are laminated cortical components, are, in birds, either nuclear or nuclear-like structures.

Shimizu and Karten (chapter 6) elaborate a hypothesis, first formulated by Karten (1969), which may resolve this contradiction. They assume that the appropriate comparisons were not between avian nuclear regions and mammalian cortical areas, but between specific cell populations that could be either lumped together in nuclear structures, as in birds, or distributed in laminar form, as in mammals. The beauty of this assumption is twofold; it resolves some of the existing contradictions of previous comparative approaches and at the same time provides important clues to the phylogeny of the cortex. If birds and mammals share a large part of their connectivity patterns, but not their pattern of forebrain organization, the evolution of the neocortex must have proceeded in two independent and sequential steps: first the generation of specific neuronal populations and their basic connectivity in all amniotes, and second the reorganization of these cell groups into a laminar cortical pattern in mammals.

Although comparisons between birds and mammals may provide insights into the functional anatomy of both classes, important specializations may be overlooked if hypotheses emerging from studies with cats and monkeys are too quickly generalized to birds. Thus, in mammals, it was widely assumed that the geniculate and extrageniculate systems had different and complementary roles. The extrageniculostriate pathway was assumed to transform visual information into motor commands that rapidly fixate the object of interest with the fovea. The geniculostriate pathway was assumed to analyze subtle details within the frontal visual field and to estimate depth by stereoscopic vision. Most avian neurobiologists assumed that the avian visual system has a similar pattern of organization, with the thalamofugal system homologous in function to the geniculostriate, while the tectofugal was assumed to be homologous to the extrageniculate system. This assumption was reinforced by the elegant electrophysiological studies of Pettigrew (1979) in owls, which suggested a geniculostriate-like role for the thalamofrontal system of owls. However, a large number of behavioral experiments in pigeons failed to reveal a substantial contribution of the thalamofugal pathway to frontal vision (Hodos, chapter 4).

This conflict is gradually being resolved by recognizing that neural systems are constrained by natural selection and thus reflect the specific ecological demands of a species. These demands have to be different in frontally oriented predators like owls and in panoramic and laterally oriented prey like pigeons. As reviewed by Güntürkün, Miceli, and Watanabe (chapter 7), the avian thalamofugal pathway seems to be specialized to only one visual field, either frontal or lateral. The frontal specialization seems to prevail in birds of prey, which have to precisely specify the target distance while moving with high speed. The lateral specialization then probably dominates in fruit- and seed-eating birds, which constantly have to monitor their environment for predators.

The lateral specialization of the thalamofugal pathways in nonpredators creates the unexpected constraint that binocular vision has to be carried out by the tectofugal pathway. Until recently this possibility would have been denied simply because of lack of sufficient commissural connections, which could integrate both halves of the visual world within this system. But as shown by Engelage and Bischof (chapter 8) new anatomical and electrophysiological data demonstrate that the commissural tectofugal crosstalk is much larger than previously assumed. Additionally the ectostriatum, which is the primary telencephalic target of the tectofugal projection, seems to be composed of laminae in which ipsilateral and contralateral inputs are distinctly represented. These results open the possibility that it is the tectofugal system that provides the neural substrate for binocular integration and depth perception in pigeons (McFadden, chapter 3). The neural algorithms to perform stereoscopic vision are then probably not bound to a specific visual pathway but can be implemented in any visual system that represents the partly overlapping inputs of both eyes.

Casini, Fontanesi, and Bagnoli (chapter 9) provide evidence that mechanisms for stereoscopic vision require a neural substrate, which precisely aligns the input from both eyes. They demonstrate that the visual thalamus of owls indeed possesses a complex organization that could subserve the alignment of retinal maps and the segregation of the thalamic input into the Wulst. The intra- and extratelencephalic output of the Wulst seems additionally to be organized in columns, an anatomical pattern well known from the geniculostriate system of mammals. Are these similarities a product of homologous evolutionary traits, or do they reflect a nice example of convergent evolution as suspected by Casini, Fontanesi, and Bagnoli? We presently do not know, but we have obviously come a long way from Rolando's "mess of fibers."

REFERENCES

Karten, H. J., The organization of the avian telencephalon and some speculations on the phylogeny of the amniote telencephalon. In C. Noback and J. Petras (Eds.), *Comparative and Evolutionary Aspects of the Vertebrate Central Nervous System. Ann. N.Y. Acad, Sci.* 167 (1969), 146–179.

Pettigrew, J. D., Binocular visual processing in the owl's telencephalon. *Proc. Royal Soc. London* 204 (1979), 435–455.

Rolando, L. Saggio sopra da vera struttura del cervetto e sopra de fonzioni del sistema nervoso, Sassari, 1809. Partly translated and reprinted as: Expériences sur les fonctions du système nerveux. *J. Physiol. Exp.* 3 (1823), 95–113.

6 The Avian Visual System and the Evolution of the Neocortex

Toru Shimizu and Harvey J. Karten

As the contents of this book testify, the visual system of birds has been the subject of intensive investigation over the past two decades. These studies have provided both fundamental information about avian visual behavior and the visual brain, and theoretical insights about the evolution of the vertebrate central nervous system. The present chapter outlines an hypothesis about the evolutionary relationships between avian telencephalic structures and mammalian neocortex (Karten, 1969; Nauta and Karten, 1970; Karten and Shimizu, 1989; Karten, 1991). This hypothesis has proven heuristically useful in organizing a large body of data and in stimulating further investigations.

The origin of the neocortex is a persistent problem in the history of comparative neuroanatomy. The nonmammalian telencephalon—particularly that of reptiles and birds—consists mainly of nuclear structures with only a thin cortical shell, and lacks the layered organization characteristic of the mammalian neocortex. Consequently, it was generally assumed that the neocortex is found only in mammalian brains (e.g., Ariëns Kappers et al., 1936). Accordingly, the nuclear structures of the nonmammalian telencephalon were homologized with components of the subcortical striatum of mammals, a conclusion evident in the nomenclature of the major telencephalic structures of nonmammalian vertebrates: paleo*striatum*, archi*striatum*, ecto*striatum*, neo*striatum*, and hyper*striatum*.

This nomenclature remains in current use, even though contemporary studies employing anatomical, physiological, neurochemical, and behavioral techniques have shown that only a small portion of the sauropsid telencephalon (i.e., the paleostriatum in birds) directly corresponds to the mammalian striatum (review by Reiner et al., 1984). This leaves us with the question, With what mammalian forebrain structures may the other components of the nonmammalian telencephalon be homologous?

In birds, studies of the visual system have indicated that at least some of these telencephalic "nuclear" components correspond to mammalian pallial structures. These findings have led to a reevaluation of established assumptions about neocortical evolution and have raised questions as to the evolutionary origin and functional utility of lamination in the mammalian telencephalon.

TWO VISUAL AREAS IN BIRDS AND MAMMALS

About 300 million years ago, the common ancestors of all modern amniotes (reptiles, birds, and mammals) were primitive tetrapods called "stem reptiles." The lines of modern reptiles, birds, and mammals departed from the stem reptiles at least 280 million years ago, and have evolved independently since then. The relationships among living amniotes are thus quite distant (Hodos and Campbell, 1969; Macphail, 1982). Nevertheless, the basic patterns of forebrain organization among amniotes appear strikingly similar (e.g., Northcutt, 1981).

In all amniotes thus far studied, retinal information is conveyed to the telencephalon by two distinct major pathways. One travels from the retina directly to a cell group in the thalamus then to the telencephalon. This route is often designated as the *thalamofugal pathway* in sauropsids and is presumed to correspond to the *geniculostriate pathway* in mammals. The other pathway runs from the retina to the mesencephalon (optic tectum/superior colliculus) to a cell group in the thalamus and then to the telencephalon. This pathway is designated as the *tectofugal pathway* in birds, corresponding, putatively, to the *colliculothalamocortical* pathway in mammals (figure 6.1).

In birds, the thalamofugal pathway terminates in a region of the dorsal telencephalon within the hyperstriatum, called the visual "Wulst" (bulge), because it forms a noticeable protuberance on the surface of the hemisphere. The visual Wulst is often compared to the striate cortex in mammals for a number of reasons. It is organized in a laminar fashion (Pettigrew, 1979), exhibits a comparable pattern of afferent and efferent connections (Karten et al., 1973; Bagnoli and Burkhalter, 1983; Miceli et al., 1987), and retinotopic organization of the receptive fields (Miceli et al., 1979). It should be noted, however, that there are important differences in microcircuitry (Reiner and Karten, 1983) and chemistry (Shimizu and Karten, 1990; see Güntürkun, Miceli, and Watanabe, this volume).

The telencephalic target of the avian tectofugal pathway is a region called the ectostriatum (specifically its "core" region), which is located ventrally within the dorsal ventricular ridge (DVR) of the lateral telencephalon. If we assume an equivalence between the avian tectofugal and the mammalian colliculothalamocortical pathways, the ectostriatum should correspond to the thalamo-recipient regions of the temporal visual cortex in mammals. However, such an equivalence is not easy to establish. The DVR, including the ectostriatum, is organized in a nonlaminar nuclear fashion, complicating comparisons with the laminated mammalian neocortex. Moreover, unlike the temporal cortex, which is

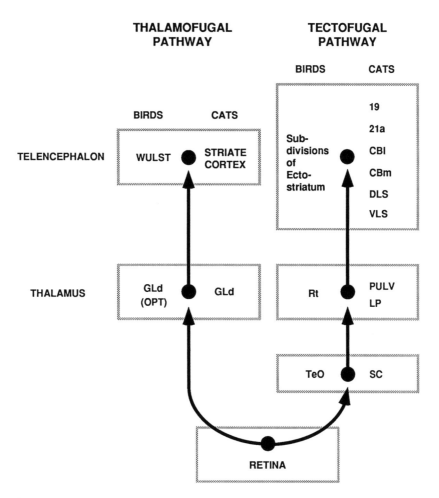

THALAMOFUGAL
PATHWAY

TECTOFUGAL
PATHWAY

Figure 6.1 A schematic drawing of the two pathways from the retina to the telencephalon in birds and in cats: 19 and 21a, areas 19 and 21a; CBl and CBm, lateral and medial divisions of the Clare-Bishop complex; DLS and VLS, dorsal and ventral lateral suprasylvian visual areas; GLd, lateral geniculate nucleus pars dorsalis; LP, lateral posterior nucleus; PUL, pulvinar; OPT, opticus principalis thalami; Rt, nucleus rotundus; SC, superior colliculus; TeO, optic tectum.

the source of extratelencephalic projects, neurons of the ectostriatum tend to terminate in the surrounding areas ("belt" region) of the ectostriatum (Shimizu et al., 1989), rather than in extratelencephalic structures.

HYPOTHESIS 1: NONLAMINAR CORTICAL EQUIVALENTS

This apparent contradiction may be resolved if we assume that the appropriate comparisons are not between nonmammalian nuclear regions and mammalian cortex as a whole, but between specific nuclear regions in nonmammalian vertebrates and specific neuronal populations within individual laminae of mammalian neocortex. The assumption derives from a hypothesis about the evolution of the vertebrate brain originally formulated by Karten (1969) and recently restated and elaborated (Karten and Shimizu, 1989; Karten, 1991). These authors have suggested that the basic microcircuitry of telencephalic processing is common to reptiles, birds, and mammals. "In birds, the various components corresponding to neurons within individual laminae of mammalian neocortex are segregated into discrete nuclear groupings within the DVR of the telencephalon. In mammals, these nuclear grouping are stretched out horizontally in apposition to each other, with greater interlaminar organization" (Karten, 1991, p. 267). In other words, neurons corresponding to those in the mammalian temporal cortex are present in the avian brain, but they form nonlaminar nuclei instead of layers.

This hypothesis may also provide a possible explanation for the apparent lack of correspondence in the efferent projection patterns of the avian ectostriatum and the mammalian temporal cortex. In mammals, neurons in layer IV receiving thalamic input do not send their axons to extratelencephalic targets, but to neurons in adjacent layers II and III. Similarly, the core portion of ectostriatum that receives the thalamic input does not contribute to a descending extratelencephalic output but projects upon the "belt" region of the ectostriatum, which might then be viewed as corresponding to cortical layers II and III.

Recent studies on the avian brain have further suggested that not only the ectostriatum, but other nuclei in the DVR may correspond to different layers or components of the neocortex. The belt region of ectostriatum projects to surrounding areas in the DVR (Ritchie and Cohen, 1979; Shimizu et al., 1989). Neurons in some of these regions in turn project directly or indirectly to another restricted region in the archistriatum. This region of the archistriatum projects on layers 10–13 of the ipsilateral optic tectum (Brecha et al., 1976; Karten et al., 1992). These sequential projections from thalamic input areas to extratelencephalic output areas are reminiscent of the interlaminar circuitry of the neocortex (figure 6.2). Thus, although a laminar configuration is not present in the avian forebrain, equivalent circuitry appears to be maintained through the connections of different nuclei of the DVR.

HYPOTHESIS 2: ORIGINS OF THE NEOCORTEX

It has been suggested (Karten and Shimizu, 1989) that comparisons between putatively equivalent avian and mammalian cell groups might provide some clues to the origin of neocortex. In the absence of definitive information, it is often assumed that the stem reptiles and perhaps the early mammals possessed a forebrain organization similar to that of primitive reptiles and birds. Thus, if neurons of the neocortical equivalents are present in the nonmammalian brain, the precursors of these

A. CIRCUITRY IN MAMMALIAN CORTEX

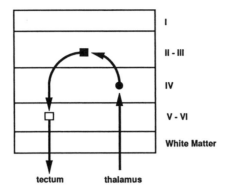

I

II - III

IV

V - VI

White Matter

tectum   thalamus

B. EQUIVALENT CIRCUITRY IN AVIAN DVR

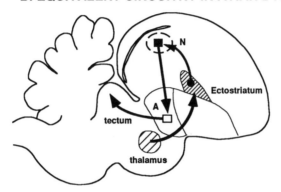

N

Ectostriatum

tectum

A

thalamus

Figure 6.2 (A) A schematic drawing of a typical pattern of neural circuitry in the sensory cortical areas. (B) A schematic drawing of the organization of the tectofugal pathway in a sagittal section of the avian brain: A, archistriatum; N, neostriatum.

neurons might have already existed over 280 million years ago. In the case of central visual structures, for example, the hypothesis postulates that ancestral reptiles had cell populations that were precursors of both the nonmammalian Wulst and the mammalian striate cortex. That there should be both similarities and differences between the two regions is therefore not surprising (see below).

This hypothesis challenges the prevalent notion that the neocortex is a result of recent evolutionary events unique to the mammalian brain. Instead, the theory proposes that the evolution of the vertebrate brain involved two independent and sequential steps; first, the origin of constituent neuronal populations and their occurrence as precursors of cortical neurons in the telencephalon of nonmammals; and second, the development of a laminar cortical organization in mammals (figure 6.3).

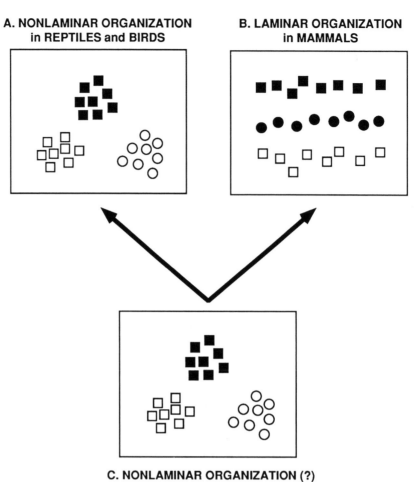

Figure 6.3 Schematic representations of the organization of cortical and cortical-equivalent cells in the sauropsid (A), mammalian (B), and stem reptiles (C).

Such a theory accounts parsimoniously for the organization of both the nonmammalian telencephalon and the mammalian neocortex.

ONTOGENETIC CONSIDERATIONS

Although the nonlaminar DVR in adult birds is quite different in appearance from the laminar organization of mammalian cortex (e.g., lateral pallium/temporal cortex) there have been reports suggesting that neurons of DVR and lateral pallium originally migrated from similar proliferative regions. The critical area in mammals was described by Källén (1962) and later named a subventricular zone (SVZ) by Stensaas and Gilson (1972), who studied rat and rabbit embryos. According to these authors, SVZ is located at the dorsolateral angle of the striatum and the ventricle (figure 6.4). This location corresponds topographically

A. MIGRATORY COURSE OF SVZ CELLS IN MAMMALS

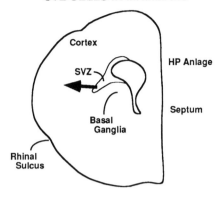

B. MIGRATORY COURSE OF DVR CELLS IN BIRDS

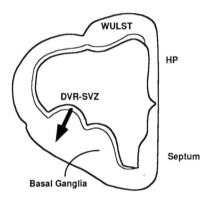

Figure 6.4 Schematic drawings of the transverse section of the mammalian (A) and avian (B) telencephalon. Arrows indicate possible migratory routes of cells during embryonic development. HP, hippocampus.

to that of DVR in birds and reptiles. During embryogenesis, mitotic cells in SVZ seem to be astrocytes and neuron-like cells. These cells migrate into the lateral pallium, and then SVZ disappears shortly after birth. Another similarity between SVZ and DVR is the migratory pattern of their cells during development. The migratory course of the SVZ cells is rather "unusual" in the mammalian cerebral cortex, and similar to that observed in the developing DVR. In the mammalian cortex, neurons that have common characteristics in function are organized in distinct cortical columns. Many cortical cells are known to migrate *radially* along these vertical columns, from the pallial ependyma to their final destination (e.g., Rakic, 1988). In contrast, cells from SVZ migrate along *tangential* routes to form distinct columns in the cortex, the tem-

Shimizu & Karten: The Evolution of the Neocortex

poral region in particular. In birds, a similar pattern of nonradial migration is observed in DVR during embryonic development (Balaban et al., 1988). The implications of the embryological data have been explored in more detail by Karten (1991).

NEUROCHEMICAL CONSIDERATIONS

The immunohistochemical techniques, which have proven such powerful tools for examining the distribution of different neurochemicals within the mammalian neocortex (e.g., Foote and Morrison, 1987), have recently been applied to the avian Wulst. Shimizu and Karten (1990) found that there are at least three important similarities between these avian and mammalian telencephalic structures. First, a wide variety of transmitters, peptides, and receptors are common to both structures. These include choline acetyltransferase (ChAT), nicotinic acetylcholine receptor (nAChR), tyrosine hydroxylase (TH), serotonin (5-HT), glutamic acid decarboxylase (GAD), γ-aminobutyric acid A receptor (GABA$_A$R), cholecystokinin (CCK), substance P (SP), leucine-enkephalin (L-ENK), neurotensin (NT), neuropeptide Y (NPY), somatostatin (SRIF), corticotropin-releasing factor (CRF), and vasoactive intestinal polypeptide (VIP). Significantly, the classical neurotransmitters (i.e., cholinergic, catecholaminergic, serotonergic, and GABAergic systems) are extensively distributed in both Wulst and neocortex.

Second, in the Wulst, as in mammalian neocortex, the distribution of many transmitter-related compounds parallels the laminar organization of the region. The most superficial layer of the Wulst, the hyperstriatum accessorium (HA), contains many SP-stained cells, a moderate number of GAD- and SRIF-stained cells, and a low density of nAChR- and L-ENK-positive cells. In the layer ventral to HA, the hyperstriatum intercalatus superior (HIS), there are a moderate number of GAD- and CCK-immunoreactive cell bodies, and a few cells containing nAChR-, SP-, and L-ENK-like immunoreactivities. The deepest layer of the Wulst, the hyperstriatum dorsale (HD), contains many CCK-, GAD-, SP-, and L-ENK-stained cell bodies. The distribution of neuropil immunoreactivity also reflects the laminar organization. The highest densities of TH-, 5-HT-, SP-, NPY-, SRIF-, CRF-, and VIP-positive neuropil in the Wulst are observed in HA, while the highest density of CCK- and NT-stained neuropil is found in HD.

Finally, in both the Wulst and mammalian neocortex, there is a characteristic distribution of some neuroactive substances *within* specific layers. At least two such regions are found within HA: a dorsorostral portion characterized by dense TH-immunoreactive neuropil, and a ventrocaudal portion, with dense SP staining. Similarly, HD contains a ventromedial portion characterized by GABAAR-, SP-, CCK-, L-ENK-, and NT-positive neuropil or cell bodies, whereas little immunoreactivity for these compounds is seen in a dorsolateral portion. Finally, a specific pattern of immunoreactivity is found in the most dorsolateral portion of the Wulst near the vallecula (hyperstriatum laterale), which, in addition to being the only region containing NPY-positive cells, also contains the highest densities of ChAT- and L-ENK-stained fibers, and high densities of 5-HT-, TH-, GAD-, SP-, and CCK-positive neuropil.

Despite these similarities, there are also significant differences between avian Wulst and mammalian neocortex with respect to the distribution of some peptides. For example, NPY-immunoreactivity, which is common in the neocortex, is minimal in the Wulst. Conversely, immunoreactivity to NT is minimal in the mammalian neocortex, but moderately intense in Wulst. It should be noted, however, that even in mammals there are marked species differences in the distribution patterns of these and other compounds.

Such comparisons provide important data bearing on the evolutionary history of these compounds and thus on the evolution of cortex and Wulst. Thus, similarities between the innervation patterns of classical neurotransmitters in the avian Wulst and mammalian neocortex suggest that these chemical characteristics are less open to modification and thus phylogenetically conservative. Their conservation over time probably reflects their general role in a variety of critical functions common to both the avian and mammalian telencephalic neural circuits. On the other hand, the variability of peptide distribution patterns among different vertebrates implies that these characteristics are more plastic and the observed differences between classes and species may be the result of modifications through evolutionary history and adaptation. Their role in the telencephalic circuits is, therefore, likely to be associated with neural functions that are species-specific rather than common to all vertebrates.

BEHAVIORAL CONSIDERATIONS

An often unstated corollary of neocortical uniqueness was the widely held assumption that the behavior of birds was less complex, less plastic, in a word, less "intelligent" than that of mammals. In a classic example of circular reasoning, the presumed cognitive inferiority of birds was then explicitly correlated with the absence of a neocortex. Recent reassessments of the cognitive abilities of birds (Macphail, 1982) have rendered such positions untenable. Birds are demonstrably capable of exhibiting behaviors, many of them visually guided, which, when found in mammals, have been categorized as "cognitive" (see part V, this volume). The complexity of auditory and vocal capacities in song birds is also well established (see a review by Konishi, 1985). It is clear from such studies that the nonlaminated telencephalon of birds mediates behaviors rivaling in their complexity mammalian behaviors previously assumed to be uniquely correlated with the possession of a laminated telencephalon. Indeed, in reviewing such studies one wonders about the functional contribution of lamination as an alternate means of organizing populations of vertebrate neurons.

BRAIN MECHANISMS AND VISUAL FUNCTION IN BIRDS AND MAMMALS

Despite the lack of any convincing empirical evidence, a highly laminated structure has often been implicitly considered a prerequisite for the optimal functioning of neural networks. Hence the prevailing view that the laminar organization of the mammalian striate cortex provides the most efficient neural substrate for analyzing visual information.

It is therefore noteworthy that visual performance (e.g., acuity, color discrimination) in many birds equals or excels that exhibited by many mammals, including primates (see Martin, chapter 1). This performance is accomplished by neural circuits hodologically and functionally comparable to those of the neocortex, but without laminar organization. What then, we may ask, are the benefits of lamination in the neocortex?

Answers to that question are likely to come from careful comparisons between the structure and function of individual cortical laminae in mammals and specific telencephalic nuclear regions in nonmammalian forms. Previous studies of the avian visual system have helped to bring the problem of cortical lamination to the forefront of comparative neuroanatomy. Future studies of that system should contribute to its resolution.

REFERENCES

Ariëns Kappers, C. U., Huber, G. C., and Crosby, E. C. (1936). *The Comparative Anatomy of the Nervous System of Vertebrates, Including Man.* Republished in 1960. New York: Hafner.

Bagnoli, P., and Burkhalter, A. (1983). Organization of the afferent projections to the Wulst in the pigeon. *J. Comp. Neurol.* 214: 103–113.

Balaban, E., Teillet, M. A., and Le Douarin, N. (1988). Application of the quail-chick chimera system to the study of brain development and behavior. *Science 241:* 1339–1342.

Brecha, N., Hunt, S. P., and Karten, H. J. (1976). Relations between the optic tectum and basal ganglia in the pigeon. *Soc. Neurosci. Abstr.* 1:95.

Foote, S. L., and Morrison, J. H. (1987). Extrathalamic modulation of cortical function. *Annu. Rev. Neurosci.* 10:67–95.

Hodos, W., and Campbell, C. B. G. (1969). *Scala nature:* Why there is no theory in comparative psychology. *Psychol. Rev.* 76:337–350.

Källén, B. (1962). Embryogenesis of brain nuclei in the chick telencephalon. *Ergebnisse Anat. Entwick.* 36:62–82.

Karten, H. J. (1969). The organization of the avian telencephalon and some speculations on the phylogeny of the amniote telencephalon. In C. Noback and J. Petras (Eds.), *Comparative and Evolutionary Aspects of the Vertebrate Central Nervous System. Annals New York Academy of Sciences* 167:146–179.

Karten, H. J. (1991). Homology and evolutionary origin of the "neocortex." *Brain Behav. Evol.* 38:264–272.

Karten, H. J., and Shimizu, T. (1989). The origins of neocortex: Connections and laminations as distinct events in evolution. *J. Cog. Neurosci.* 1:291–301.

Karten, H. J., and Shimizu, T. (1991). Are visual hierarchies in the brains of the beholders? Constancy and variability in the visual system of birds and mammals. In P. Bagnoli and W. Hodos (Eds.), *The Changing Visual System: Maturation and Aging in the Central Nervous System.* NATO ASI Series. New York: Plenum Press.

Karten, H. J., Hodos, W., Nauta, W. J. H., and Revzin, A. M. (1973). Neural connections of the "visual Wulst" of the avian telencephalon. Experimental studies in the pigeon (*Columba livia*) and owl (*Speotyto cunicularia*). *J. Comp. Neurol.* 150:253–277.

Karten, H. J., Cox, K., and Shimizu, T. (1992). "Extrastriate" visual pathways in the pigeon: Descending projections upon the optic tectum. *Soc. Neurosci.* 18:1031.

Konishi, M. (1985). Birdsong: From behavior to neuron. *Annu. Rev. Neurosci.* 8:125–170.

Konishi, M., Emlen, S. T., Ricklefs, and Wingfield, J. C. (1989). Contributions of bird studies to biology. *Science* 246:465–472.

Macphail, E. M. (1982). *Brain and Intelligence in Vertebrates.* New York: Oxford University Press.

Miceli, D., Gioanni, H., Repérant, J., and Peyrichoux, J. (1979). The avian visual wulst: I. An anatomical study of afferent and efferent pathways. II. An electrophysiological study of the functional properties of single neurons. In A. M. Granda and J. H. Maxwell (Eds.), *Neural Mechanisms of Behavior in the Pigeon,* pp. 223–254. New York: Plenum Press.

Miceli, D., Repérant, J., Villalobos, J., and Dionne, L. (1987). Extratelencephalic projections of the avian Wulst. A quantitative autoradiographic study in the pigeon *Columba livia. J. Hirnforschung* 28:45–57.

Nauta, W. J. H., and Karten, H. J. (1970). A general profile of the vertebrate brain with sidelights on the ancestry of the cerebral cortex. In F. O. Schmitt (Ed.), *The Neurosciences: Second Study Program.* New York: Rockefeller Press.

Northcutt, R. G. (1981). Evolution of the telencephalon in nonmammals. *Annu. Rev. Neurosci.* 4:301–350.

Pettigrew, J. D. (1979). Binocular visual processing in the owl's telencephalon. *Proc. Roy. Soc. (London), Ser. B* 204:435–454.

Rakic, P. (1988). Specification of cerebral cortical areas. *Science* 241:170–176.

Reiner, A., and Karten, H. J. (1983). The laminar source of efferent projections from the avian Wulst. *Brain Res.* 275:349–354.

Reiner, A., Brauth, S. E., and Karten, H. J. (1984). Evolution of the amniote basal ganglia. *Trends Neurosci.* 7:320–325.

Ritchie, T. L. C., and Cohen, D. H. (1979). The avian tectofugal visual pathway: Projections of its telencephalon target ectostriatal complex. *Soc. Neurosci. Abstr.* 2:119.

Shimizu, T., and Karten, H. J. (1990). Immunohistochemical analysis of the visual wulst of the pigeon (*Columba livia*). *J. Comp. Neurol.* 300:346–369.

Shimizu, T., and Karten, H. J. (1991). Central visual pathways in reptiles and birds: Evolution of the visual system. In J. Cronly-Dillon and R. Gregory (Eds.), *Vision and*

Visual Dysfunction, vol. 2: Evolution of the Eye and Visual System, pp. 421–441. London: Macmillan Press.

Shimizu, T., Woodson, W., Karten, H. J., and Schimke, J. B. (1989). Intratelencephalic connections of the visual areas in birds (*Columba livia*). *Soc. Neurosci. Abstr.* 15:1398.

Stensaas, L. J., and Gilson, B. C. (1972). Ependymal and subependymal cells of the caudate-pallial junction in the lateral ventricle of the neonatal rabbit. *Zeit. Zellforschung* 132:297–322.

7 Anatomy of the Avian Thalamofugal Pathway

Onur Güntürkün, Dom Miceli, and
Masami Watanabe

The most impressive aspect of the avian brain is the enormous degree of development of its visual system. Although the volume of, for instance, the pigeon brain barely reaches 0.15% of that of humans, the pigeon's optic nerve contains about 2.5 times more fibers than the optic nerve of man (pigeon: Binggeli and Paule, 1969; human: Curcio and Allen, 1990). Most of these fibers project to the optic tectum, so that the majority of the early studies on the avian visual system concentrated on the tectally projecting optic axons. Bellonci (1888) was the first to also recognize some fibers in the dorsolateral thalamic area as being of retinal origin but was not sure whether they ended there or passed through to terminate at the midbrain level. Eleven years later Edinger and Wallenberg (1899) reported that after enucleation degenerating terminals were detected in the dorsolateral aspect of the thalamus, an observation that was repeatedly replicated in the following decades (Huber and Crosby, 1929; Cowan et al., 1961; Hirschberger, 1967). Karten and Nauta (1968) demonstrated first that this retinorecipient nuclear complex projects onto the visual Wulst in the forebrain, and introduced the term "thalamofugal pathway" to describe this retinothalamo-Wulst projection. Since most people have come to agree that the avian thalamofugal pathway corresponds to the mammalian geniculostriate system (Shimizu and Karten, this volume), we will use in this chapter the term n. geniculatis lateralis pars dorsalis (GLd) to describe the retinorecipient part of the avian diencephalon that projects on the visual Wulst. The following survey gives an account of the present state of knowledge regarding the retinal projections onto the dorsolateral thalamus, the various subdivisions of the GLd, the thalamofugal projection onto the forebrain, and the internal organization and projections of the Wulst.

THE RETINAL PROJECTION ONTO THE GLd

In cats, retinal alpha, beta, and gamma cells project differentially onto GLd and tectum, with the GLd being mainly characterized by its beta cell input (Illing and Wässle, 1981; Kelly and Gilbert, 1975). For birds, a comparable retinal ganglion cell classification does not exist (but see Hayes, 1981). However studies in owls (Bravo and Pettigrew, 1981) and pigeons (Remy and Güntürkün, 1991) demonstrated that the avian GLd receives most of its retinal afferents from medium-sized ganglion cells and from a small number of very large retinal neurons, a situation similar to mammals. These results open the possibility that the avian thalamofugal pathway could be characterized by afferents from retinal neurons, which are comparable to beta cells. It should, however, cautiously be remarked that this assumption rests only on comparisons of soma diameters and does not include any data on dendritic morphology or axonal diameters. There is now evidence that cholecystokinin and neurotensin/LANT 6 (Güntürkün and Karten, 1991) are involved as transmitters/modulators in this projection.

While the GLd of both owls and pigeons seems to receive afferents from similar retinal ganglion cell classes, the retinal location of these neurons is completely different. In birds of prey, injections of horseradish peroxidase (HRP) into the GLd labels ganglion cells in the temporal retina (Bravo and Pettigrew, 1981; Bravo and Inzunza, 1983). The temporal retina subserves frontal vision and is thought to be essential to establish binocular convergence in the forebrain. This assumption is supported by results of Pettigrew and Konishi (1976a, b), Pettigrew (1978, 1979), and Porciatti et al. (1990) who demonstrated that large numbers of neurons in the visual Wulst of owls, kestrels, and vultures possess binocular visual fields with retinal disparity. However, injections of retrograde tracers into the GLd of pigeons mainly label ganglion cells in the central, nasal, and inferior retina, while only a very small number of labeled neurons are found in the superiotemporal part, the so-called "red field" (Remy and Güntürkün, 1991) (figure 7.1).

The pigeon's red field has been suggested as the source of visual information from the frontal binocular visual field, situated mainly below the eye-beak axis (Martinoya et al., 1981; Hayes et al., 1987; Nalbach et al., 1990). The paucity of afferents from the red field should render the thalamofugal pathway of pigeons largely frontally blind. Indeed the single unit study of Miceli et al. (1979) found that none of the recorded 170 units from the pigeon's Wulst had their receptive fields in the frontal binocular area. Thus, while the GLd of several birds of prey seems to be specialized for the frontal binocular visual field, the GLd of pigeons mainly receives afferents representing the lateral monocular field. This functionally important difference seems not to be the result of the laterally placed eyes of pigeons, since the kestrel (*Falco sparverius*), a diurnal raptor, which has lateral eyes, is also characterized by an overrepresentation of the frontal binocular visual field within its thalamofugal pathway (Pettigrew, 1978).

What could be the functional relevance of this thalamofugal specialization to only one visual field? Pigeons and many other seed- or fruiteating birds fixate novel or complex and distant stimuli laterally and

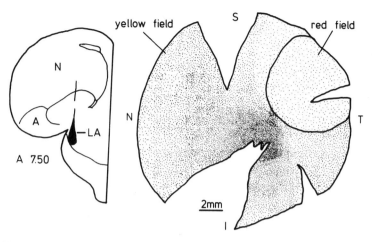

Figure 7.1 Fast Blue-labeled retinal ganglion cells contralateral to an injection into the n. lateralis anterior (LA) of the pigeon. Each dot on the retina represents one labeled neuron. Note the paucity of labelings in the red field. Abbreviations: A, archistriatum; I, inferior; N, neostriatum; S, superior; T, temporal.

switch to frontal binocular vision only to peck the scrutinized object (Friedman, 1975; Bischof, 1988; Bloch et al., 1988; Kirmse, 1990). Thus, in these species visual detection and analysis of food objects, conspecifics, and enemies are mainly performed by those parts of the neural apparatus that represent the lateral visual field. The frontal binocular area is involved only during the last visually guided sequences before and within pecking bouts (Bischof, 1988). The lateral specialization of the thalamofugal pathway in pigeons could therefore be related to the fact that it is mainly the lateral visual field that requires fine analysis of the visual scenery. This assumption is supported by psychophysical experiments that reveal that the lateral visual field of pigeons has high acuity values (Hahmann and Güntürkün, 1993) and electrophysiological recordings that generally demonstrate neurons with small stationary receptive fields within GLd and Wulst (pigeon: Revzin, 1969; Britto et al., 1975; Gusel'nikov et al., 1976; Jassik-Gerschenfeld et al., 1976, 1979; Miceli et al., 1979; Britten, 1987; chick: Wilson, 1980; Pateromichelakis, 1981).

However, behavioral data seem to contradict the notion that the thalamofugal system is involved in fine visual analysis. Lesions of the GLd or the Wulst produce only minimal deficits in a variety of visual discrimination tasks (Güntürkün, 1991; Hodos, this volume). However, all of these studies used pigeons and employed tasks requiring discriminative pecking responses to patterns presented on response keys. Pigeons pecking a key fixate it with their red field (Goodale, 1983). Since the red field has only limited projections onto the GLd, thalamofugal lesions are likely to produce minimal deficits when tested with this procedure. This assumption is supported by a recent behavioral study

(Hahmann and Güntürkün, 1993) in which the visual acuity of head-fixed pigeons was determined before and after GLd lesions. While the animals were postoperatively unimpaired in their frontal acuity, they were unable to discriminate even coarse grating patterns in the lateral field.

The frontal specialization of the thalamofugal system in birds of prey could be related to their more complex feeding habits, which require them to specify the distance of objects with great precision while moving with high speed. This is probably achieved through depth cues such as binocular disparity or through flow-field variables (Davies and Green, 1990). Although, for example, eagles and falcons fixate distant objects mainly laterally (Reymond, 1985; Kirmse, 1990) they switch to frontal vision when approaching prey. The combination of high frontal acuity (Fox et al., 1976; Reymond, 1985, 1987) with the need for complex and fast visual information analysis could explain the specialization of the thalamofugal pathway to the frontal visual field in birds of prey.

THE INTERNAL ORGANIZATION OF THE GLd

Hirschberger (1967) demonstrated that the GLd did not consist of a single homogeneous cell group, but could be subdivided into two retinorecipient nuclei. Subsequent authors further delineated the GLd into components of different topological positions and numbers (Karten and Hodos, 1967; Repérant, 1973; Meier et al., 1974; Ehrlich and Mark, 1984), (table 7.1). Discrepancies in these studies are due mainly to difficulties in delimiting boundaries between individual cell groups, which differ only minimally in their cytoarchitectonic properties. Only a covert lamination of the GLd is partially indicated by differential output of subnuclear components to the ipsilateral and the contralateral Wulst (Meier et al., 1974; Miceli et al., 1975; Miceli and Repérant, 1982). Miceli et al. (1990) used this projectional lamination in combination with the regional variations in the density of the retinal input to subdivide the GLd into four components. Güntürkün and Karten (1991) further delineated the GLd according to the biochemical contents of the various cell groups (figure 7.2).

According to an integrated view of these different attempts, the lateral geniculate complex can be subdivided from dorsal to ventral into three main components: the n. geniculatus lateralis pars, dorsalis (GLd), the n. marginalis tractus optici (nMOT, probably equivalent to the intergeniculate leaflet of mammals), and the n. geniculatus lateralis, pars ventralis (GLv, equivalent to the mammalian GLv). The GLd itself seems to consist of six components, of which only four constitute the core portion, since they are retinorecipient and project onto the visual Wulst. The four main structures are the n. dorsolateralis anterior thalami, pars lateralis (DLL), the n. dorsolateralis anterior thalami, pars magnocellularis (DLAmc), the n. lateralis dorsalis nuclei optici principalis thalami

Table 7.1. Nomenclatures Used to Describe the Subcomponents of the GLd, together with Projections and Chemically Defined Cell Groups of Each Subnucleus

	Nomenclature					Projections	Chemically defined cell groups
Güntürkün and Karten (1991) (pigeon)	Karten and Hodos (1967) (pigeon)	Repérant (1973) (pigeon)	Meier et al. (1974) (pigeon)	Ehrlich and Mark (1984) (chick)			
LA	LA	LA	LA	LA	?	GABA
SPC	SPC	SP	SPC	—	Visual and somatosensory Wulst, APH	ACh CCK SP
DLAmc	DLAmc	DLAlm	DLAmc	DLAmc	Bilaterally to visual Wulst	ACh GABA
DLL	DLL and DLA	DLAlp and medial DLAlr	Medial DLLd and dorsal DLLv	DLL, zones B, C, and rostral A	Bilaterally to visual Wulst	ACh CCK GABA
LdOPT	—	Lateral part of DLAlr	Lateral part of DLLd	DLAlr	To visual Wulst	SP
SpRt	—	—	Ventral DLLv (DLLvv)	Caudoventral zone A of DLL	Ipsilaterally to visual Wulst	CCK GABA
nMOT	—	—	—	—	To ipsilateral superficial tectal layers	NPY
GLv	GLv	GL	GLv	GLv	Tectum, area pretectalis	Oxytocin GABA

See list of abbreviations at the end of the chapter for definitions.

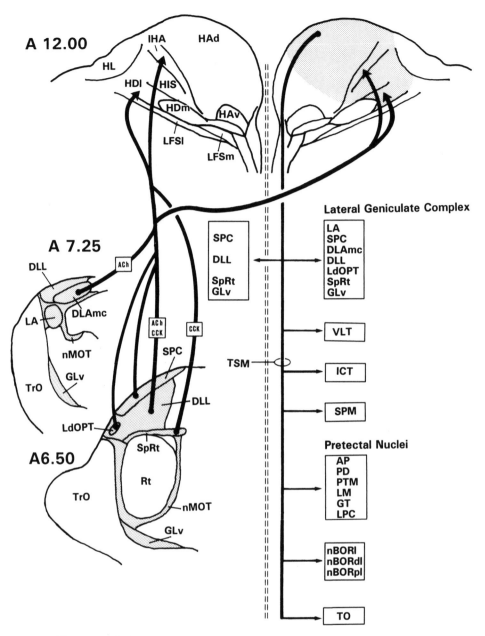

Figure 7.2 Schematic view of the thalamofugal pathway of the pigeon. To the left the various subcomponents of the lateral geniculate complex are depicted (dotted structures) together with the ascending projections onto the ipsilateral and the contralateral Wulst and the neurotransmitters/modulators of the relay neurons. Note that the SpRt projects only ipsilaterally. At the top of the subdivisions of the Wulst are given with the nomenclature to the left and the presumed extent of the visual components to the right (dotted areas). Only IHA and HDl represent input layers. To the right the descending Wulst projections via the TSM are depicted. The broken double line is the partition between the hemispheres. Abbreviations are given in the list of abbreviations.

Functional Anatomy of the Avian Visual System

(LdOPT), and the n. suprarotundus (SpRt). The two additional noncore subcomponents are the n. lateralis anterior (LA) and the n. superficialis parvocellularis (SPC).

The DLL and the DLAmc constitute the two largest GLd subcomponents. In all avian species studied, the retinal innervation covers only parts of these two structures (pigeon: Miceli et al., 1975; Güntürkün and Karten, 1991; chick: Ehrlich and Mark, 1984; quail: Watanabe, 1987; dove: Norgren and Silver, 1989). This intranuclear heterogeneity is matched in the DLL by the uneven distribution of cholinergic, GABAergic, and cholecystokinergic perikarya (Güntürkün and Karten, 1991). At least a part of the cholinergic and cholecystokinergic cells project onto the visual Wulst and thus constitute relay neurons, while probably most or all of the GABAergic perikarya belong to interneurons (Bagnoli et al., 1981; Güntürkün and Karten, 1991) (figure 7.3). The majority of these chemically specified structures are distributed along the dorsolateral part of the DLL where retinal endings reach their highest density.

Watanabe (1987) demonstrated in quails that a part of the retinal fibers end in synaptic glomeruli where they make asymmetric, and thus probably excitatory, contacts with dendrites and somata of relay neurons. But retinal terminals synapse also on dendrites of nonrelay neurons. These postsynaptic dendrites are in turn presynaptic to relay neuron dendrites on which they make symmetric, and thus probably inhibitory, contacts (figure 7.4). This "triadic relation" is also typical for X cells of the GLd of cats and is supposed to be responsible for the feedfoward inhibition of geniculate relay cells (Sherman and Koch, 1986). GABA has been identified in mammals to be the inhibitory interneuronal transmitter within this triad (Pasik et al., 1990). Iontophoretic applications of GABA or its antagonist bicuculline demonstrated that the inhibitory interneurons are responsible for a sharpening of the receptive field center-surround antagonism, an increase of the orientation bias to moving lines, and an increase of the slope of the contrast response curve (Sillito and Kemp, 1983; Vidyasagar, 1984; Berardi and Morrone, 1984). Altogether these effects narrow the tuning characteristics of the mammalian GLd relay neurons. Avian GLd neurons are also characterized by relatively small receptive fields (1° in owls, 2–4° in pigeons, 3° in chicks; these numbers give the smallest values encountered and not the average), center-surround organization, and low adaptation to stimulus repetition (Britto et al., 1975; Jassik-Gerschenfeld et al., 1976, 1979; Pettigrew, 1979; Pateromichelakis, 1981; Britten, 1987). While these similarities to mammals are pronounced in owls, pigeons and chicks demonstrate important differences in having additionally many directionally selective cells with large receptive fields (Britto et al., 1975; Wilson, 1980; Britten, 1987).

The LdOPT is the smallest subnucleus within the GLd and is characterized by a dense innervation of cholecystokinin- and neurotensin-

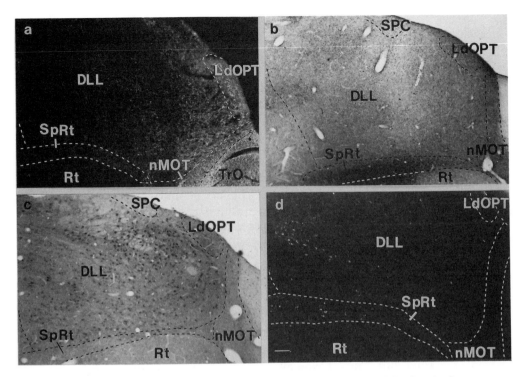

Figure 7.3 Afferents, chemoarchitectonics, and projections of the dorsal subcomponents of the pigeon's lateral geniculate complex as revealed in four different experiments. In (a) the contralateral retinal afferents are labeled with an intraocular injection of RITC. Note the paucity of fibers in medial DLL; (b) serotonergic brainstem afferents innervating all subcomponents with a diffuse network of fibers. The ventromedial border of SpRt is difficult to delineate, since the n. triangularis and the dorsomedial aspect of Rt are also densely innervated by serotonergic fibers; (c) ChAT-labeled cells in DLL from which all or at least a large part represent relay neurons; (d) retrogradely labeled neurons in DLL and SpRt after a Fluorogold injection into the medial aspect of the visual Wulst. Note that the majority of labeled cells are clustered in the medial part of both structures. All sections correspond about to the level A 6.50 of the pigeon brain atlas (Karten and Hodos, 1967); dorsal is upward and medial is to the left. Abbreviations are given in the list of abbreviations. The bar (100 μm) in (d) applies to all micrographs.

positive presynaptic endings of retinal origin. A large number of GABAergic perikarya from the lateral DLL have processes that penetrate the LdOPT (Güntürkün and Karten, 1991). All or at least most of the perikarya within LdOPT are substance P-positive and seem to project to the visual Wulst (Miceli et al., 1990). The SpRt consists of a thin sheet of cholecystokinergic and GABAergic neurons at the dorsal border of the n. rotundus. Both chemically defined neuronal populations seem to project to the visual Wulst (Bagnoli et al., 1983; Güntürkün and Karten, 1991). Previous authors defined the SpRt as the n. dorsolateralis anterior thalami pars lateralis pars ventroventralis (DLLvv) and recognized an exclusively ipsilateral projection from this structure to the

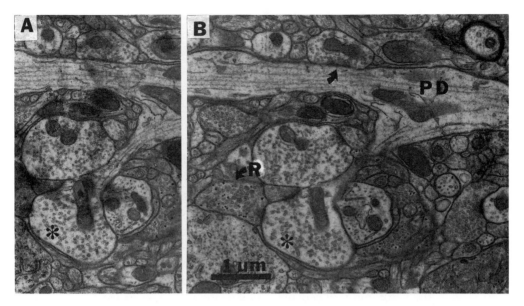

Figure 7.4 Serial section through a synaptic glomerulus of the dorsolateral part of the quail DLL. (B) A terminal (asterisks) that derives from a shaft of a presynaptic dendrite (PD) is postsynaptic to a retinal (R) and a nonretinal terminal (arrow). (A) The neck of the terminal of the presynaptic dendrite.

Wulst (Hunt and Webster, 1972; Miceli et al., 1975, 1979; Nixdorf and Bischof, 1982).

Both LA and SPC are probably not subcomponents of the GLd. LA is densely innervated by the retina but lacks projections onto the forebrain, a key feature of the GLd (Miceli et al., 1975, 1979; Nixdorf and Bischof, 1982; Bagnoli and Burkhalter, 1983; Miceli and Reperant, 1985; Ehrlich and Stuchberry, 1986). SPC projects topographically onto the visual Wulst, but is reached by only a small number of retinal fibers (Repérant, 1973; Miceli and Repérant, 1985; Miceli et al., 1990; Güntürkün and Karten, 1991). However some recent evidence indicates that these few retinal fibers arborize in the region of the Wulst-projecting cells (Miceli et al., unpublished observations) and could thus mediate some visual responses (Maxwell and Granda, 1979).

MODULATORY BRAINSTEM AFFERENTS

Electrophysiological studies demonstrate that the receptive field properties of most GLd neurons are not remarkably different from those of retinal ganglion cells. Since an important elaboration of visual information seems not to take place, the diencephalic component of the thalamofugal pathway is often seen as a rather simple relay to the forebrain. But it seems to be more likely that one of the primary functions of the GLd is not to process visual information as such but to gate and modify it in the context of the nonvisual information flow. In cats this is exemplified in the fact that 80–90% of synapses within the GLd are of nonretinal origin (Guillery, 1971). Comparable data do not exist for birds, but as in mammals, the avian GLd is also innervated by four major transmitter-specific brainstem systems, which are probably involved in gating visual information according to the arousal level of the animal and the attention it pays to speciffc sensory cues.

All GLd subcomponents of pigeons are innervated by serotonergic fibers that are distributed with high densities in DLAmc and SpRt and intermediate densities in DLL and LdOPT (Güntürkün and Karten, 1991). According to Vischer et al. (1982) the pigeon's GLd is characterized by medium levels of 5-HT$_1$ receptors. The activity of the serotonergic system of mammals is modulated according to the sleep–waking cycles with high activity levels during waking states and low levels during slow wave sleep (Jouvet, 1972). Release of serotonin leads to an inhibition of spontaneous and evoked activity of rat GLd relay neurons (Kayama et al., 1989). Pape and McCormick (1989) demonstrated that the serotonin-induced hyperpolarization of mammalian GLd neurons enhances a cAMP-mediated sodium/potassium ion current. This enhancement reduces the ability of GLd neurons to generate rythmic burst firing, which is characteristic for slow-wave sleep. It thus promotes a state of excitability during periods of waking.

The avian GLd is also characterized by a dense cholinergic fiber network and by intermediate levels of muscarinic acetylcholine receptors (Vischer et al., 1982; Wächtler, 1985; Wächtler and Ebinger, 1979; Güntürkün and Karten, 1991). Acetylcholine directly excites cat GLd relay neurons due to a nicotinic receptor-mediated increase in cation conductance followed by a muscarinic M$_1$-receptor-mediated decrease in potassium conductance. At the same time GABAergic GLd interneurons are inhibited through an increase of potassium conductance via muscarinic M$_2$-receptors (Francesconi et al., 1988). McCormick (1989) suggests that the transition from synchronized thalamic activity during slow-wave sleep to desynchronized activity during arousal is associated with the activation of the cholinergic brainstem system.

All GLd subnuclei are innervated by tyrosine hydroxylase (TH) positive fibers (Bagnoli and Casini, 1985; Güntürkün and Karten, 1991). The presence of this enzyme was until recently interpreted as an indication for a noradrenergic input. Since a dopaminergic fiber plexus could also be visualized within the GLd, it seems likely that only parts of TH-positive fibers represent noradrenaline. Kitt and Brauth (1986) traced a projection from the noradrenergic locus coeruleus to the pigeon's GLd and Balthazart et al. (1989) demonstrated the existence of a high density of α_1-receptors within this structure. Application of noradrenaline or stimulation of the locus coeruleus increases the excitability of rat GLd relay neurons (Kayama et al., 1982). This facilitatory effect is due to an α_1-adrenoceptor coupled decrease in potassium conductance. This generates a slow depolarization, which brings the membrane potential closer to single spike firing threshold (McCormick, '89).

Dopaminergic fibers, which probably originate from the n. tegmenti pedunculo-pontinus, pars compacta (TPc) and the area ventralis tegmentalis (AVT) of the midbrain, are present with low densities throughout all GLd subcomponents (Güntürkün, unpublished observations). In rats, dopaminergic terminals seem to terminate preferentially on dendrites of GABAergic interneurons (Papadopoulos and Parnavelas, 1990). Since dopamine acts in an inhibitory manner in most systems studied, the activation of the dopaminergic afferents of the GLd could result in an inhibition of interneurons and thus an excitation of GLd relay neurons.

THALAMO-WULST PROJECTIONS

Karten and Nauta (1968) were the first to demonstrate that GLd neurons project to the visual Wulst ("bulge"), an elevation in the frontodorsal forebrain. These findings were replicated and extended in different avian species (pigeons: Hunt and Webster, 1972; Karten et al., 1973; Miceli et al., 1975; Bagnoli and Burkhalter, 1983; Miceli and Repérant, 1985; zebra finches: Nixdorf and Bischof, 1982; falcons: Bravo and Inzunza, 1983; quails: Watanabe et al., 1983; chicks: Ehrlich and Stutchberry, 1986; owls: Karten et al., 1973; Bagnoli et al., 1990).

The thalamo-Wulst projection is bilateral in all species studied, but the relative contribution of both sides seems to depend on the species-typical position of the eyes. In owls with their essentially frontal eyes the ipsilateral and the contralateral sides contribute about comparable number of fibers to the forebrain projection (Bagnoli et al., 1990). In lateral-eyed birds like pigeons the ipsilateral side clearly predominates (Miceli et al., 1990). These species also differ with respect to the degree of lamination of ipsilaterally and contralaterally projecting neurons within GLd subnuclei. While relay cells are arranged in several segregated bands within the DLL of owls, only a coarse differentiation seems to be present in pigeons, with the contralaterally projecting neurons being located in the dorsal, and the ipsilaterally projecting ones in the ventral DLL (Miceli et al., 1990).

Different investigators disagree as to the projectional topography of the GLd subnuclei. According to Miceli et al. (1990) medial DLL projects to rostral and lateral DLL to intermediate Wulst, whereas DLAmc and SpRt innervate all Wulst regions. According to Güntürkün and Karten (in prep.), however, DLL, DLAmc, and SpRt projections are independent from each other but are all organized such that lateral thalamic neurons connect to the lateral, and rostral neurons to the rostral Wulst. Hopefully these contradictions will be clarified within the near future.

THE INTERNAL ORGANIZATION AND THE PROJECTIONS OF THE VISUAL WULST

The Wulst can be subdivided into a rostral somatosensory (Funke, 1989), a medial hippocampal (Casini et al., 1986), and a caudal visual division (Shimizu and Karten, 1990). The following account will deal only with the visual component, which is organized from dorsal to ventral in four laminae: hyperstriatum accessorium (HA), intercalated nucleus of the hyperstriatum accessorium (IHA), hyperstriatum intercalatus superior (HIS), and hyperstriatum dorsale (HD). In the barn owl the molecular IHA layer can additionally be differentiated into an external and an internal component (figure 7.5). These subdivision are based on the cytoarchitectonics of the Wulst and do not reflect the full complexity of the structure, since Shimizu and Karten (1990) were able to distinguish at least 8 subdivisions using immunocytochemical techniques (see figure 7.2). The granular IHA and probably also lateral HD are the major recipients of the GLd input (Karten et al., 1973; Watanabe et al., 1983). Possibly due to the cholinergic nature of a large part of GLd relay neurons, many IHA cells positive for nicotinic acetylcholine receptors can be detected (Shimizu and Karten, 1990). All Wulst laminae are additionally characterized by cholinergic, catecholaminergic, and sero-tonergic fibers, which probably represent modulatory afferents similar to those found in the GLd (Bagnoli and Casini, 1985; Shimizu and Karten, 1991). Electrophysiological studies demonstrated similarities between the visual Wulst of birds and the striate cortex of mammals. In the visual Wulst of raptors most neurons are primarily concerned with binocular visual processing, are selectively tuned to stereoscopic depth cues, are sensitive to visual experience during the neonatal period, and have small receptive fields of about 1° (Pettigrew and Konishi, 1976a, b; Pettigrew, 1979). This is not the case for species such as pigeons, chicks, and zebra finches in which binocular neurons are rare or in which ipsilaterally evoked visual responses are very weak and irregular (Miceli et al., 1979; Wilson, 1980; Bredenkötter and Bischof, 1990a, b). Additionally the receptive fields encountered are considerably larger in nonraptors (pigeons: 2°, Revzin, 1969; chicks: 10°–20°, Wilson, 1980).

The intratelencephalic projections of the visual Wulst arise from the supra- and infragranular layers and lead ipsilaterally to the medial hyperstriatum ventrale, the lateral lobus parolfactorius, the area para-hippocampalis, the neostriatum caudolaterale, the archistriatum, the ectostriatal belt, and the neostriatum intermediale at the medial edge of the ectostriatum (Ritchie, 1979). The thalamofugal pathway thus modulates neural processes within the projection areas of the first and the second tectofugal pathways (Gamlin and Cohen, 1986), and within nonsensory, associational areas such as the neostriatum caudolaterale (Waldmann and Güntürkün, 1993).

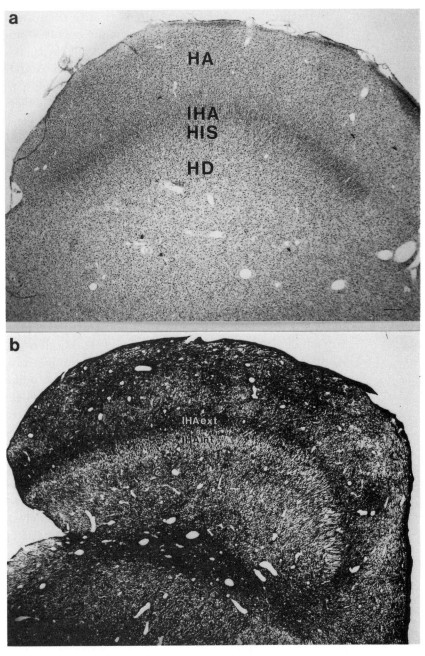

Figure 7.5 (a) Cresyl violet and (b) Gallyas stained frontal section of the Wulst of the barn owl. The fiber staining clearly reveals the distinction between the external (ext) and internal (int) IHA. Dorsal is upward and lateral is to the left. Abbreviations are given in the list of abbreviations. Bar = 500 μm.

Güntürkün et al.: Anatomy of the Thalamofugal Pathway

The extratelencephalic Wulst efferents arise from the supragranular hyperstriatum accessorium and lead via the tractus septomesencephalicus (TSM) primarily to GLd, GLv, pretectal nuclei, basal optic root nucleus, and tectum opticum (Karten et al., 1973; Bagnoli et al., 1980; Miceli et al., 1987). Within GLd, the terminal fields partially overlap with those areas in the subnuclei DLL and SpRt, which both receive direct retinal input and project to the visual Wulst. Degenerating terminals from the lesioned visual Wulst make asymmetric contacts with dendritic spines and partly also with presynaptic dendrites but do not contribute to synaptic glomeruli (Watanabe, 1987). Since electrical stimulation of the Wulst is known to activate DLL relay neurons, TSM fibers probably act via direct excitation of relay neuron dendrites or by inhibition of the GABAergic interneurons (Britto, 1978).

The Wulst projection onto the tectum is probably of great importance for our understanding of the functional circuitries within the avian visual system. All authors agree that most TSM fibers terminate within layers 12 to 13 of the ipsilateral tectum and may thus be able to modulate the ascending output to the n. rotundus and the descending projections to rhombencephalic motor and premotor structures (Karten et al., 1973; Bagnoli et al., 1980; Reiner and Karten, 1982; Miceli et al., 1979, 1987). Although there are contradictions regarding the extent of innervation of the superficial tectal laminae, a part of the data indicate that TSM terminals overlap with retinorecipient layers (Karten et al., 1973; Miceli et al., 1987). Consequently Leresche et al. (1983) could demonstrate that a large proportion of visually responsive cells in the superficial layers of the optic tectum depend for their receptive field properties on input from an intact Wulst. Cryogenic block of the Wulst caused a reversible response depression of a majority of tectal cells and drastically diminished the directional tuning of half of the directionally selective neurons. Thus, the visual properties of tectal cells are not solely a reflection of the retinal afferents and the intratectal circuitry, but also depend on the thalamofugal input.

ABBREVIATIONS

A	archistriatum
ACh	acetylcholine
AP	area pretectalis
APH	area parahippocampalis
CCK	cholecystokinin
ChAT	choline acetyltransferase
DLA	n. dorsolateralis anterior thalami
DLAlm	n. dorsolateralis anterior thalami, pars lateralis magnocellularis

DLAlp	n. dorsolateralis anterior thalami, pars lateralis principalis
DLAlr	n. dorsolateralis anterior thalami, pars lateralis rostralis
DLAmc	n. dorsolateralis anterior thalami, pars magnocellularis
DLL	n. dorsolateralis anterior thalami, pars lateralis
DLLd	n. dorsolateralis anterior, pars lateralis pars dorsalis
DLLv	n. dorsolateralis anterior, pars lateralis pars ventralis
DLLvv	n. dorsolateralis anterior, pars lateralis pars ventroventralis
GABA	γ-aminobutyric acid
GL	n. geniculatus lateralis
GLd	n. geniculatus lateralis, pars dorsalis
GLv	n. geniculatus lateralis, pars ventralis
GT	griseum tectale
HAd	dorsal portion of the hyperstriatum accessorium
HAv	ventral portion of the hyperstriatum accessorium
HD	hyperstriatum dorsale
HDl	lateral portion of the hyperstriatum dorsale
HDm	medial portion of the hyperstriatum dorsale
HIS	hyperstriatum intercalatus superior
HL	hyperstriatum laterale
ICT	n. intercalatus thalami
IHA	n. intercalatus hyperstriati accessorii
LA	n. lateralis anterior
LdOPT	n. lateralis dorsalis nuclei optici principalis thalami
LFSl	lateral portion of the lamina frontalis superior
LFSm	medial portion of the lamina frontalis superior
LM	n. lentiformis mesencephali
LPC	n. laminaris precommisuralis
N	neostriatum
nBORdl	n. of the basal optic root, pars dorsalis pars lateralis
nBORl	n. of the basal optic root, pars lateralis
nBORpl	n. of the basal optic root, pars principalis pars lateralis
nMOT	n. marginalis tractus optici
NPY	neuropeptide Y
NT	neurotensin
OPT	n. principalis opticus thalami
PD	n. pretectalis diffusus
PTM	n. pretectalis medialis

RITC	rhodamine-β-isothiocyanate
Rt	n. rotundus
S	serotonin
SP	n. superficialis parvocellularis (Repérant)
SP	substance P
SPC	n. superficialis parvocellularis
SPM	n. spiriformis medialis
SpRt	n. suprarotundus
T	n. triangularis
TH	tyrosine hydroxylase
TO	tectum opticum
TrO	tractus opticus
TSM	tractus septomesencephalicus
Va	valeculla
VLT	n. ventrolateralis thalami

REFERENCES

Bagnoli, P., and Burkhalter, A. Organization of the afferent projections to the Wulst in the pigeon. *J. Comp. Neurol.* 214 (1983), 103–113.

Bagnoli, P., and Casini, G. Regional distribution of catecholaminergic terminals in the pigeon visual system. *Brain Res.* 337 (1985), 227–286.

Bagnoli, P., Grassi S., and Magni, F. A direct connection between visual Wulst and tectum opticum in the pigeon (*Columba livia*) demonstrated by horseradish peroxidase. *Arch. Ital. Biol.* 118 (1980), 72–88.

Bagnoli, P., Beaudet, A., Stella, M., and Cuénod, M. Selective retrograde labelling of cholinergic neurons with 3H-choline. *J. Neurosci.* 1 (1981), 691–695.

Bagnoli, P., Burkhalter, A., Streit, P., and Cuénod, M. 3H-GABA selective retrograde labeling of neurons in the pigeon thalamo-Wulst pathway. *Arch. Ital. Biol.* 121 (1983), 47–53.

Bagnoli, P., Fontanesi, G., Casini, G., and Porciatti, V. Binocularity in the little owl, *Athene noctua*. I. Anatomical investigation of the thalamo-Wulst pathway. *Brain Beh. w. Evol.* 35 (1990), 31–39.

Balthazart, J., Ball, G. F., and McEwen, B. S. An autoradiographic study of alpha-adrenergic receptors in the brain of the Japanase quail (*Coturnix coturnix japonica*). *Cell Tissue Res.* 258 (1989), 563–568.

Bellonci, J. Über die centrale Endigung des Nervus opticus bei den Vertebraten. *Zeitschrift wissensch. Zool.* 47 (1888), 1–46.

Berardi, N., and Morrone, M. D. The role of gamma-aminobutyric acid mediated inhibition in the response properties of cat lateral geniculate neurones. *J. Physiol. (London)* 357 (1984), 505–524.

Binggeli, R. L., and Paule, W. J. The pigeon retina: Quantitative aspects of the optic nerve and ganglion cell layer. *J. Comp. Neurol.* 137 (1969), 1–18.

Bischof, H.-J. The visual field and visually guided behaviour in the zebra finch (*Taeniopygia guttata*). *J. Comp. Physiol. A.* 163 (1988), 329–337.

Bloch, S., Jäger, R., Lemeignant, M., and Martinoya, C. Correlations between ocular saccades and headmovements in walking pigeons. *J. Physiol. (London)* 406 (1988), 173.

Bravo, H., and Pettigrew, J. D. The distribution of neurons projecting from the retina and visual cortex to the thalamus and tectum opticum of the barn owl, *Tyto alba,* and the burrowing owl, *Speotyto cunicularia. J. Comp. Neurol.* 199 (1981), 419–441.

Bravo, H., and Inzunza, O. Estudio anatomico en las vias visuales parallelas en falconiformes. *Arch. Biol. Med. Exp.* 16 (1983), 283–289.

Bredenkötter, M., and Bischof, H.-J. Differences between ipsilaterally and contralaterally evoked potentials in the visual Wulst of the zebra finch. *Vis. Neurosci.* 5 (1990a), 155–163.

Bredenkötter, M., and Bischof, H.-J. Ipsilaterally evoked responses of the zebra finch visual Wulst are reduced during ontogeny. *Brain Res.* 515 (1990b), 343–346.

Britten, K. H. Receptive fields of neurons of the principal optic nucleus of the pigeon (*Columba livia*). Ph. D. thesis, SUNY, Stony Brook, 1987.

Britto, L. R. G. Hyperstriatal projections to primary visual relays in pigeons: Electrophysiological studies. *Brain Res.* 153 (1978), 382–386.

Britto, L. R. G., Francesconi, W., Brunelli, M., and Magni, F. Visual response pattern of thalamic neurons in the pigeon. *Brain Res.* 97 (1975), 337–343.

Casini, G., Bingman, V. P., and Bagnoli, P. Connections of the pigeon dorsomedial forebrain studied with WGA-HRP and 3H-proline. *J. Comp. Neurol.* 245 (1986), 454–470.

Cowan, W. M., Adamson, L., and Powell, T. P. S. An experimental study of the avian visual system. *J. Anat.* 95 (1961), 545–563.

Curcio, C. A., and Allen K. A. Topography of ganglion cells in human retina. *J. Comp. Neurol.* 300 (1990), 5–25.

Davies, M. N. O., and Green, P. R. Optic flow-field variables trigger landing in hawk but not in pigeons. *Naturwissenschaften* 77 (1990), 142–144.

Edinger, L., and Wallenberg, A. Untersuchungen über das Gehirn der Taube. *Anat. Anz. 15 (1899), 245–271.*

Ehrlich, D., and Mark R. An atlas of the primary visual projections in the brain of the chick *Gallus gallus. J. Comp. Neurol.* 223 (1984), 592–610.

Ehrlich, D., and Stuchberry, J. A note on the projection from the rostral thalamus to the visual hyperstriatum of the chicken (*Gallus gallus*). *Exp. Brain Res.* 62 (1986), 207–211.

Fox, R., Lehmkuhle, S. W., and Westendorf, D. H. Falcon visual acuity. *Science* 192 (1976), 263–265.

Francesconi, W., Müller, C. M., and Singer, W. Colinergic mechanisms in the reticular control of transmission in the cat lateral geniculate nucleus. *J. Neurophysiol.* 59 (1988), 1690–1718.

Friedman, M. B. How birds use their eyes. In Wright, P., Caryl, P. G., and Vowles, D. M. (Eds.), Neural and Endocrine Aspects of Behaviour in Birds. Elsevier, Amsterdam, 1975, pp. 181–204.

Funke, K. Somatosensory areas in the teencephalon of the pigeon II. Spinal pathways and afferent connections. *Exp. Brain Res.* 76 (1989), 620–638.

Gamlin, P. D. R., and Cohen, D. H. Second ascending visual pathway from the optic tectum to the telencephalon in the pigeon (*Columba livia*). *J. Comp. Neurol.* 250 (1986), 296–310.

Goodale, M. A. Visually guided pecking in the pigeon (*Columba livia*). *Brain Behav. Evol.* 22 (1983), 22–41.

Guillery, R. W. Patterns of synaptic interconnections in the dorsal lateral geniculate nucleus of the cat and monkey: A brief review. *Vision·Res. Suppl.* 3 (1971), 211–227.

Güntürkün, O. The functional organization of the avian visual system. In Andrew, R. J. (Ed.), *Neural and Behavioural Plasticity: The Use of the Domestic Chick as a Model*. Oxford University Press, Oxford, 1991, pp. 92–105.

Güntürkün, O., and Karten, H. J. An immunocytochemical analysis of the lateral geniculate complex in the pigeon (*Columba livia*). *J. Comp. Neurol.* 314 (1991), 721–749.

Gusel'nikov, V. I., Morenkov, E. D., and Do Cong Hunh. Responses and properties of receptive fields of neurons in the visual projection zone of the pigeon hyperstriatum. *Neirofiziologiya* 8 (1976), 230–236.

Hahmann, U., and Güntürkün, O. The visual acuity for the lateral visual field of the pigeon (*Columba livia*) *Vision Res.* 33 (1993), 1659–1664.

Hayes, B. P. The structural organization of the pigeon retina. *Progr. Ret. Res.* 1 (1981), 197–226.

Hayes, B. P., Hodos, W., Holden, A. L., and Low, J. C. The projection of the visual field upon the retina in the pigeon. *Vision Res.* 27 (1987), 31–40.

Hirschberger, W. Histologische Untersuchungen an den primären visuellen Zentren des Eulengehirns und der retinalen Repräsentation in ihnen. *J. Orn.* 108 (1967), 187–202.

Huber, G. C., and Crosby, E. C. The nuclei and fibre paths of the avian diencephalon, with consideration of telencephalic and certain mesencephalic centres and connexions. *J. Comp. Neurol.* 48 (1929), 1–225.

Hunt, S. P., and Webster, K. E. Thalamo-hyperstriate interrelations in the pigeon. *Brain Res.* 44 (1972), 647–651.

Illing, R. B., and Wassle, H. The retinal projection to the thalamus in the cat: A quantitative investigation and a comparison with the retinotectal pathway. *J. Comp. Neurol.* 202 (1981), 265–285.

Jassik-Gerschenfeld, D., Teulon, J., and Ropert, N. Visual receptive field types in the nucleus dorsolateralis anterior of the pigeon's thalamus. *Brain Res.* 108 (1976), 295–306.

Jassik-Gerschenfeld, D., Teulon J., and Hardy, O. Spatial interactions in the visual receptive fields of the nucleus dorsolateralis anterior of the pigeon thalamus. In Granda, A. M., and Maxwell, J. H. (Eds.), *Neural Mechanisms of Behavior in the Pigeon*. Plenum Press, New York (1979), pp. 145–164.

Jouvet, M. The role of monoamines and acetylcholine containing neurons in the regulation of the sleep-waking cycle. *Ergebn. Physiol.* 64 (1972), 166–307.

Karten, H. J., and Hodos, W. A Stereotaxic Atlas of the Brain of the Pigeon (*Columba livia*). The Johns Hopkins Press, Baltimore, 1967.

Karten, H. J., and Nauta, W. J. H. Organization of retinothalamic projections in the pigeon and owl. *Anat. Rec.* 160 (1968), 373.

Karten, H. J., Hodos, W., Nauta W. J. H., and Revzin, A. L. Neural connections of the "visual Wulst" of the avian telencephalon. Experimental studies in the pigeon (*Columba livia*) and the owl (*Speotyto cunicularia*) *J. Comp. Neurol.* 150 (1973), 253–277.

Kayama, Y., Negi, T., Sugitani, M., and Iwama, K. Effects of locus coeruleus stimulation on neuronal activities of dorsal lateral geniculate nucleus and perigeniculate reticular nucleus of the rat. *Neuroscience* 7 (1982), 655–666.

Kayama, Y., Shimada, S., Hishikawa, Y., and Ogawa, T. Effects of stimulating the dorsal raphe nucleus of the rat on neuronal activity in the dorsal lateral geniculate nucleus. *Brain Res.* 489 (1989), 1–11.

Kelly, J. P., and Gilbert, C. D. The projections of different morphological types of ganglion cells in the cat retina. *J. Comp. Neurol.* 163 (1975), 65–80.

Kirmse, W. Kritische Übersicht zur selektiven Sensomotorik des Blickens und multifoveates Spähen bei Vögeln. *Zool. Jb. Physiol.* 94 (1990), 217–228.

Kitt, C. A., and Brauth, S. E. Telencephalic projections from midbrain and isthmal cell groups in the pigeon. I. Locus coeruleus and subcoeruleus. *J. Comp. Neurol.* 247 (1986), 69–91.

Leresche, N., Hardy, O., and Jassik-Gerschenfeld, D. Receptive field properties of single cells in the pigeon's optic tectum during cooling of the 'visual Wulst.' *Brain Res.* 267 (1983), 225–236.

Martinoya, C., Rey, J., and Bloch, S. Limits of the pigeon's binocular field and direction for best binocular viewing. *Vision Res.* 21 (1981), 1197–1200.

Maxwell, J. H., and Granda, A. M. Receptive fields of movement-sensitive cells in the pigeon thalamus. In Granda, A. M., and Maxwell, J. H. (Eds.), *Neural Mechanisms of Behavior in the Pigeon*. Plenum, New York, 1979, pp. 177–197.

McCormick, D. A. Cholinergic and noradrenergic modulation of thalamocortical processing. *Trends Neurosci.* 12 (1989), 215–221.

Meier, R. E., Mihailovic, J., and Cuénod, M. Thalamic organization of the retino-thalamo-hyperstriatal pathway in the pigeon (*Columba livia*). *Exp. Brain Res.* 19 (1974), 351–364.

Miceli, D., Peyrichoux, J., and Repérant, J. The retino-thalamo-hyperstriatal pathway in the pigeon. *Brain Res.* 100 (1975), 125–131.

Miceli, D., and Repérant, J. Thalamo-hyperstriatal projections in the pigeon as demonstrated by retrograde double-labeling with fluorescent tracers. *Brain Res.* 245 (1982), 365–371.

Miceli, D., and Repérant, J. Telencephalic afferent projections from the diencephalon and brainstem in the pigeon. A retrograde multiple-label fluorescent study. *Exp. Biol.* 44 (1985), 71–99.

Miceli, D., Gioanni, H., Repérant, J., and Peyrichoux, J. The avian visual Wulst: I. An anatomical study of afferent and efferent pathways. II. An electrophysiological study of the functional properties of single neurons. In Granda, A. M., and Maxwell, J. H. (Eds.), *Neural Mechanisms of Behavior in Birds*. Plenum Press, New York, 1979.

Miceli, D., Repérant, J., Villalobos, J., and Dionne, L. Extratelencephalic projections of the avian visual Wulst. A quantitative autoradiographic study in the pigeon *Columba livia*. *J. Hirnforsch.* 28 (1987), 45–57.

Miceli, D., Marchand, L., Repérant, J., and Rio, J.-P. Projections of the dorsolateral anterior complex and adjacent thalamic nuclei upon the visual Wulst in the pigeon. *Brain Res.* 518 (1990), 317–323.

Nalbach, H.-O., Wolf-Oberhollenzer, F., and Kirschfeld, K. The pigeon's eye viewed through an ophtalmoscopic microscope: Orientation of retinal landmarks and significance of eye movements. *Vision Res.* 30 (1990), 529–540.

Nixdorf, B. E., and Bischof, H. J. Afferent connections of the ectostriatum and visual Wulst in the zebrafinch (*Taeniopygia guttata castanotis* Gould)—an HRP study. *Brain Res.* 248 (1982), 9–17.

Norgren, R. B. Jr., and Silver, R. Retinal projections in quail (*Coturnix coturnix*). *Visual Neurosci.* 3 (1989), 377–387.

Papadopoulos, G. C., and Parnavelas, J. G. Distribution and synaptic organization of dopaminergic axons in the lateral geniculate nucleus of the rat. *J. Comp. Neurol.* 294 (1990), 356–361.

Pape, H.-J., and McCormick, D. A. Noradrenaline and serotonin selectively modulate thalamic burst firing by enhancing a hyperpolarizing-activated cation current. *Nature (London)* 340 (1989), 715–718.

Pasik, P., Molinar-Rode, R., and Pasik, T. Chemically specified systems in the dorsal lateral geniculate nucleus of mammals. In Cohen, B., and Bodis-Wollner, I. (Eds.), *Vision and the Brain*. Raven, New York, 1990, pp. 43–83.

Pateromichelakis, S. Response properties of visual units in the anterior dorsolateral thalamus of the chick (*Gallus domesticus*). *Experientia* 37 (1981), 279–280.

Pettigrew, J. D. Comparison of the retinotopic organization of the visual Wulst in nocturnal and diurnal raptors, with a note on the evolution of frontal vision. In Cool, S. J., and Smith, E. L. (Eds.), *Frontiers of Visual Science*, New York, Springer, 1978, pp. 328–335.

Pettigrew, J. D. Binocular visual processing in the owl's telencephalon. *Proc. Royal Soc. London* 204 (1979), 435–455.

Pettigrew, J. D., and Konishi, M. Neurons selective for orientation and binocular disparity in the visual Wulst of the barn owl (*Tyto alba*). *Science* 193 (1976a), 675–678.

Pettigrew, J. D., and Konishi, M. Effects of monocular deprivation on binocular neurons in the owl's visual Wulst. *Nature (London)* 264 (1976b), 753–754.

Porciatti, V., Fontanesi, G., Rafaelli, A., and Bagnoli, P. Binocularity in the little owl, *Athene noctua*. II. Properties of visually evoked potentials from the Wulst in response to monocular and binocular stimulation with sine wave gratings. *Brain Behav. Evol.* 35 (1990), 40–48.

Reiner, A., and Karten, H. J. Laminar distribution of cells of origin of the descending tectofugal pathway in the pigeon (*Columba livia*). *J. Comp. Neurol.* 204 (1982), 165–187.

Remy, M., and Güntürkün, O. Retinal afferents to the tectum opticum and the n. opticus principalis thalami in the pigeon. *J. Comp. Neurol.* 305 (1991), 57–70.

Repérant, J. Nouvelles données sur les projections visuelles chez le Pigeon (*Columba livia*). *J. Hirnforsch.* 14 (1973), 151–187.

Revzin, A. M. A specific visual projection area in the hyperstriatum of the pigeon. *Brain Res.* 15 (1969), 246–249.

Reymond, L. Spatial visual acuity of the eagle Aquila audax: A behavioral, optical and anatomical investigation. *Vision Res.* 25 (1985), 1477–1491.

Reymond, L. Spatial visual acuity of the falcon, *Falco berigora*: A behavioral, optical and anatomical investigation. *Vision Res.* 27 (1987), 1859–1874.

Ritchie, T. L. C. Intratelencephalic visual connections and their relationship to the archistriatum in the pigeon (*Columba livia*). Ph. D. Thesis, University of Virgina, 1979.

Sherman, S. M., and Koch, C. The control of retinogeniculate transmission in the mammalian lateral geniculate nucleus. *Exp. Brain.* 73 (1986), 1–20.

Shimizu, T., and Karten, H. J. Immunohistochemical analysis of the visual Wulst of the pigeon (*Columba livia*). *J. Comp. Neurol.* 300 (1990), 346–369.

Sillito, A. M., and Kemp, J. A. The influence of GABAergic inhibitory processes of the receptive field structure of X and Y cells in the cat dorsal lateral geniculate nucleus (DLGN). *Brain Res.* 277 (1983), 63–77.

Vidyasagar, T. R. Contribution of inhibitory mechanisms to the orientation sensitivity of cat dLGN neurones. *Exp. Brain Res.* 55 (1984), 192–195.

Vischer, A., Cuénod, M., and Henke, H. Neurotransmitter receptor ligand binding and enzyme regional distribution in the pigeon visual system. *J. Neurochem.* 38 (1982), 1372–1382.

Wächtler, K. Regional distribution of muscarinic acetylcholine receptors in the telencephalon of the pigeon (*Columba livia f. domestica*). *J. Hirnforsch.* 26 (1985), 85–89.

Wächtler, K., and Ebinger, P. The pattern of muscarinic acetylcholine receptor binding in the avian forebrain. *J. Hirnforsch.* 30 (1989), 409–414.

Waldmann, C., and Güntürkün, O. The dopaminergic innervation of the pigeon caudolateral forebrain: Immunocytochemical evidence for a "prefrontal" in birds? *Brain Res.* 600 (1993), 225–234.

Watanabe, M. Synaptic organization of the nucleus dorsolateralis anterior thalami in the Japanese quail (*Coturnix coturnix japonica*). *Brain Res.* 401 (1987), 279–291.

Watanabe, M., Ito, H., and Masai, H. Cytoarchitecture and visual receptive neurons in the Wulst of the Japanese quail (*Coturnix coturnix japonica*). *J. Comp. Neurol.* 213 (1983), 188–198.

Wilson, P. The organization of the visual hyperstriatum in the domestic chick. II. Receptive field properties of single units. *Brain Res.* 188 (1980), 333–345.

8 The Organization of the Tectofugal Pathway in Birds: A Comparative Review

Jürgen Engelage and Hans-Joachim Bischof

In higher vertebrates visual information is processed by two prominent parallel pathways: the geniculocortical and extrageniculocortical pathways of mammals and the thalamofugal and tectofugal pathway in birds (e.g., Polyak, 1957 and see chapter 6; figure 8.1). The geniculocortical pathway includes the lateral geniculate nucleus (LGN) of the thalamus, area 17 (primary visual cortex, V1) of the striate cortex, and areas 18 and 19 in the extrastriate cortex. The extrageniculocortical pathway includes the superior colliculus (mesencephalon), the thalamic nucleus lateralis posterior (diencephalon), and telencephalic projection areas including the lateral suprasylvian cortex (reviews in Hubel and Wiesel, 1977; Creutzfeldt, 1988). Its avian counterpart, the tectofugal pathway, includes the optic tectum (mesencephalon), thalamic nucleus rotundus (diencephalon), and ectostriatum (telencephalon). The thalamofugal pathway (retino-lateral geniculate nucleus-Wulst) was reviewed in chapter 7. This chapter reviews the anatomy and physiology of the tectofugal pathway within a comparative perspective.

A substantial body of anatomical, physiological, and neurobehavioral (lesion) data, gathered over the past few decades, suggests that the dual sets of pathways in birds and mammals are homologous (Karten, 1969; Revzin and Karten, 1966; Revzin 1969, 1970, 1979; Kimberly et al., 1979; Miceli et al., 1979; Hodos et al., 1986; Wilson, 1980b; Denton, 1981; Shimizu and Karten, 1990). Perhaps, because that same period saw an explosion of research on the geniculostriate pathway (Hubel, 1982; Wiesel, 1982), studies in birds have focused primarily on the geniculocortical homologue: the thalamofugal pathway. The discovery by Pettigrew and Konishi (1976a,b) of some striking similarities between the visual Wulst of owls and mammalian visual cortex reinforced the thalamofugal focus.

However, owls, unlike most birds, have frontally placed eyes, resulting in significant overlap of the left and right hemifields and allowing binocular vision in a large region in front of the birds. In mammals like cats, monkeys, and man, binocular vision has been shown to allow precise distance estimation by neurons, which are sensitive to the dis-

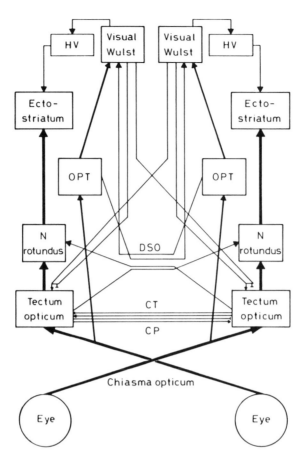

Figure 8.1 Main projections of the tectofugal and the thalamofugal pathway. Thick lines, tectofugal pathway; medium lines, thalamofugal pathway; thin lines, interhemispheric connections (DSO, CT, and CP) and connections between the two main pathways (HV → ectostriatum). DSO, decussatio supraoptica; CT, commissura tectalis; CP, commissura posterior; OPT, nucleus opticus principalis thalami; HV, hyperstriatum ventrale.

parity of the images on both eyes (e.g., Pettigrew, 1978), and has been presumed to facilitate detection of camouflaged objects. Both features would be especially useful for diurnal and nocturnal raptors. Thus, binocular vision in owls, and other diurnal raptors like falcons and kestrels, may be adaptive specializations to the demands of hunting prey. Several studies (Stingelin, 1958; Henke, 1983) have concluded that the relative size of the thalamofugal pathway and the degree of organization of the visual Wulst are related to the degree of binocular overlap, and this conclusion is supported by the comparative data of Pettigrew and his colleagues (Bravo and Pettigrew, 1981; Bravo and Inzunza, 1983).

Unlike owls, most birds have laterally placed eyes and a much less well-developed thalamofugal pathway. Indeed, it has long been evident that the tectofugal pathway is the most prominent pathway in birds

(Karten, 1969, Karten et al., 1973; Cohen and Karten, 1974). Moreover, the visual Wulst of lateral-eyed birds such as chicks, pigeons, and finches does not process ipsilateral or binocular visual information to a significant extent (Perisic et al., 1971; Wilson 1980b; Denton, 1981; Bredenkötter and Bischof, 1990). Neurobehavioral studies of the two pathways in pigeon—a lateral-eyed bird—indicate that tectofugal lesions produce severe discrimination deficits, while thalamofugal pathway lesions show obvious effects only if combined with lesions of the tectofugal pathway (Hodos et al., 1982; Watanabe et al., 1984, 1986). Finally, a rapidly growing body of data suggests that, in laterally eyed birds, the tectofugal pathway mediates some visual processes performed in mammals primarily by the geniculocortical pathway and by the thalamofugal pathway in frontal-eyed birds. Specifically, these data indicate that in laterally eyed birds simultaneous processing of visual information from both eyes and binocular interaction is carried out by the tectofugal visual pathway.

ANATOMICAL ORGANIZATION OF THE TECTOFUGAL VISUAL PROJECTIONS

In both birds and mammals, the optic nerves project in a highly ordered manner onto their primary visual target areas in the mesencephalon and diencephalon. The visual space of the external world is represented as an array of receptive fields on a map in the visual target areas in birds and mammals. The representation of visual information in a topographical order is probably maintained up to the primary sensory target areas of the telencephalon and in many cases even up to the secondary projection areas of the visual pathways.

In most mammals, the decussation of the optic nerve is only partial, the proportion of uncrossed fibers varying as little as 10% in the rabbit to 50% in primates and man (Polyak, 1957). In contrast, the optic nerves of adult birds are virtually completely crossed (see, e.g., McLoon, 1982; McLoon and Lund, 1982; Bagnoli et al., 1987). The retinal projection on the contralateral tectum is probably retinotopically organized (Hamdi and Whitteridge, 1954). While there is no clear evidence for a topographic projection of the retinogeniculate (GLd) projection, it is known that in owls and falcons the temporal retina, representing the binocular visual field, projects heavily on GLd (Bravo and Pettigrew, 1981; Bravo and Inzunza, 1983). In contrast, the dorsotemporal retina (red field) of lateral-eyed birds projects almost exclusively on the optic tectum, while the much larger yellow field of the central retina projects on both tectum and GLd. Moreover, the retinal projection on GLd is generally much smaller than its projection on the tectum (Remy and Güntürkün, 1991). Even in more frontal-eyed birds, more than 60% of the retinal efferents terminate in the optic tectum (Bravo and Pettigrew, 1981).

The optic tectum is a highly laminated structure within which 6 (Cowan et al., 1961) to 15 (Cajal, 1891) layers may be distinguished. Retinal efferents form the superficial layers (mainly the stratum opticum) of the optic tectum. The projection is topographically organized. Tectal efferents arise from the deeper layers, mainly the stratum griseum centrale (SGC). The optic tectum is also the recipient of thalamofugal efferents from the visual Wulst (Bagnoli et al., 1980), providing a link between the two visual pathways. Electrophysiological studies indicated that the tectal projection on the thalamic nucleus rotundus projection may also be topographically organized (Revzin and Karten, 1966); and anatomical analysis reveals four or five subdivisions of rotundus, whose functional significance is not known (Benowitz and Karten, 1976; Nixdorf and Bischof, 1982; Bischof and Niemann, 1990; Martinez-de-la-Torre et al., 1990).

The nucleus rotundus projects ipsilaterally on the ectostriatum, a telencephalic structure divisible into "core" and "belt" regions, but little is known of the organization of the projection (Karten and Hodos, 1970; Benowitz and Karten, 1976; Nixdorf and Bischof, 1982). It is generally assumed that thalamic input reaches the "core" region, which then projects on the ectostriatal "belt," which may also receive Wulst efferents (Ritchie and Cohen, 1977; Watanabe et al., 1985). The subsequent intratelencephalic connections of the tectofugal pathway include a projection from ectostriatal "belt" to the neostriatum intermediale laterale (NIL), which, in turn, projects on the archistriatum intermedium (AI). AI projects on the optic tectum, completing a tectofugal loop made up of linked tectal–thalamic–telencephalic structures. Karten and Shimizu (1991) suggested that this nuclear circuitry resembles, in its general organizational pattern, the connectivity pattern of mammalian cortical layers (see chapter 6).

A "second" tectofugal pathway (Gamlin and Cohen, 1986) originates in the tectum, relays in the caudal dorsolateral posterior nucleus of the thalamus (DLPc), and terminates in specific areas of the intermediate and caudal neostriatum (NI, NC). The existence of still another telencephalic visual projection area was suggested by the finding of visual evoked potentials in the caudolateral telencephalon, with response latencies shorter than those recorded from Wulst and ectostriatum, but its input source has not been identified (Güntürkün, 1984).

RESPONSE PROPERTIES OF NEURONS IN THE TECTOFUGAL PATHWAY

Despite the relative paucity of physiological studies of the visual pathways in birds (see Granda and Maxwell, 1979), there are some data on the response properties of neurons at several levels of the tectofugal pathway. It has long been known, for example, that avian retinal ganglion cells can perform complex analyses of visual properties such as horizontal edge detection and direction selectivity (Maturana and Frenk, 1963). Early studies of tectal neurophysiology (e.g., Hamdi and Whitteridge, 1954) demonstrated a point-to-point representation of the pigeon's visual space on the optic tectum. The upper half of the left visual field is represented on the upper surface of the right optic tectum and the horizontal meridian is projected onto the lateral edge of the optic tectum. Within this projection, the spatial extension of the horizontal meridian is magnified in the tectal map. Bilge (1971) reported an increase in receptive field size from about $2°-3°$ in the superficial layers to up to $70° \times 180°$ in the deeper layers (namely the SGC). A substantial proportion (ca. 70%) of tectal neurons is sensitive to moving stimuli and about 30% of these show a high degree of directional specificity, i.e., stimulation in the preferred direction of movement increases spontaneous firing rate, stimulation in the "null direction" leads to a reduction in firing rate (Jassik-Gerschenfeld and Guichard, 1972). However, most tectal units are only broadly tuned for direction and the majority prefer forward or downward directions of movement (Frost and DiFranco, 1976). Subsequent studies (Frost et al., 1981) have shown that tectal neurons are inhibited if the stimuli (e.g., white disks) and a structured background were moved in phase, but facilitated if the stimuli were moved in a direction opposite to the background. In addition to these properties, about 30% of tectal cells showed clear chromatic responses in their action spectra as well, i.e., they may be involved in color vision (Varela et al., 1983).

It appears that the responses of tectal neurons may be modulated by thalamofugal inputs relayed via visual Wulst efferents to the optic tectum (e.g., Bagnoli et al., 1982). Bagnoli et al. (1977, 1979) showed that both single unit activity and the prominent P wave of the tectal slow field potential (Holden, 1968) are reduced by concurrent activation of the optic tectum and the visual Wulst. This effect is time locked, i.e., the P wave completely disappears only if the visual Wulst is stimulated 30 msec prior to the optic tectum. Leresche et al. (1983) found that while the responses of most tectal cells to visual stimulation are clearly reduced during cooling of the visual Wulst, some direction-selective tectal units increase their responses. Thus visual Wulst input sharpens and facilitates neuronal responses in some cases and suppresses them in other cases. Neither the mechanism nor the functional significance of this observation is known.

The receptive fields of rotundal neurons are larger than those of tectal units but have similar characteristics, including preferential responses to moving stimuli with a clear directional, but no orientation, selectivity (Revzin, 1979; Maxwell and Granda, 1979). Revzin (1979) suggested a functional differentiation of the nucleus into a posterior third (responding to anything that moves, an anterior two-thirds (responding selectively to "abstract" stimulus characteristics such as size, direction, and velocity), and a ventral part, concerned primarily with brightness responses. Recently, Wang and Frost (1992) displayed computer-generated images of stimuli moving in spatial three-dimensional trajectories and found neurons in pigeon that apparently signal the time to collision with objects by simultaneously coding the speed and distance of a visual target. Finally, rotundal units also appear to have a selective response to the wavelength of light stimuli (Granda and Yazulla,, 1971; Maxwell and Granda, 1979). Opponent color units have been found in the nucleus rotundus of the pigeon (Yazulla and Granda, 1973) and in the nucleus geniculatus laterale pars ventrale (GLv), another thalamic nucleus receiving direct tectal input (Varela et al., 1983).

The few published studies of ectostriatal units have found (1) that most units were responsive to visual stimuli, (2) that they all had very large receptive fields, and (3) that the proportion of directionally selective cells is increased by comparison with retina, tectum, and rotundus. Most units prefer upward/downward or fore/aft movements, but none was selectively responsive to orientation (Revzin, 1970; Kimberly et al., 1971). Revzin (1979) suggested that the functional organization of the nucleus rotundus is simply relayed to the ectostriatal core. However, from the single unit data available, neither the existence nor nature of that organization is clear.

Using the methods of current source-density (CSD) analysis (e.g., Nicholson and Freeman 1975; for review see: Mitzdorf, 1985), Engelage and Bischof (1989) recorded contralateral and ipsilateral flash-evoked slow field potentials in the ectostriatum of the zebra finch. They found that the time course of macroscopic current sinks, indicating sites of excitatory synaptic activity; the negative wave of visual evoked potentials and single unit responses to the same stimulus match exactly (Figure 8.2). The most characteristic feature of the current source density depth profiles is an early prominent current sink (8.3:a) in the ectostriatal core, with corresponding dorsal and ventral current sources. A delayed sink (8.3:b)–source–sink (8.3:c) sequence located within the core region is also detectable in contralateral and ipsilateral CSD depth profiles. This clearly shows that the generators for the contralateral and ipsilaterally evoked visual potentials are located within the ectostriatal core (figure 8.3). Contralaterally and ipsilaterally evoked responses commonly show the same basic pattern of alternating sinks and sources in their CSD depth profiles (Engelage and Bischof, 1989). Macroscopic sinks and sources as shown above emerge only if during activation of the system neuronal assemblies become active concomitantly. The data therefore suggest that despite its homogeneous anatomical organization, the ectostriatum may have a high degree of physiological parcellation, reflecting the existence of distinct functional subdivisions.

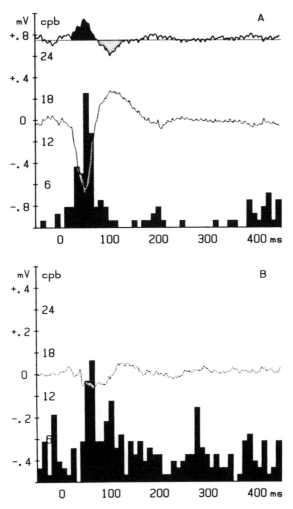

Figure 8.2 Flash-evoked slow field potential (VEP), current source-density profile (CSD), and single unit activity at an identical recording site in the ectostriatum of the zebra finch. (A) Contralateral stimulation; (B) ipsilateral stimulation. The stimulus is delivered at 0 msec. For the VEP response bin width is 500 μsec, average 64 ×, and the ordinate scale is in mV. Signals are filtered only by a 4-Hz highpass filter. CSDs are calculated according to the formula developed by Nicholson and Freemann (1975). As the differentiation grid for ectostriatal VEPs is 500 μm, the VEP traces 250 μm above and below the recording site had to be taken into account for the calculation of the CSD profile. For the single unit response bin width is 10 msec, average 16 ×, and the ordinate scale is in spikes/bin. Signals are band pass filtered with limits at 300 Hz and 10 kHz. The most important result of this comparison is the perfect agreement in the time patterns of VEP, CSD, and single unit activity. This shows that the three methods demonstrated reflect, to a high degree, the same physiological processes in ectostriatal visual processing.

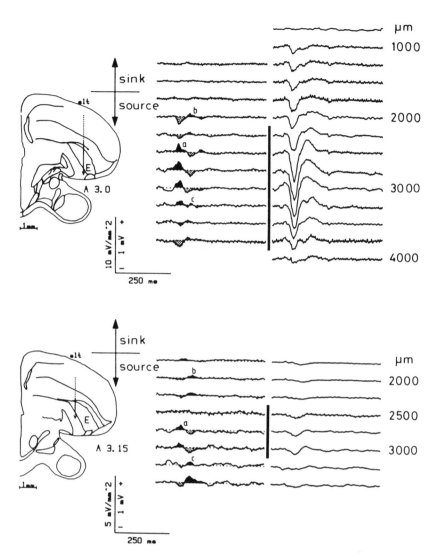

Figure 8.3 Comparison of contralateral (top) and ipsilateral (bottom) evoked potentials and related current source-density depth profiles in the ectostriatum of the zebra finch. (Left) Frontal sections (anterior 3.0 and 3.15) of the zebra finch brain with electrode tracks. (Middle) Current source-density depth profiles calculated from the VEP traces in the right column. Average 64 ×, bin width 500 μsec, step width 250 μm stimulus at 0 msec, differentiation grid for CSDs is 500 μm. Signals are filtered only by a 4 Hz highpass filter. CSDs are calculated according to the formula developed by Nicholson and Freemann (1975). The heavy bars represent the solid part of the electrode track markings in the left column. The figure clearly demonstrates that the generators for the contralateral and ipsilateral extracellularly recorded VEPS are located within the ectostriatal core region.

HEMISPHERIC INTEGRATION IN THE TECTOFUGAL PATHWAY

Because the optic chiasm is completely crossed in birds, both visual pathways in each hemisphere receive their primary visual information exclusively from the contralateral eye. Hence ipsilateral and binocular stimulus processing can be achieved only by secondary recrossing fibers connecting the visual target areas of the left and right hemispheres. Such fibers exist at several brain levels (see figure 8.1) and include the mesencephalic tectal commissure (CT) (Robert and Cuenod, 1969a) and the dorsal and ventral supraoptic decussations of the forebrain (DSOD, DSOV). In the thalamofugal pathway, recrossing fibers in DSOD connect the GLd complex to the visual Wulst of both hemispheres (Karten et al., 1973; Bagnoli and Burkhalter, 1982; Mihailovic et al., 1974). In the tectofugal pathway, recrossing fibers of the tectorotundal projection, traveling in DSOV, connect the optic tectum to the nucleus rotundus of the contralateral side (Benowitz and Karten, 1976) and have recently been shown to make a significant contribution (about 23%) to the efferent projections of the optic tectum (Bischof and Niemann, 1990).

For the thalamofugal pathway, the only known source for hemispheric interactions is the recrossing bilateral GLd–visual Wulst projection (Karten et al., 1973; Bagnoli et al., 1982). In lateral-eyed birds— e.g., zebra finches, pigeons, and chicks—the visual Wulst, though clearly responsive to contralaterally presented stimuli, is essentially unresponsive to ipsilateral or binocular stimuli (Parker and Delius, 1972; Denton, 1981; Wilson, 1980b; Bredenkötter and Bischof, 1990). For the tectofugal pathway, in contrast, multiple potential sources of hemispheric interaction have been demonstrated. At caudal levels, an inhibitory role for the tectal commissure is suggested by the report that about 25% of tectal neurons driven via the CT were inhibited during electrical stimulation of the contralateral optic tectum (Robert and Cuenod, 1969b), a finding later confirmed by intracellular studies in pigeon (Hardy et al., 1984, 1985) and evoked potential analyses in the zebra finch (Engelage and Bischof, 1988).

The early studies of thalamic and telencephalic tectofugal structures provided no evidence with respect to the processing of ipsilateral and bilateral stimuli (e.g., Revzin, 1966; 1970; Maxwell and Granda, 1979; Kimberly et al., 1971; Parker and Delius, 1972). However, Engelage and Bischof argued that the capacity for panoramic vision, seen in all lateral-eyed birds, must imply central access to ipsilateral (and binocular) visual inputs. Using visual evoked potential (VEP) methods, these investigators systematically examined thalamofugal and tectofugal structures in the visual system of the zebra finch, a lateral-eyed bird with only a small binocular visual field (Bischof, 1988). Their studies showed that, in contrast with the Wulst (Bredenkötter and Bischof, 1990), the ectostriatum is clearly responsive to contralaterally *and* ipsilaterally presented flashed stimuli (figure 8.4). The ipsilaterally evoked potentials reached

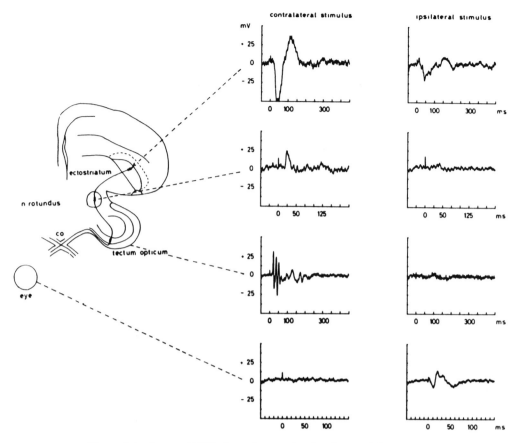

Figure 8.4 Averaged VEPs from the tectofugal pathway of the zebra finch. (Left) Simplified diagram (compare figure 8.1) of the pathway. (Right) Diagrams from bottom to top: recordings from eye, optic tectum nucleus, rotundus, and ectostriatum. (Left column) Contralateral stimulation. (Right column) Ipsilateral stimulation. Average 64 ×, bin width 200–500 μsec (see variations of the time scale), stimulus at 0 msec. Signals are filtered only by a 4 Hz highpass filter. The figure clearly shows that the ectostriatum receives information from the ipsilateral eye.

amplitudes up to 50% of contralaterally evoked responses (Engelage and Bischof, 1988).

Supporting evidence for tectofugal ipsilateral processing comes from some unexpected results of VEP recordings in unilaterally enucleated subjects. Ipsilaterally evoked ectostriatal VEPs in these birds were dramatically enhanced, with their highest amplitudes comparable to those of contralaterally evoked VEPs in normal zebra finches (figure 8.5). In contrast with the significant differences in amplitudes and latencies reported for normal birds, there were no significant differences in either parameter between ipsilaterally evoked VEPs in enucleated birds and contralaterally evoked VEPs in normal birds (Engelage and Bischof, 1988). Interestingly, ipsilaterally evoked VEPs could also be detected in the nucleus rotundus of enucleated but not of normal birds, but no

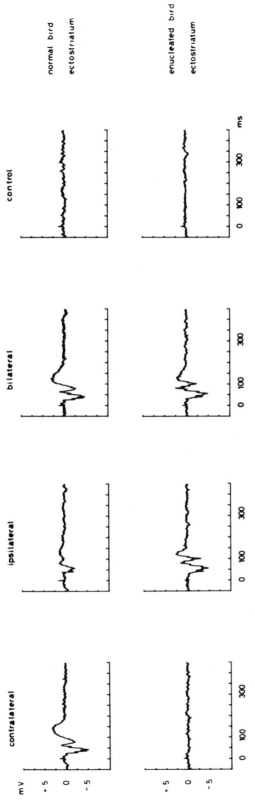

Figure 8.5 Summary of the effects of enucleation on responses of the ectostriatum in a bird enucleated 3 days prior to the recordings. In normal birds (upper row) contralateral and bilateral stimulus responses are very similar. Ipsilateral VEPs are about 50% smaller than contralaterally and bilaterally evoked VEPs. In enucleated birds (lower row) the situation is clearly changed. Ipsilateral VEPs reach amplitudes similar to contralateral VEPs in normal birds and are as high as bilaterally evoked VEPs. This clearly shows that ipsilateral stimulus responses are not due to light spreading from one eye to the other. As ipsilaterally evoked VEPs in enucleated birds are clearly enhanced, it is concluded that ipsilateral stimulus responses in normal birds are severely inhibited. Average 64 ×, bin width 500 μsec, stimulus at 0 msec. Signals are filtered only by a 4 Hz highpass filter.

ipsilateral VEPs were detected in the optic tectum. Experiments in the thalamofugal and tectofugal pathway compared the effects of an acute unilateral injection of tetrodotoxin (a substance blocking EPSPs) into the eye while recording from ipsilateral visual Wulst and ipsilateral ectostriatum. The facilitatory effects on VEPs seen in ectostriatum were not seen in the visual Wulst. Engelage and Bischof (1988) concluded that visual information is conveyed from the ipsilateral eye to the contralateral optic tectum, recrosses to the ipsilateral nucleus rotundus, and is finally conveyed to the ipsilateral ectostriatum, a conclusion consistent with the connectivity pattern of these structures (Karten et al., 1973; Benowitz and Karten, 1976; Hunt and Künzle, 1976; Nixdorf and Bischof, 1982; Bischof and Niemann, 1990).

These findings are also consistent with a major role for inhibitory mechanisms in ipsilateral stimulus processing in the ectostriatum. From a comparison of VEPs in different target areas in enucleated birds, Engelage and Bischof (1988) concluded that the spontaneous activity of retinal ganglion cells severely suppresses responsiveness in the ipsilateral ectostriatum of normal birds. This inhibition is probably generated by tectal crosstalk via the tectal commissure and intrinsic tectal circuits.

This "mutual inhibition" hypothesis was supported by experiments in which inhibitory synapses in the optic tectum were blocked by the application of picrotoxin. When applied to the optic tectum ipsilateral to the recording site in the ectostriatum, ipsilaterally and contralaterally evoked responses were substantially enhanced, but the enhancement was greatest for the ipsilateral responses. This shows that ipsilateral information must, to some extent, be conveyed from one optic tectum to the other. Picrotoxin injection into the optic tectum contralateral to the ectostrial recording site enhanced ipsilaterally, but not contralaterally evoked responses, demonstrating that ipsilateral stimulus responses are selectively inhibited in the optic tectum contralateral to the recording site (figure 8.6). The results are in agreement with those of the enucleation experiments.

Finally, experiments in which the neuronal activity of either the visual Wulst or the optic tectum was suppressed by either cooling or "spreading depression" (Leao, 1944) showed that the ipsilateral evoked responses observed in the ectostriatum are not primarily mediated by inputs relayed through the visual Wulst to the tectofugal ectostriatum. Ipsilaterally evoked ectostriatal potentials were significantly reduced but not abolished during suppression of ipsilateral Wulst activity. In contrast suppression of optic tectum activity ipsilateral to the ectostriatal recording site led to a decrease in ipsilateral responses and a severe reduction of contralateral responses. These experiments, while confirming an important role for tectal inhibitory processes, also suggest that the visual Wulst may have a significant excitatory influence on the processing of contralaterally evoked visual information in the ectostriatum (figure 8.7). Thus it cannot be excluded that both the recrossing

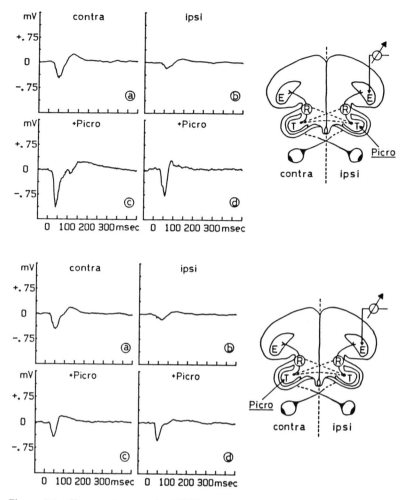

Figure 8.6 Changes in ectostriatal VEP responses during picrotoxin-induced disinhibition of the optic tectum contralateral and ipsilateral to the recording site in the ectostriatum. (Upper panel, a and b) Responses to contralateral and ipsilateral stimulation before picrotoxin injection; (c and d) responses after picrotoxin injection into the optic tectum ipsilateral to the recording site. (Lower panel, a and b) Responses to contralateral and ipsilateral stimulation before picrotoxin injection; (c and d) responses after picrotoxin injection into the optic tectum contralateral to the recording site. Injection into the ipsilateral optic tectum enhances ipsilateral and contralateral responses; injections into the contralateral optic tectum selectively enhances ipsilateral responses. Average 64 ×, bin width 500 μsec, stimulus at 0 msec. Signals are filtered only by a 4 Hz highpass filter. The results show the major importance of the tectal circuitry for the selective suppression of ipsilateral stimulus responses. The observed changes are also in perfect agreement with the results from the enucleation experiments reported above.

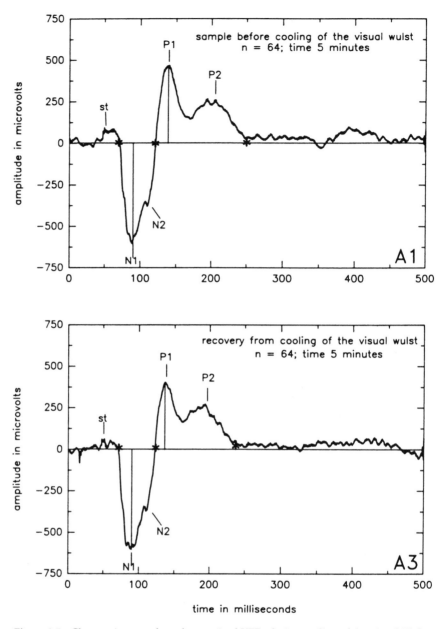

Figure 8.7 Changes in contralateral ectostriatal VEPs during cooling of the visual Wulst ipsilateral to the recording site. (A1) before cooling; (A2) during cooling; (A3) recovery from cooling; (A4) computer simulated amplitude enhancement of VEP wave. Amplitude enhancement was achieved by multiplication of each bin with the quotient from maximal amplitude of the negative wave from recovery divided by maximal amplitude of the negative wave during cooling. Superimposed (thin line) is the VEP recorded after recovery (A3). The arrows indicate the major differences between the VEPs recorded during and

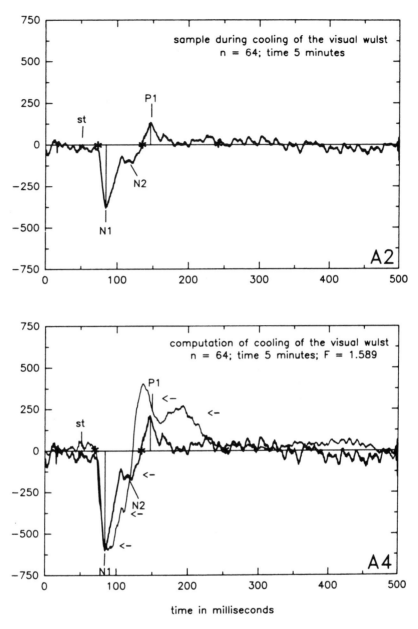

after cooling of the visual Wulst. Thin horizontal lines mark the zero line and thin vertical lines mark the locations of amplitude measurements. Average 64 ×, bin width 500 μsec, stimulus at 50 msec. Signals are filtered only by a 4 Hz highpass filter. Note the severe amplitude reduction of N1 and P1 and the almost complete diminution of N2 and P2 due to the suppression of visual Wulst activity indicating an excitatory contribution of visual Wulst efferents to ectostriatal visual stimulus processing.

optic tectum, nucleus rotundus projections, and the visual Wulst, optic tectum projections, make some contribution to the marked inhibition of ipsilateral stimulus responses.

NEUROBEHAVIORAL STUDIES OF THE TECTOFUGAL PATHWAY

In contrast to the minimal effects of the thalamofugal pathway lesions, it has been repeatedly found that damage restricted to one or more tectofugal structures produced significant deficits on a variety of visually guided tasks, including color, brightness, pattern, and size discriminations. Particularly in spatial resolution tasks, combined thalamotectofugal pathway lesions produce significantly more severe deficits than lesions restricted to the tectofugal pathway alone (Macko and Hodos, 1984; Hodos et al., 1984). The finding of deficits in line orientation after rotundal lesions (Mulvanny, 1979) suggests the existence of orientation-selective units in the tectofugal pathway despite the absence of supporting electrophysiological evidence. Moreover, the tectofugal, rather than the thalamofugal pathway is critical for the mediation of interocular transfer of visual discrimination learning (Watanabe et al., 1986; Remy and Watanabe, this volume). Finally, Hodos et al. (1982) showed that following rotundal lesions (which normally produce substantial brightness discrimination deficits), a second lesion in the ventrolateral geniculate nucleus (a tectofugal fiber recipient) virtually diminished the deficits produced by the first lesion. These investigators discussed their findings in the context of parallel processing of visual information and a modulatory contribution of the different visual target areas to information processing.

The contribution of the second tectofugal pathway remains unclear. Single unit recordings (Korzeniewska and Güntürkün 1990) showed that its nuclear component (DLP) is multimodal, responding to both somatosensory and visual inputs. Lesion studies (Hodos et al., 1986; Kertzmann and Hodos, 1988) revealed the same pattern as observed in the thalamotectofugal comparisons. Only if combined with lesions in the "first" tectofugal pathway, lesions in thalamic and telencephalic targets of the "second" tectofugal pathway led to significant deficits in visual discrimination tasks.

Taken together, the results of all these studies are consistent with (1) a dominant role for the tectofugal pathway in visual discriminations of colors, brightness, and patterns, (2) a supportive role for thalamofugal structures in mediating spatial resolution, and (3) the importance of interaction between the two major visual pathways. The tectofugal pathway, acting in isolation, appears capable of mediating a substantial part of the visual processing carried out by birds. A similar view is gradually coming to be held with respect to the homologous visual pathways in mammals (Creutzfeldt, 1988).

CONCLUSIONS

The functional contribution of the tectofugal pathway to the processing of visual information is far from clear. The optic tectum receives a point-to-point projection from the retina, and the receptive fields of the outer tectal layers are small enough to allow for a precise localization of objects within visual space. However, because the subsequent targets of tectal projections to diencephalic and telencephalic structures have large receptive fields (as well as the inner tectal layers), these structures may be more concerned with the analysis of directionality, orientation, and velocity of moving objects, and the processing of colors, contours, and other more general features of the visual scene. Paradoxically, however, lesion studies indicate that despite their large receptive fields, higher levels of the tectofugal pathway may also be involved in the analysis of fine visual detail. This could be achieved by small subunits within the large receptive fields or by additional modulatory inputs from the thalamofugal pathway. Whatever the mechanism, the tectofugal pathway is probably involved in almost all types of visual information processing. Even the processing of binocular information, which until recently was thought to be an exclusive domain of the thalamofugal pathway, is, in lateral-eyed birds, performed mainly by the tectofugal pathway.

A persistent problem for investigators concerns the functional significance of the physiologically and morphologically defined subdivisions of rotundus. It is not known whether these subdivisions comprise independent topographical maps or not and how they project to the ectostriatum. More information is needed on the intrinsic organization and neostriatal projections of ectostriatum, and the role of the Wulst projection on its "belt" region. A second problem is raised by the existence of an anatomically defined tectothalamic–telencephalic–tectal feedback loop. One of its possible functions may be the modulation of incoming information flow by descending telencephalic inputs. Another would be the comparison, at tectal levels, of incoming visual information with inputs from higher centers, its integration with other tectal sensory inputs, and its projection on final common path behavioral mechanisms. Finally, given the emerging picture of a dominant tectofugal pathway, and a pattern of information flow from thalamofugal to tectofugal structures, but not vice versa, what role is left for the thalamofugal pathway in lateral-eyed birds?

Investigations with 2-deoxyglucose suggest that the visual Wulst is active only in awake, aroused birds, while the ectostriatum shows a high level of spontanous activity under almost all conditions (Bischof and Herrmann, 1986). The functional implications of this observation are presently obscure. Moreover, because both pathways are likely to be involved simultaneously in almost any task, e.g., binocular processing, the determination of their separate functions in isolation is likely to be both empirically difficult and conceptually erroneous. Finally, the function of different parts of the visual system appears to have changed during evolution. Despite such difficulties, this review testifies to the progress that has been made in clarifying the role of tectofugal structures in visual processing by birds.

REFERENCES

Bagnoli, P., and Burkhalter, A. Organisation of the afferent projections to the Wulst in the pigeon. *J. Comp. Neurol.* 214 (1983), 103–113.

Bagnoli, P., Francesconi, W., and Magni, F. Visual Wulst influences on the optic tectum of the pigeon. *Brain. Behav. Evol.* 14 (1977), 217–237.

Bagnoli, P., Francesconi, W., and Magni, F. Interaction of optic tract and visual Wulst impulses on single units of the pigeon's optic tectum. *Brain Behav. Evol.* 16 (1979), 19–37.

Bagnoli, P., Grassi, S., and Magni, F. A Direct connection between visual Wulst and optic tectum in the pigeon (*Columba livia*) demonstrated by horseradish peroxidase. *Arch. Ital. Biol.* 118 (1980), 72–88.

Bagnoli, P., Francesconi, W., and Magni, F. Visual Wulst–optic tectum relationships in birds: A comparison with the mammalian corticotectal system. *Arch. Ital. Biol.* 120 (1982), 212–235.

Bagnoli, P., Porciatti, V., Fontanesi, G., and Sebastiani, L. Morphological and functional changes in the retinotectal system of the pigeon during the early posthatching period. *J. Comp. Neurol.* 256 (1987), 400–411.

Benowitz, L. J., and Karten, H. J. Organization of the tectofugal visual pathway in the pigeon: A retrograde transport study. *J. Comp. Neurol.* 167 (1976), 503–520.

Bilge, M. Electrophysiological investigations on the pigeon's optic tectum. *Q. J. Exp. Physiol.* 56 (1971), 242–249.

Bischof, H. J. The visual field and visually guided behaviour in the zebra finch (*Taeniopygia guttata*). *J. Comp. Physiol. A* 163 (1988), 329–337.

Bischof, H. J., and Herrmann, K. Arousal enhances [14C] 2-deoxyglucose uptake in four forebrain areas of the zebra finch. *Behav. Brain. Res.* 21 (1986), 215–221.

Bischof, H. J., and Niemann, J. Contralateral projections of the optic tectum in the zebra finch (*Taeniopygia guttata castanotis*). *Cell. Tissue. Res.* 262 (1990), 307–313.

Bravo, H., and Inzunza, O. Estudio Anatomico en las Vias Visuales Paralelas en Falconiformes. Anatomical studies of the parallel visual pathway in falconiformes. *Arch. Biol. Med. Exp.* 16 (1983), 283–289.

Bravo, H., and Pettigrew, J. D. The distribution of neurons projecting from the retina and visual cortex to the thalamus and tectum opticum of the barn owl *Tyto alba* and the burrowing owl *Speotyto cunnicularia*. *J. Comp. Neurol.* 199 (1981), 419–441.

Bredenkötter, M., and Bischof, H. J. Differences between ipsilaterally and contralaterally evoked potentials in the visual Wulst of the zebra finch. *Visual. Neurosci.* 5 (1990), 155–163.

Cajal, S. R. Sur la Fine Structure du Lobe Optique des Oiseaux et sur l'Origine Reelle des Nerfes Optique. *Int. Mschr. Anat. Physiol. B* 8 (1891), 337–366.

Cohen, D. H., and Karten, H. J. The structural organization of the avian brain: An overview. In I. J. Goodman and M. W. Schein (Eds.), *Birds Brain and Behavior*. Academic Press, New York, 1974, pp. 29–73.

Cowan, W. M., Adamson, L., and Powell, T. P. An experimental study of the avian visual system. *J. Anat.* 95 (1961), 545–563.

Creutzfeldt, O. D. Extrageniculo-striate visual mechanisms: Compartimentalization of visual functions. In T. P. Hicks and G. Benedek (Eds.), *Vision within Extrageniculo-Striate Systems*. Elsevier, Amsterdam, 1988, pp. 307–320.

Denton, C. J. Topography of the hyperstriatal visual projection area in the young domestic chicken. *Exp. Neurol.* 74 (1981), 482–498.

Engelage, J., and Bischof, H. J. Enucleation enhances ipsilateral flash evoked responses in the ectostriatum of the zebra finch (*Taeniopygia guttata Castanotis* Gould). *Exp. Brain. Res.* 70 (1988), 79–89.

Engelage, J., and Bischof, H. J. Flash evoked potentials in the ectostriatum of the zebra finch: A current-source-density analysis. *Exp. Brain. Res.* 74 (1989), 563–572.

Frost, B. J., and DiFranco, D. E. Motion characteristics of single units in the pigeon optic tectum. *Vision. Res.* 16 (1976), 1229–1234.

Frost, B. J., Scilley, P. L., and Wong, S. C. P. Moving backround patterns reveal double-opponency of directionally specific pigeon tectal neurons. *Exp. Brain. Res.* 43 (1981), 173–185.

Gamlin, P. D. R., and Cohen, D. H. A second ascending visual pathway from the optic tectum to the telencephalon in the pigeon (*Columba livia*). *J. Comp. Neurol.* 250 (1986), 296–310.

Granda, A. M., Maxwell, J. H. (Eds.) *Neural Mechanisms of Behavior in the Pigeon.* New York, Plenum Press, 1979.

Granda, A. M., and Yazulla, S. The spectral sensitivity of single units in the nucleus rotundus of pigeon, *Columba livia. J. Gen. Physiol.* 57 (1971), 363–384.

Güntürkün, O. Evidence for a third primary visual area in the telencephalon of the pigeon. *Brain. Res.* 294 (1984), 247–254.

Hamdi, F. A., and Whitteridge, D. The representation of the retina on the optic tectum of the pigeon. *Q. J. Exp. Physiol.* 39 (1954), 11–119.

Hardy, O., Leresche, N., and Jassik-Gerschenfeld, D. Postsynaptic potentials in neurons of the pigeon's optic tectum in response to afferent stimulation from the retina and other visual structures: An intracellular study. *Brain. Res.* 311 (1984), 65–74.

Hardy, O., Leresche, N., and Jassik-Gerschenfeld, D. Morphology and laminar distribution of electrophysiologically identified cells in the pigeon's optic tectum: An intracellular study. *J. Comp. Neurol.* 233 (1985), 390–404.

Henke, H. The central part of the avian visual system. In G. Nistica and L. Bolis (Eds.), *Progress in Nonmammalian Brain Research.* CRC Press, Boca Raton, FL, 1983, pp. 113–158.
Hodos, W., Macko, K. A., and Sommers, D. I. Interactions between components of the avian visual system. *Behav. Brain. Res.* 5 (1982), 157–173.

Hodos, W., Macko, K. A., and Besette, B. B. Near field acuity changes after visual system lesions in pigeons. II. Telencephalon. *Behav. Brain. Res.* 13 (1984), 15–30.

Hodos, W., Weiss, S. R. B., and Bessette, B. B. Size threshold changes after lesions of the visual telencephalon in pigeons. *Behav. Brain. Res.* 21 (1986), 203–214.

Hodos, W., Weiss, S. R. B., and Bessette, B. B. Intensity difference thresholds after lesions of ectostriatum in pigeons. *Behav. Brain. Res.* 30 (1988), 43–53.

Holden, A. L. The field potential profile during activation of the avian optic tectum. *J. Physiol.* 194 (1968), 75–90.

Hubel, D. H. Evolution of the ideas on the primary visual cortex 1955–1978: A biased historical account. In NPF (Ed.), *The Nobel Prizes 1981*. The Nobel Prize Foundation, Stockholm, 1982, pp. 220–256.

Hubel, D. H., and Wiesel, T. N. The Ferrier lecture functional architecture of Macaque monkey visual cortex. *Proc. R. Soc. London Ser. B* 198 (1977), 1–59.

Hunt, S. P., and Kunzle, H. Observations on the projections and intrinsic organisation of the pigeon optic tectum: An autoradiographic study based on anterograde and retrograde, axonal and dendritic flow. *J. Comp. Neurol.* 170 (1976), 153–172.

Jassik-Gerschenfeld, D., and Guichard, J. Visual receptive fields of single cells in the pigeon's optic tectum. *Brain. Res.* 40 (1972), 303–317.

Karten, H. J. The organisation of the avian telencephalon and some speculations on the phylogeny of the amniote telencephalon. *Ann. N. Y. Acad. Sci.* 167 (1969), 164–179.

Karten, H. J., and Hodos, W. Telencephalic projections of the nucleus rotundus in the pigeon (*Columba livia*). *J. Comp. Neurol.* 140 (1970), 33–52.

Karten, H. J., and Shimizu, T. Are visual hierarchies in the brains of the beholders? Constancy and variability in the visual system of birds and mammals. In P. Bagnoli and W. Hodos (Eds.), *The Changing Visual System: Maturation and Aging in the Central Nervous System*. Plenum Press, New York, 1991, pp. 51–59.

Karten, H. J., Hodos, W., Nauta, W. J. H., and Revzin, M. A. Neuronal connections of the visual Wulst of the avian telencephalon. Experimental studies in the pigeon (*Columba livia*) and owl (*Speotyto cunicularia*). *J. Comp. Neurol.* 150 (1973), 253–278.

Kertzmann, C., and Hodos, W. Size-difference threshold after lesions of thalamic visual nuclei in pigeons. *Visual Neurosci.* 1 (1988), 83–92.

Kimberly, R. K., Holden, A. L., and Bamborough, P. Response characteristics of pigeon forebrain cells to visual stimulation. *Vision. Res.* 11 (1971), 475–478.

Korzeniewska, E., and Güntürkün, O. Sensory properties and afferents of the N. dorsolateralis posterior thalami of the pigeon. *J. Comp. Neurol.* 292 (1990), 457–479.

Leao, A. A. P. Spreading depression of activity in cerebral cortex. *J. Neurophysiol.* 7 (1944), 359–390.

Leresche, N., Hardy, O., and Jassik-Gerschenfeld, D. Receptive field properties of single cells in the pigeon's optic tectum during cooling of the 'visual Wulst'. *Brain Res.* 267 (1983), 225–236.

Macko, K. A., and Hodos, W. Near-field acuity after visual system lesions in pigeons. I. Thalamus. *Behav. Brain. Res.* 13 (1984), 1–14.

Martinez-de-la-Torre, M., Martinez, S., and Puelles, L. Acetylcholinesterase-histochemical differential staining of subdivisions within the nucleus rotundus in the chick. *Anat. Embryol.* 181 (1990), 129–135.

Maturana, H. R., and Frenk, S. Directional movement and horizontal edge detectors in the pigeon retina. *Science* 142 (1963), 977–979.

Maxwell, J. H., and Granda, A. M. Receptive fields of movement-sensitive cells in the pigeon thalamus. In A. M. Granda and J. H. Maxwell (Eds.), *Neural Mechanisms of Behavior in the Pigeon*. Plenum Press, New York, 1979, pp. 177–197.

McLoon, S. C. Alterations in precision of the crossed retinotectal projection during chick development. *Science* 215 (1982), 1418–1420.

McLoon, S. C., and Lund, R. D. Transient Retinofugal Pathways in the Developing Chick. *Exp. Brain. Res.* 45 (1982), 277–284.

Miceli, D., Gioanni, H., Reperant, J., and Peyrichoux, J. The avian visual Wulst: I. An anatomical study of afferent and efferent pathways. II. An electrophysiological study of the functional properties of single neurons. In A. M. Granda and J. H. Maxwell (Eds.), *Neural Mechanisms of Behavior in the Pigeon.* Plenum Press, New York, 1979, pp. 223–254.

Mihailovic, J., Perisic, M., Bergonzi, R., and Meier, E. R. The dorsolateral thalamus as a relay in the retino-Wulst pathway in pigeon (*Columba livia*). *Exp. Brain. Res.* 21 (1974), 229–240.

Mitzdorf, U. Current source-density method and application in cat cerebral cortex: Investigation of evoked potentials and EEG phenomena. *Physiology* 65 (1985), 37–100.

Mulvanny, P. Discrimination of line orientation by pigeons after lesions of thalamic visual nuclei. In A. M. Granda and J. H. Maxwell (Eds.), *Neural Mechanisms of Behavior in the Pigeon.* Plenum Press, New York, 1979, pp. 199–222.

Nicholson, C., and Freeman, J. A. Theory of current-source-density analysis and determination of conductivity tensor for annuran cerebellum. *J. Neurophysiol.* 38 (1975), 366–368.

Nixdorf, B. E., and Bischof, H. J. Afferent connections of the ectostriatum and visual Wulst in the zebra finch (*Taeniopygia guttata castanotis* Gould): An HRP study. *Brain. Res.* 248 (1982), 9–17.

Parker, D. M., and Delius, J. D. Visual evoked potentials in the forebrain of the pigeon. *Exp. Brain. Res.* 14 (1972), 198–209.

Perisic, M., Mihailovic, J., and Cuenod, M. Electrophysiology of contralateral and ipsilateral visual projections to the Wulst in pigeon (*Columba livia*). *J. Neurosci.* 2 (1971), 7–14.

Pettigrew, J. D. Comparison of the retinotopic organization of the visual Wulst in nocturnal and diurnal raptors, with a note on the evolution of frontal vision. In S. J. Cool and E. C. Smith (Eds.), *Frontiers in Visual Science.* Springer, New York, 1978, pp. 328–335.

Pettigrew, J. D., and Konishi, M. Effect of monocular deprivation on binocular neurons in the owl's visual Wulst. *Nature (London)* 264 (1976a), 753–754.

Pettigrew, J. D., and Konishi, M. Neurons selective for orientation and binocular disparity in the visual Wulst of the barn owl (*Tyto alba*). *Science* 193 (1976b), 675–678.

Polyak, S. *The Vertebrate Visual System.* University of Chicago Press, Chicago, 1957.

Remy, M., and Güntürkün, O. Retinal afferents to the tectum opticum and the nucleus opticus principalis thalami in the pigeon. *J. Comp. Neurol.* 305 (1991), 57–70.

Revzin, A. M. A specific visual projection area in the hyperstriatum of the pigeon. *Brain. Res.* 15 (1969), 246–249.

Revzin, A. M. Some characteristics of wide-field-units in the brain of the pigeon. *Brain. Behav. Evol.* 3 (1970), 195–204.

Revzin, A. M. Functional localization in the nucleus rotundus. In A. M. Granda and J. H. Maxwell (Eds.), *Neural Mechanisms of Behavior in the Pigeon.* Plenum Press, New York, 1979, pp. 165–175.

Revzin, A. M., and Karten, H. J. Rostral projections of the optic tectum and the nucleus rotundus in the pigeon. *Brain. Res.* 3 (1966), 264–276.

Ritchie, T. C., and Cohen, D. H. The avian tectofugal visual pathway: Projections of its telencephalic target the ectostriatal complex. *Soc. Neurosci. Abstr.* 3 (1977), 94.

Robert, F., and Cuenod, M. Electrophysiology of the intertectal comissures in the pigeon. I. Analysis of the pathways. *Exp. Brain. Res.* 9 (1969a), 119–122.

Robert, F., and Cuenod, M. Electrophysiology of the intertectal comissures in the pigeon. II. Inhibitory interaction. *Exp. Brain. Res.* 9 (1969b), 123–136.

Shimizu, T., and Karten, H. J. Multiple origins of neocortex: Contributions of the dorsal ventricular ridge. In B. L. Finlay et al. (Eds.), *The Neocortex*. Plenum Press, New York, 1990, pp. 75–86.

Singelin, W. *Vergleichend Morphologische Untersuchungen am Vorderhirn der Vogel auf Cytolog.* Heltnig und Lichtenhahn, Basel, 1958.

Varela, F. J., Letelier, J. C., Marin, G., and Maturana, H. R. The neurophysiology of avian color vision. *Arch. Biol. Med. Exp.* 16 (1983), 291–303.

Wang, Y., and Frost, B. J. Time to collision is signalled by neurons in the nucleus rotundus of the pigeon. *Nature (London)* 356 (1992), 236–238.

Watanabe, S., Hodos, W., and Bessette, B. B. Two eyes are better than one: Superior binocular discrimination learning in pigeons. *Physiol. Behav.* 32 (1984), 847–850.

Watanabe, M., Ito, H., and Ikushima, M. Cytoarchitecture and ultrastructure of the avian ectostriatum: Afferent terminals from the dorsal telencephalon and some nuclei in the thalamus. *J. Comp. Neurol.* 236 (1985), 241–257.

Watanabe, S., Hodos, W., Bessette, B. B., and Shimizu, T. Interocular transfer in parallel visual pathways in pigeons. *Brain. Behav. Evol.* 29 (1986), 184–195.

Wiesel, T. N. The postnatal development of the visual cortex and the influence of the environment. In NPF (Ed.), *The Nobel Prizes 1981*. The Nobel Prize Foundation, Stockholm, 1982, pp. 258–283.

Wilson, P. The organization of the visual hyperstriatum in the domestic chick. I. Topology and topography of the visual projection. *Brain Res.* 188 (1980a), 319–332.

Wilson, P. The organization of the visual hyperstriatum in the domestic chick. II. Receptive field properties of single units. *Brain Res.* 188 (1980b), 333–345.

Yazulla, S., and Granda, A. M. Opponent-color units in the thalamus of the pigeon (*Columba livia*). *Vision. Res.* 13 (1973), 1555–1563.

9 Binocular Processing in Frontal-Eyed Birds

G. Casini, G. Fontanesi, and P. Bagnoli

Despite the total decussation of the optic nerve axons, binocular integration occurs in the avian telencephalon by means of the bilateral projections from the thalamic visual relays (Engelage and Bischof, 1988, 1989; Karten et al., 1973). As noted by McFadden (chapter 3), the presence of binocular vision allows an animal to derive a three-dimensional visual world from a two-dimensional retinal array. In birds as in mammals, there are considerable differences in the degree of binocular overlap. Because the presence of frontal eyes provides a large binocular overlap, binocular vision is probably most highly developed in frontal-eyed birds, including diurnal and nocturnal raptors (e.g., owl, falcon).

In both birds and mammals the presence of binocular vision is associated with the existence of certain structural and functional properties of specific telencephalic regions. Numerous similarities have been found between the visual Wulst of raptors and the striate cortex of mammals. Common features of the two regions include a high degree of binocular interaction, selectivity for stimulus orientation and direction of movement, as well as binocular disparity (Pettigrew and Konishi, 1976a; Pettigrew, 1979). Functional parallels also extend to the phenomenon of plasticity, since binocular neurons in the Wulst of the owl are extremely sensitive to monocular deprivation during a critical developmental period (Pettigrew and Konishi, 1976b).

STRUCTURAL AND FUNCTIONAL FEATURES UNDERLYING BINOCULAR VISION IN OWLS

Recent studies have shown that the strongly binocular visual system of owls displays a higher degree of morphological and functional complexity than the visual pathways of lateral-eyed birds. The visual thalamus of the owl possesses a complex organization that subserves the alignment of retinal maps and the segregation of thalamic input into the Wulst, thus allowing a precise representation of the binocular visual space (Bagnoli et al., 1990; Porciatti et al., 1990). Despite some differences in the organization of visual pathways in birds and mammals, it appears that the two classes employ similar mechanisms to achieve higher visual capacities and binocularity. In both classes, highly organized visual thalamic relays seem to be a common feature of species that rely on a rapid evaluation of spatial cues including depth perception. In terms of convergent evolution, therefore, common evolutionary trends toward binocularity and stereopsis can account for similarities in the organization of the thalamocortical pathways of binocular mammals and birds.

This hypothesis is further supported by the close resemblance of the Wulst-TeO projections in owls to the mammalian corticocollicular pathway (Casini et al., 1992). In owls, Wulst projections on TeO appear to be organized in laminae, with labeled terminal fields distributed in patches of dense reaction product (figure 9.1A). This distribution is similar to that described in frontal-eyed mammals and allows cortical neurons related to a particular retinal hemifield to project to that part of the superior colliculus connected to the same hemifield (see Sparks,

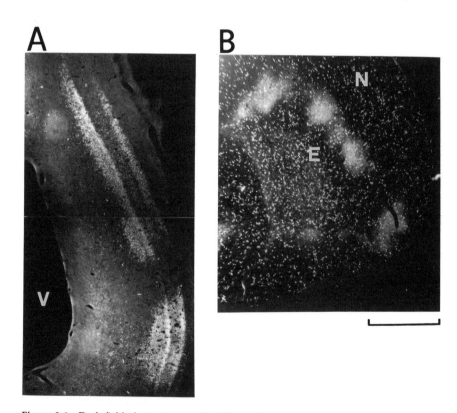

Figure 9.1 Dark-field photomicrographs of frontal sections through the owl mesencephalon (A) and telencephalon (B). This animal had received a series of WGA-HRP injections in the ipsilteral visual Wulst. Anterogradely labeled terminal fields are organized in patches or columns of dense reaction product in both superficial optic tectum and ectostriatum. Modified from Casini et al. (1992). Calibration bar: 410 μm (A); 1250 mm (B).

1988, for review). If we assume that, as in mammals, properties of tectal cells are dependent on binocular input from the thalamofugal system, e.g., the Wulst, then the TeO of (frontal-eyed) raptors appears to be a more complex and finely tuned structure for the utilization of visual cues than the TeO of lateral-eyed birds.

A complex and precisely organized intratelencephalic circuitry is also present in both nocturnal and diurnal raptors. In owls, the terminal fields of Wulst projections on the ipsilateral ectostriatum are organized in columns (Casini et al., 1992), suggesting the existence of complex connection patterns that could subserve possible interactions between tectofugal and thalamofugal visual pathways (figure 9.1B). In the owl, ocular dominance columns can also be detected in the visual Wulst, although they are seen only after monocular deprivation (Pettigrew and Gynther, 1989). In the falcon (figure 9.2) stimulation of one eye leads to the asymmetrical activation of the Wulst, which displays ocular dominance columns on the brain side contralateral to the stimulated side (Bagnoli and Francesconi, 1984).

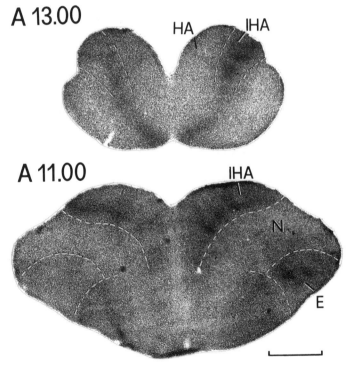

Figure 9.2 2-[^{14}C]Deoxyglucose autoradiographs from the brain of a restrained falcon in which the left eye was covered during visual stimulation. In the telencephalon contralateral to the exposed eye, increased metabolic activity results in columnar organization of labeling in the visual Wulst and the ectostriatum (E). HA, hyperstriatum accessorium; IHA, nucleus intercalatus hyperstriati accessorii. Modified from Bagnoli and Francesconi (1984). Calibration bar: 3.3 mm.

Casini et al.: Binocular Processing

In both mammals and birds the relative contribution of the crossed and uncrossed thalamocortical and corticocollicular projections as well as the complexity of the intratelencephalic circuitry appear to be closely correlated with the position of the eyes. Substantial ipsilateral projections are present in rats (Sefton et al., 1981), hamsters (Lent, 1982), and rabbits (Hofbauer and Hollander, 1986) as well as in chicks and pigeons (Mestres and Delius, 1982; Bagnoli and Burkhalter, 1983; Miceli et al., 1987). Bilateral projections are found in animals with extremely good binocularity such as cats, monkeys (Huerta and Harting, 1984), and owls. Figure 9.3 presents a schematic representation of the organization of visual pathways in cats and owls. Taken together, these findings suggest that despite the presence of completely crossed retinofugal projections, the organization of visual pathways in frontal-eyed birds provides a substrate for the highly developed binocularity critical for a visually guided prey-hunting raptor.

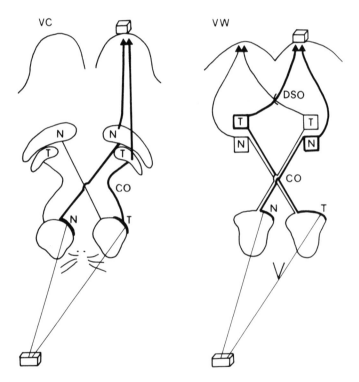

Figure 9.3 Schematic representation of the ascending pathways originating from the nasal and the temporal retina in cats (left) and owls (right). Half-field stimulation is also represented. The partial recrossing of retinofugal fibers, typical of mammals, allows the thalamic relay to represent different hemifields of both eyes. In owls, despite the total decussation of retinal fibers, the partial recrossing of thalamic fibers allows the segregation of thalamic inputs to the visual Wulst, which receives complementary information from the nasal and the temporal retina of both eyes. N, nasal; T, temporal; VC, visual cortex; VW, visual Wulst; CO, chiasma opticum; DSO, decussatio supraoptica. Modified from Pettigrew and Konishi (1976a).

Immunohistochemical analysis indicates that the structural complexity of visual pathways in frontal-eyed birds is also characteristic of the distribution of neurotransmitters and neuropeptides in their central visual relays. The distribution of specific immunoreactivity within somata and neuropil is generally similar to that of pigeons, although some characteristics seem to be peculiar to the owl. Along the tectofugal pathway, different neurotransmitters are segregated in specific layers of TeO (figure 9.4). Pretectal nuclei show a transmitter distribution comparable to that in pigeons. A discrete aggregate of CCK-positive cell bodies is found in the dorsolateral thalamus, while cholinergic cells, which are numerous in the pigeon visual thalamus, are completely absent. In the telencephalon, regional variations in transmitter distribution are found within the Wulst layers with a particularly high density of CCK-, NPY-, and SP-positive neuropilar processes (figure 9.5A). Numerous peptidergic cell bodies are also present in the ectostriatum, which in pigeons generally shows scarse peptide immunoreactivity (figure 9.5B). This distribution suggests that the owl's visually guided behavior may rely both on an extremely well-differentiated thalamofugal pathway (such as is also present in mammals) and on a tectofugal system, which shows a high eterogeneity in transmitter content, but which, in mammals, plays only a minor role in visual information processing. Thus, in addition to some characteristics common to both frontal-eyed and lateral-eyed birds, transmitter distribution in the owl's visual system shows some properties that may be uniquely correlated with its species-typical, visually guided predatory behavior.

There are some suggestive similarities in transmitter distribution in the visual systems of owls and mammals. These include the lack of cholinergic transmission in the owl's thalamocortical pathway, although such transmission is characteristic of lateral-eyed birds. Interestingly, most of the cholinergic innervation of the mammalian striate cortex originates from neurons in the basal forebrain. In mammals, cholinergic neurons represent only a minor cell population in visual thalamus, which is transiently expressed during early development. According to recent studies, the geniculocortical pathway may utilize excitatory amino acids (Johnson and Burkhalter, 1992) and a relation between those substances and binocular function is postulated. Indeed activation of NMDA receptors during development is important for the establishment of the neuronal circuitry subserving binocularity (Shatz, 1990). The evolutionary significance of the absence of cholinergic transmission in the thalamocortical connections of frontal-eyed birds will remain unclear until a possible transmitter candidate is found in raptors and compared with putative transmitters in mammals. On the other hand, differences in the chemical anatomy of the thalamocortical connections in different bird species may be related to the different functional de-

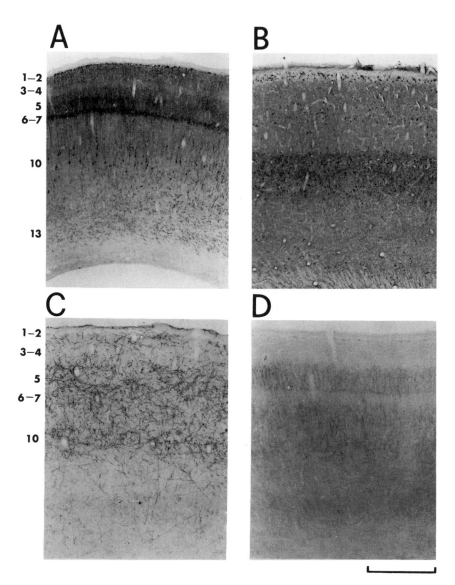

Figure 9.4 Photomicrographs illustrating the distribution of immunoreactive cells and processes in transverse sections of the owl optic tectum. ChAT, SS, NPY, and L-ENK immunostaining are shown in A, B, C and D, respectively. Note the laminar distribution of immunoreactivity in the different tectal layers. Main differences with immunostaining distribution in the pigeon optic tectum include the highly organized layering pattern, the presence of ChAT-positive cells in the superficial tectal layers, and the absence of L-ENK-positive cells in the deeper layers. Nomenclature of tectal layers are taken from Ramón y Cajal (1891). Calibration bar: 750 µm.

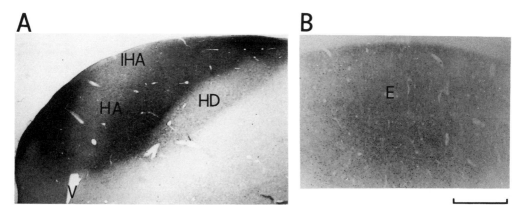

Figure 9.5 (A) Distribution of SP immunoreactivity in the owl telencephalon. In the visual Wulst, intensely immunostained cells and processes show a regional distribution. HA, hyperstriatum accessorium; HD, hyperstriatum dorsale; IHA, nucleus intercalatus hyperstriati accessorii; V, ventriculus. (B) Numerous immunolabeled cells can be observed in the ectostriatum (E). Calibration bar: (A) 1.0 mm; (B) 1.0 mm.

mands on their visual systems. Taken together, our results suggest that there are substantial differences in the morphological, functional, and neurochemical organization of the avian visual system, which are likely to be related to the diversity in the visually guided behavior typical of birds.

CONCLUSION

Although the mammalian visual system has traditionally been considered as the most efficient among vertebrates for analyzing visual information, birds are capable of an excellent and, in some cases, superior visual performance. Their visual capabilities, including binocular integration, are achieved through information processing mechanisms different from, but at least as efficient as those of mammals. Better understanding of the differential organization of the parallel processing of visual information in this nonmammalian system may provide a useful new approach to the analysis of visual processing in mammals.

ACKNOWLEDGMENTS

Preliminary results on transmitter distribution were obtained in collaboration with J. T. Erichsen (SUNY at Stony Brook). Supported by the C. N. R. Target Project on Biotechnology and Bioinstrumentation (Ct 92. 01167. PF70 to P. Bagnoli). The owls used in this study were obtained from a national institution, which collects protected birds with severe wing or leg damage. Anatomical nomenclature after the stereotaxic atlas of Karten and Hodos (1967).

REFERENCES

Bagnoli P., and A. Burkhalter. (1983). Organization of the afferent projections to the Wulst in the pigeon. *J. Comp. Neurol.* 214:103–113.

Bagnoli P., and W. Francesconi. (1984). Mapping of functional activity in the falcon visual system with 14C 2-deoxyglucose. *Exp. Brain Res.* 53:217–222.

Bagnoli P., G. Fontanesi, G. Casini, and V. Porciatti. (1990). Binocularity in the little owl, Athene noctua. I. Anatomical investigation of the thalamo-Wulst pathway. *Brain Behav. Evol.* 35:31–39.

Casini G., V. Porciatti, G. Fontanesi, and P. Bagnoli. (1992). Wulst efferents in the little owl Athene noctua: An investigation of projections to the optic tectum. *Brain Behav. Evol.* 39:101–115.

Engelage J., and H. J. Bischof. (1988). Enucleation enhances ipsilateral flash evoked responses in the ectostriatum of the zebra finch (*Taeniopygia guttata castanotis,* Gould). *Exp. Brain Res.* 70:79–89.

Engelage J., and H. J. Bischof. (1989). Flash evoked potentials in the ectostriatum of the zebra finch: A current source density analysis. *Exp. Brain Res.* 74:563–572.

Hofbauer A., and H. Hollander. (1986). Synaptic connections of cortical and retinal terminals in the superior colliculus of the rabbit: A electron microscopic double labeling study. *Exp. Brain Res.* 65:145–155.

Huerta M. F., and J. K. Harting. (1984). The mammalian superior colliculus: Studies of its morphology and connections. In H. Vanegas (Ed.), Comparative Neurology of the Optic Tectum. Plenum Press, New York, pp. 687–783.

Johnson, R. R., and A. Burkhalter. (1992). Evidence for excitatory amino acid neurotransmitters in the geniculo-cortical pathway and local projections within rat primary visual cortex. *Exp. Brain Res.* 89:20–30.

Karten, H. J., and W. Hodos. (1967). A Stereotaxic Atlas of the Brain of the Pigeon *Columba livia.* Johns Hopkins University Press, Baltimore.

Karten, H. J., W. Hodos, and W. J. H. Nauta. (1973). Neural connections of the "visual Wulst" of the avian telencephalon: Experimental studies in the pigeon (*Columba livia*) and owl (*Speotyto cunicularia*). *J. Comp. Neurol.* 150:253–278.

Lent R. (1982). The organization of subcortical projections of the hamster's visual cortex. *J. Comp. Neurol.* 206:227–242.

Mestres P., and J. P. Delius. (1982). A contribution to the study of the afferents to the pigeon optic tectum. *Anat. Embryol.* 165:415–423.

Miceli D., J. Reperant, J. Villalobos, and L. Dionne. (1987). Extratelencephalic projections of the avian visual Wulst. A quantitative autoradiographic study in pigeon Columba livia. *J. Hirnforsch.* 28:45–47.

Pettigrew J. D. (1979). Binocular visual processing in the owl's telencephalon. *Proc. R. Soc. London Ser. B* 204:435–454.

Pettigrew J. D., and I. C. Gynther. (1989). Cytoarchitecture of ocular dominance columns in owl visual cortex. *Neurosci. Abstr.* 15:316.10.

Pettigrew J. D., and M. Konishi. (1976a). Neurons selective for orientation and binocular disparity in the visual Wulst of the barn owl *Tito alba. Science* 193:675–678.

Pettigrew J. D., and M. Konishi. (1976b). Effect of monocular deprivation on binocular neurones in the owl's visual Wulst. *Nature (London)* 264:753–754.

Porciatti V., G. Fontanesi, A. Raffaelli, and P. Bagnoli. (1990). Binocularity in the little owl, *Athene noctua*. II. Properties of visually evoked potentials from the Wulst in response to monocular and binocular stimulation with sine wave gratings. *Brain Behav. Evol.* 35:40–48.

Ramon Y Cajal S. (1891). Sur la fine structure du lobe optique des oiseaux et sur l'origine reelle des nerfs optiques. *Int. Mschr. Anat. Physiol.* 8:337–366.

Sefton A. J., A. Mackay-Sim, and L. J. Baur La Cotte. (1981). Cortical projections to visual centers in the rat: A HRP study. *Brain Res.* 215:1–13.

Shatz C. J. (1990). Impulse activity and the patterning of connections during CNS development. *Neuron* 5:745–756.

Sparks D. L. (1988). Neural cartography: Sensory and motor maps in the superior colliculus. *Brain Behav. Evol.* 31:49–56.

III Development of the Avian Visual System

Introduction

Hans-Joachim Bischof

Birds are particularly ideal subjects for developmental studies. The development of avian embryos to adulthood is very rapid compared to that of most mammalian species. Birds may reach their adult size and weight within 1% of their total life expectancy, in contrast to the 30% or more for many of the higher primates. Even more important is the fact that the avian embryo develops totally extra utero, and is therefore easily accessible at each stage of development. It was this second feature that attracted the first researchers of developmental processes, particularly those who wished not only to examine morphological changes, but also to study the physiological and behavioral development of the animal. One of the first researchers to take advantage of the avian model was Kuo (1932), who described the behavioral development of the chick embryo. Victor Hamburger and his colleagues (Hamburger, 1973; Hamburger and Oppenheim, 1967) greatly expanded our knowledge of the mechanisms of embryonic development by experiments involving immobilization or deafferentation of avian embryos. These studies also helped to reconcile the nature-nurture controversy, which for some decades had split the scientific community into two parts. They provided clear evidence for the currently held (epigenetic) view that every neuronal organization and behavior is developed by an interplay of genetic instructions and environmental cues (Oppenheim, 1982). Gilbert Gottlieb then showed that prenatal experience has an important impact on postnatal behavior. Species recognition in ducklings develops normally only if the embryos are exposed to certain acoustic stimuli (Gottlieb, 1976). His studies made it clear that not everything that is apparent at birth is inherited, and thus reinforced the notion of a permanent interplay of genetic and environmental cues during development.

The postnatal development of birds was for many years a domain of behavioral studies. Following Konrad Lorenz' investigations of the phenomenon of imprinting, numerous studies were performed to examine the fine details of this early learning process (Bolhuis, 1991; Immelmann and Suomi, 1980). Although it is clear that imprinting, at least in its classical cases of sexual and filial imprinting, is based on visual cues, only a few investigations were published concerning the postnatal development of visual performance of birds and of the postnatal development of the visual system (Bischof and Lassek, 1985; Bischof et al., 1991). In recent years, the embryonic development of the visual system of birds, especially chicks, has proved to be an excellent paradigm for the more general question of neuronal pathfinding and the development of order in the brain. Retinal ganglion cells are distributed evenly over the whole retina, and they project topographically to another layered structure on the surface of the brain, the tectum opticum. Thus, it is very easy to examine whether the topographical relationships between ganglion cells are preserved in the topographical map of the tectum. Likewise, it is easy to manipulate this connection and to observe the effects caused by these manipulations. Chapter 10, by Mey and Thanos, provides a survey of such experiments, and a report of recent findings and theories in this field.

In contrast to the large body of work on embryonic development, there has been relatively little research on the *postnatal* development of the avian visual system. Chapter 11, by Fontanesi, Casini, Cioccetti, and Bagnoli, provides information about the postnatal maturation of transmitter types within the visual system and shows that the ipsilateral component of the retinotectal projection, which is apparent at birth in altricial birds, is retracted within the first few posthatching days. It also provides evidence that this retraction is regulated by sensory input. This suggests that the competitive interaction between active synapses postulated by Hebb (1949) and frequently shown in mammals (e.g., Singer, 1989) also plays a role in the development of the avian visual system. Its role is further substantiated in chapter 12 by Herrmann and Bischof, who studied the development and plasticity of the tectofugal pathway. They show that the development of the visual system in birds, as in mammals, is characterized by an interplay of progressive and regressive events. They also show that monocular deprivation affects the development of the tectofugal pathway, but in a way that is slightly different from the effects found in mammals. However, their data provide evidence that competition also occurs in higher stations of the tectofugal pathway, indicating that both hemispheres interact during development. As in mammals, effects of monocular deprivation seem to occur only during a sensitive phase in early development; the visual system of adult birds is not altered by monocular deprivation. This section's final chapter, by Rogers and Adret, deals with a feature that was, until recently, attributed only to human brains: the lateralization of function (see also chapter 18). These authors found that food identification is lateralized, and that the visual pathways of the left and the right side develop differentially. Their experiments indicate that this lateralization is due to differential exposure of the eyes to light in the egg: one eye, which is covered by a wing, receives less light during the embryonic phase, and its associated visual pathway shows less development.

The chapters in this section clearly demonstrate that the development of the avian brain has become an attractive model system for the study of developmental processes in general. Moreover, comparisons between avian and mammalian brain developent should also be of interest to students of brain evolution.

REFERENCES

Bischof, H, J., and Lassek, R. The gaping reaction and the development of fear in young zebra finches (*Taeniopygia guttata castanotis*). *Z. Tierphysiol.* 69 (1985), 55–65.

Bischof, H. J., Herrmann, K., and Engelage, J. Development and plasticity of the tecto-fugal visual pathway in the zebra finch. In P. Bagnoli and W. Hodos (Eds.), *The Changing Visual System*. Plenum Press, New York, 1991, pp. 199–208.

Bolhuis, J. J. Mechanisms of avian imprinting: A review. *Biol. Rev.* 66 (1991), 303–345.

Gottlieb, G. Early development of species-specific auditory perception in birds. In G. Gottlieb (Ed.), *Neural and Behavioral Specificity*. Academic Press, New York, 1976, pp. 237–280.

Hamburger, V. Anatomical and physiological basis of embryonic motility in birds and mammals. In G. Gottlieb (Ed.), *Behavioral Embryology*. Academic Press, New York, 1973, pp. 52–76.

Hamburger, V., and Oppenheim, R. Prehatching motility and hatching behavior in the chick. *J. Exp. Zool.* 166 (1967), 171–204.

Hebb, D. O. *The Organisation of Behavior*. Wiley, New York, 1949.

Immelmann, K., and Suomi, S. Sensitive phases in development. In K. Immelmann, G. W. Barlow, L. Petrinovich, and M. Main (Eds.), *Behavioral Development*. Cambridge University Press, New York, 1981, pp. 395–431.

Kuo, Z.-Y. Ontogeny of embryonic behavior in aves: I. The chronology and general nature of the behavior of the chick embryo. *J. Exp. Zool.* 61 (1932), 395–430.

Oppenheim, R. Die Neuroembryologie des Verhaltens. In K. Immelmann, G. W. Barlow, L. Petrinovich, and M. Main (Eds.), *Verhaltensentwicklung bei Mensch und Tier*. Parey, Berlin, 1982, pp. 222–270.

Singer, W. Developmental self organization as a special case of learning. In H. Rahmann (Ed.), *Fundamentals of Memory Formation: Neuronal Plasticity and Brain Function*. Gustav Fischer Verlag, Stuttgart, 1989, pp. 272–282.

10 Developmental Anatomy of the Chick Retinotectal Projection

Jörg Mey and Solon Thanos

Retina and optic tectum are the first organs to receive and process visual information and comprise the largest part of the avian visual system. The structures are connected by the optic nerve, chiasm, and optic tract, together referred to as the primary visual pathway, whose development will be discussed in this chapter. The outstanding complexity of this system is revealed by its cytoarchitectonic differentiation and by the bare number of its cellular elements. The ganglion cell layer of the chick retina, for instance, contains about 2.4 million ganglion cells (Rager and Rager, 1978) of at least eight different morphological types (Thanos et al., 1992), more than in any other class of vertebrates.

In the chick, the development of the visual system starts around 30 hours of incubation, when the prosencephalic neural tube bulges out to form the optic vesicles. As in other precocial birds, development is completed at the time of hatching (LaVail and Cowan, 1971; Patten, 1971). The mature retinotectal connection projects the retinal surfaces onto the surfaces of the contralateral tecta in a topological order, thereby preserving neighborhood relationships between ganglion cells in the distribution of their central terminals. Since this is similar to the visual projection in other vertebrates and also to other sensory projections, and since the chick has always been a classical model in developmental biology, the avian retinofugal system has been thoroughly investigated since the nineteenth century (first: Stieda, 1868; Ramón y Cajal, 1911). It still serves as a model system to tackle fundamental problems in brain development.

By what mechanisms are growing retinal fibers guided to their destination in the brain? How is a topographic map of the retina constructed over the surface of the optic tectum? Do ingrowing axons from retinal ganglion cells know the precise locations where to produce terminal arborizations and to develop synaptic connections?

This problem of the retinotectal specificity has for a long time attracted scientific attention. Despite considerable experimental effort, however, the processes that confer the necessary information for establishing specific contacts between sensory afferents and their central target cells are still unknown.

The goal of this chapter is to review the present knowledge about the development of the chick retinotectal system in order to provide an introduction for scientists new to the field. Our discussion of earlier and recent achievements focuses on questions of axonal guidance and models that can account for the development of the precise topography in the retinotectal connection.

INNERVATION OF THE OPTIC TECTUM BY RETINAL FIBERS

The innermost layer of the retina, adjacent to the vitreous body, contains the projection neurons of this organ, the retinal ganglion cells (RGC). All visual information reaches the brain through the axons of the RGC.

Of all retinal neurons the retinal ganglion cells are the earliest to differentiate, producing their axon as a first sign of morphological development (Kahn, 1973, 1974; Horder and Mashkas, 1982; Watanabe et al., 1991). After emerging from the retinal fissure, these axons grow through the optic stalk, creating the optic nerves. Both nerves cross each other at the optic chiasm, where in chicks nearly all fibers traverse to the contralateral side. After the decussation, retinal axons ascend dorsolaterally around the brainstem forming the optic tract, which innervates the thalamus and a number of other pretectal and thalamic nuclei. Already at stage 15 (embryonic days 2 to 3), well before intraretinal connections are completed, and shortly after invagination of the optic vesicle, the first ganglion cell axons appear in the central retina, 150 μm dorsal to the entrance of the optic stalk (Goldberg and Coulombre, 1972; Kahn, 1973; Horder and Mashkas, 1982). Goldberg and Coulombre (1972) examined the axonal growth pattern of the chick retina in whole mounts. From the very beginning, the axons are aligned toward the optic stalk and grow in this direction. As they elongate and encounter neighboring fibers, axons following each other become grouped into fascicles. Subsequently, more and more axons originate in the ganglion cell layer (GCL) in a central to peripheral sequence. Their oriented growth increases the number, diameter, and length of the fiber fascicles, which now constitute the optic fiber layer (OFL). Each axon joins and follows the nearest existing fiber, such that a funneling effect in the direction of the optic stalk appears. Virtually no branching of axons is visible. At the beginning, fibers frequently meander and cross each other. Later they appear more orderly and parallel, possibly due to stretching, as the retinal tissue expands (Goldberg and Coulombre, 1972; Horder and Mashkas, 1982; Nakamura and O'Leary, 1989).

Peripheral fibers in older retinas run circumferentially, i.e., parallel to the ora serrata before leaving either radially or ventrally to the optic fissure. The circumferential fibers develop first on the temporal side, and subsequently originating nasal axons diverge from a point in the dorsal periphery of the retina (Goldberg and Coulombre, 1972). Cox, Thanos, and Bonhoeffer (unpublished observations) labeled circumferential fibers by application of RITC and DiI crystals in fixed retinal wholemounts. During development, these fibers become progressively more numerous and fasciculate, indicating that the projection is not transient. The normal intraretinal fiber growth could be reproduced in cultured wholemounts when retinas where taken from embryos older than stage 17 (60 hours), although under these conditions, some axons grow in the opposite, peripheral direction (Halfter and Deiss, 1984, 1986).

After embryonic day 3, the first fibers leave the eyeball, grow along the optic stalk, reaching the chiasm around E4, and one day later advance through the contralateral optic tract toward the tectum at whose anterior pole they arrive at E6 (Thanos and Bonhoeffer, 1983). Earliest axons enter the stalk at its ventral side, and new fibers are added peripherally and ventrally such that the circular area occupied by the first RGC is transformed into a ventral crescent in the optic nerve (Navascués et al., 1987a; Rager, 1980). Parallel to fiber invasion, the development of glioblasts proceeds in a retinodiencephalic direction in the optic nerve. Axons elongate through the extracellular space, which is organized by a framework of radial glial processes from cells in the ventral wall of the stalk (Navascués et al., 1987a; Rager and v. Oeynhausen, 1979). Glioblasts then divide and migrate radially, thereby separating optic fiber fascicles. The marginal fiber growth is further supported by glial cell death in the ventral wall (Navascués et al., 1985, 1987a,b). This may be induced by enzymes secreted from advancing axonal growth cones. Applying anterograde staining with RITC, Thanos and Bonhoeffer (1983) demonstrated a separation of fibers according to their retinal origin in the optic nerve and tract. Ventral retinal fibers grow dorsomedially, whereas dorsal fibers lie ventrolaterally in the optic pathway. Also the central to peripheral order is maintained. Before crossing in the chiasm to the contralateral side, nasal fibers occupy the medial, and temporal fibers the lateral half of the nerve. In the optic tract, however, this order prevails no longer: Nasal and temporal fibers are mixed, losing their original neighborhood relationship (Thanos and Bonhoeffer, 1983; Ehrlich and Mark, 1984; Nakamura and O'Leary, 1989). In the chick, fiber crossing in the chiasm is complete, though an abortive ipsilateral projection appears during embryogenesis. But this is soon eliminated (O'Leary et al., 1983; Williams and McLoon, 1991).

At the anterior ventral poles of the tecta, fibres from the contralateral retinas arrive on the 6th day of embryonic development (DeLong and Coulombre, 1965; Goldberg, 1974; Crossland et al., 1975; McLoon, 1985; Thanos and Bonhoeffer, 1983, 1987). Between E7 and E12 a front of elongating axons advances from the anterior ventral pole of the tectum in posterior-dorsal direction over its surface, thereby forming the stratum opticum (figure 10.1). As the growing axons reach the posterior pole, they curve and intermingle to form a raphe (Goldberg, 1974; Rager and v.Oeynhausen, 1979). New axons grow on top of the existing ones and underneath the pia, always keeping contact to the endfeet of the radial glia (Vanselow et al., 1989). Similar to the pattern in the retina, the appearance of fiber fascicles becomes more orderly and parallel with time. Although they may change between fascicles, axons do not extensively branch in the stratum opticum (Goldberg, 1974). Notwithstanding, anterograde fluorescence staining revealed that retinotectal axons frequently had collaterals directed toward pretectal nuclei (Vanselow et al., 1989).

Retinal fibers do not start to invade the outer tectal layers before E9 (Crossland et al., 1975; Thanos and Bonhoeffer, 1987). In this process, axons bifurcate in the *stratum opticum* (SO) giving off a branch that perpendicularly turns down into the developing *stratum griseum et fibrosum superficiale* (SGFS) (Rager and v.Oeynhausen, 1979; Thanos and Bonhoeffer, 1987; Vanselow et al., 1989). Between E10 and E11 the number of arborizing axons increases in the anterior tectum. Investigating the development of axonal trees, Thanos and Bonhoeffer (1987) showed that their size as well as the branching frequency increase

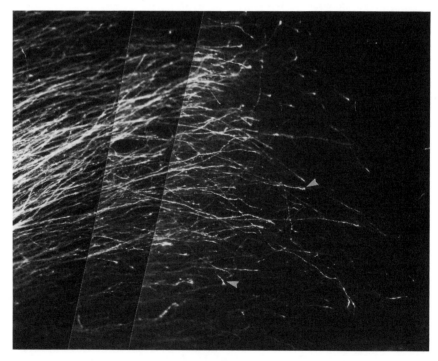

Figure 10.1 Front of retinal fibers growing over the surface of the contralateral tectum, at about embryonic day 9. To visualize the axons, crystals of the fluorescent dye D282 have been inserted into the retina. After anterograde transport of the dye in vivo, labeled axons with individual growth cones (arrowheads) are visible in the tectal wholemount.

continuously at least until E18. With respect to their terminal branching patterns, two main types of retinal axons can be distinguished in the 10-day-old embryo: One set of axons ramifies extensively in the superficial SGFS laminae, whereas fibers of the other type penetrate deeper until they start branching (Rager and v. Oeynhausen, 1979). In the adult chick, these classes seem to differentiate further, since a variety of spatially restricted terminal arbors are described that acquire characteristic configurations and end in different laminae of the SGFS (Ramón y Cajal, 1911; LaVail and Cowan, 1971; Senut and Alvarado-Mallart, 1986). Some optic terminals in laminae a–d are substance P immunoreactive (Ehrlich et al., 1987). The overall density of retinal terminals is highest in sublayers b, c, and d.

Simultaneous with the development of terminal arbors, the retinal axons are received by ascending piriform cells that accumulate below the pial surface, and by vertical neurites from deeper tectal layers (Puelles and Bendala, 1978; Rager and v. Oeynhausen, 1979). Thus, terminal arborization and segregation of the superficial tectal laminae emerge in close connection.

Investigating the process of tectal synaptogenesis, McGraw and McLaughlin (1980) found the earliest mature synapses after E8 in the rostral area. They are asymmetrical (excitatory) and axodendritic. Alluding to decreased numbers of synapses following eye enucleation, the authors suggest that some of the early contacts are made by retinal axons, and that the development of retinotectal connections follows a rostrocaudal gradient, corresponding to the other events of differentiation. Symmetrical synaptic contacts of presumably inhibitory character appear later, in the third week of embryogenesis (McGraw and McLaughlin, 1980). Correspondingly, Rager (1976) recorded the first postsynaptic potentials after optic nerve stimulation in the tectum at E11.

There is a controversy about the appearance and location of the first retinotectal connections. McLoon (1985) has detected synapses of (previously HRP-labeled) retinal fibres in the anterior tectum even earlier than McGraw and McLaughlin, namely at E7. Most authors, however, report that the first retinotectal synapses do not occur before E11 (Cantino and Sisto-Daneo, 1973; Rager, 1976; Panzica and Viglietti-Panzica, 1981). This contradiction gains relevance in light of the discussion about the way, how the correct retinotectal connections are established. This projection obeys a topographic order whereby the first arriving axons, which belong to central RGC in the retina, will be connected to the (somewhat rostroventral) area centralis of the tectum. For this reason, the question has aroused considerable interest, where the first fibers leave the SO and form synapses in the SGFS. Based on intraocular [^{3}H]proline injection and autoradiographic detection of anterogradely transported proteins, Crossland and collaborators (1975) localized a restricted, oval area near the center of the tectum, where at E10 retinal fibers first submerge into the SGFS. Concurrent with the tectal cytoarchitectonic differentiation, this area expands concentrically as fibers from more and more peripheral parts of the retina are added (Crossland et al. 1975). Experiments involving early enucleation of the optic cup indicate that the mitotic patterns and the initial differentiation of tectal neuroblasts are independent from retinal axons (Cowan et al., 1968). Retinal and tectal spatiotemporal patterns of development seem to be matched like two independent clockworks. The central tectal area, which is due to receive afferents from first central RGC, is also the first region to become receptive for axons (Crossland et al., 1975; Rager, 1980; Thanos and Bonhoeffer, 1987). These findings are contradicted by McLoon (1985), who, as mentioned, reports to have seen synapses already at E7 and in the anterior tectum. If the earliest axons immediately penetrate the rostral SGFS and form synapses, these contacts must be released subsequently, because (1) the axons will project to the central tectum in the adult chicken, and (2) by E8 the horizontal growth of the rostral tectum is completed. McLoon, therefore, postulates shifting connections, similar to the situation in frogs and fish. His claims, however, oppose all other investigations, which show that the first retinal fibres proceed over some distance of unoccupied tectal territory before reaching their destination where they form terminal arbors. This observation gains central importance for Rager's interpretation, who explains that the first fibers simply make contacts where they encounter a receptive, mature tectal area (Rager, 1980; Rager et al., 1988). These initial contacts may then be transformed into synapses (Rager, 1976; McGraw and McLaughlin, 1980; Panzica and Viglietti-Panzica, 1981; Gremo et al., 1982). So far, no further evidence for shifting connection in the chick tectum has been obtained.

EARLY INVESTIGATIONS ON THE SPECIFICITY OF THE RETINOTECTAL CONNECTION

The primary visual projection of birds like that of all other vertebrates maintains a specific, topographic order, which preserves the neighborhood relationships between retinal ganglion cells in their central connections: the retinal images are projected onto the contralateral tectal surfaces such that the dorsal tectum represents the ventral retina and the ventral tectum receives afferents from the dorsal retina. The nasal sides of each retina project to the posterior tecta, while their temporal halves are represented on the anterior tectal surfaces (figure 10.2). For birds, this pattern was first discovered in the pigeon (Hamdi and Whitteridge, 1954; McGill et al., 1966) and in the chick (DeLong and Coulombre, 1965, 1967), since then constituting a central problem for developmental biology: What are the underlying mechanisms of this specific connection between two systems that develop ontogenetically independent from each other until that connection takes place?

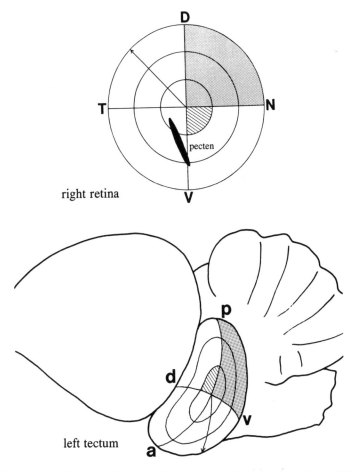

Figure 10.2 Schematic drawing of the topographic projection of the chick retina onto the contralateral tectal surface. RGC axons from the central retina terminate centrally, while cells located in the retinal periphery project to the tectal margin (indicated by the arrows from center to periphery in both organs). RGC situated in the dorsal retina are connected to the ventral tectum, while the temporal retina is represented in the anterior tectum. Ventral and nasal halves of the retina project to the dorsal and posterior parts of the tectum accordingly. Anatomical directions are designated D (dorsal, superior), N (nasal), V (ventral, inferior), and T (temporal) for the retina, and as p (posterior), v (ventral), a (anterior), and d (dorsal) for the optic tectum.

During the first period of its history in the 1960s and 1970s the research on the avian retinotectal projection was based on experimental lesions and transplantation studies (Cowan et al., 1961; DeLong and Coulombre, 1965, 1967; Crossland et al., 1974; Goldberg, 1974). DeLong and Coulombre (1965) found that after retinal lesions in 4- to 5-day-old chick embryos the 12- to 13-day-old embryonic tecta had specific defects in retinal innervation. The investigators concluded that the tectal areas, which failed to become normally innervated, corresponded to ablated retinal quadrants. To further investigate the target specificity of retinal axons, they transplanted E4 retinal fragments from known quadrants of the eye onto the tectal surface of 6- to 7-day-old host embryos. The contralateral eyes had been removed to exclude interference with the retinotectal innervation of the host, and growing axons were examined 5 days later (DeLong and Coulombre, 1967). The fibers that grew out from the grafts showed a place specificity in their orientation: Axons growing from dorsal retinal grafts were directed ventrally, ventral and ventrotemporal fibers grew dorsally, and nasal grafts extended axons in posteriordorsal direction (DeLong and Coulombre, 1967). However, the place specificity revealed by this technique was rather inaccurate and, besides, the experiments could not be reproduced (Goldberg 1974). In another approach based on partial lesions, Crossland and co-workers (1974) removed retinal segments in chicks of different embryonic stages and investigated the ensuing tectal innervation. Axons from not affected retinal areas projected to their correct targets thereby passing unoccupied territory. They also found that ganglion cells are determined with respect to their target specificity already between 45 and 52 hours of incubation. The conclusions described so far are questioned by the results obtained in a set of experiments where the transplantations and lesions were resumed and tectal wholemounts analyzed (Goldberg 1974). Goldberg found neither evidence for specific tectal innervation defects after retinal lesions nor specific orientation of fibers growing from retinal grafts on the tectum. When defects of tectal innervation occurred they were always in dorsal areas, which are the latest to receive optic projections. (Taking into account that the tectum rotates during development by 90° Goldberg redefined the tectal axes. Using the commonly accepted terminology, which defines the larger tectal axis as anterior–posterior, his dorsal innervation deficits are actually posterior.) Corroborating results are reported in tectal transplants from quail to chicks: In the presence of a supernumerary graft, the host tectum was partially deprived from retinal innervation, and the noninnervated parts lay always in the most dorsocaudal area (Alvarado-Mallart and Sotelo, 1984). These contradictions point to general difficulties when interpreting results from the in vivo experiments that were performed at that time.

The experimental uncertainties prompted various theoretical considerations about possible mechanisms, how the correct retinotectal connections arise. Several models have been proposed and partially corroborated by empirical tests. Not all of the mechanisms in discussion are mutually exclusive, but different concepts emphasize the importance of different factors. A general affinity of retinal axons to the target area and competition for receptive neurons are always assumed.

1. The topographic order of retinal axons is simply preserved in the whole retinotectal pathway. This may be accomplished by the temporal sequence of fibre arrival and tectal maturation (Rager, 1976, 1980), or

neighborhood relationships are maintained by fiber–fiber communication (Arees and DeLong, 1977).

2. Positional cues in the target area mark the place for each individual axon terminal (Sperry, 1963). The current view holds that few substances are distributed in gradients over the tectal surface, and that retinal axons have varying affinities to these molecules, depending on the location of their retinal origin (Gierer, 1981; 1987; Bonhoeffer and Gierer, 1984; Fraser and Perkel, 1990).

3. Initial connection develops either at random or is only roughly ordered by some general guidance mechanism, and the specific connectivity emerges when incorrect terminals are eliminated later (Rager and Rager, 1978; McLoon, 1982). Functional tests of neighborhood relationship, e.g., temporal correlation of activity, may be the selective forces.

MAINTENANCE OF TOPOGRAPHIC ORDER BY SEQUENTIAL MATURATION AND GROWTH

The model is based on the following assumptions: First, retinal ganglion cells are generated in a central to peripheral succession, and in that sequence their axons arrive at the optic fissure with locations and angles that also depend on the site of their cell somata. As a result, fibers are placed in the optic nerve in a chronotopic order that corresponds to the spatial order of the ganglion cells (Goldberg, 1974; Rager, 1980; Thanos and Bonhoeffer, 1983). Second, the regional maturation of the tectum proceeds in a sequence that exactly matches the retinal ganglion cell differentiation. Rager describes that the rostral-central region, which has to receive central retinal axons, is the first tectal area to develop appropriate receptive structures, concluding that the earliest fibers grow as long until they encounter mature dendrites on the tectal surface. Later, axons are added successively according to their position in the optic tract (Rager and v. Oeynhausen, 1979; Rager, 1980). It is of critical importance for this model that the retinal neighborhood relations are preserved and appropriately transformed in the optic pathway. The transformation has to provide for that specific mirror imaging of the ventral retina to dorsal tectum, temporal retina to anterior tectum, etc. Rager stresses that the precision required in the retinotectal connection only needs to be in the order of fiber fascicles, not of single cells (Rager, 1980).

What is the experimental evidence? Ehrlich and Mark (1984) made laser lesions in the retina and examined the pattern of fiber degeneration. They found that the central-peripheral RGC succession of the retina is represented along the rostrocaudal axis in the optic tract. On the other hand, temporal and nasal fibers seemed to be mixed. Rager himself and his co-workers never observed a mixing of nasal and temporal fibers, though (Rager et al., 1988). An additional, contradictory fact, namely that many fibers enter the tectum at an incorrect position along the dorsoventral axis, has been corroborated by others as well (Nakamura and O'Leary, 1989). An investigation by Rager's group of the axonal pathways along their course established that transformations of the retinotectal topography follow particular constraints: In the optic nerve head, fibers are mirrored across an axis extending from dorsotemporal to ventronasal retina. Afterward, only minor changes occur as clockwise rotation behind the chiasm, and flattening of the whole tract. This leads to an organization of fibers when they arrive at the tectum, which fulfill the requirements for Rager's model (Rager et al., 1988). Additional support for the maintenance of order may come from preferential mutual adhesion by neighboring fibers (Arees and DeLong, 1977). The rough order of the projection will be refined later (Rager, 1980).

Given the ambiguous results of the earlier works on retinotectal specificity, the concept could suffice, were it not for several experiments that demonstrate correction by retinal axons with and without disturbance of their pathway: After perturbation of neurite fasciculation with anti-N-CAM Fab', early arriving and misrouted axons made corrections and turned toward their appropriate target area (Thanos et al., 1984). Growth correction could similarly be obtained under normal conditions (see figure 10.3) and when axons were deflected by insertion of teflon barriers into the tectal tissue (Thanos and Bonhoeffer, 1986, 1987; Nakamura and O'Leary, 1989; Kobayashi et al., 1990). More than 75% of the corrections were accurate, indicating the presence of directional cues and no random branching (Nakamura and O'Leary, 1989). However, in the study using anti-N-CAM Fab' and similarly after surgical deflection of fibers in the chiasm, the later arriving axons from the peripheral retina appeared to follow other fibers, made no corrections, and projected to ectopic positions (Fujisawa et al., 1984; Thanos et al., 1984), as would be concluded from a hypothesis that relies only on maintenance of neighborhood relationships. Taken together the experiments prove some ability of early arriving fibers to recognize their position relative to a specific target in the tectum, and to correct their course appropriately.

POSITIONAL CUES PROVIDED BY CHEMICAL MARKERS ON THE TECTUM

The Chemoaffinity Hypothesis

To explain such "homing" behavior of nerve fibers, Sperry (1963) postulated a growth mechanism that would selectively establish synaptic associations independent of function and be regulated by specific cytochemical affinities. While the early articulation of the theory required literally millions of chemically distinguished cell types alone for the

Development of the Avian Visual System

retina, that postulate of biochemical labels for every individual neuron has been abandoned in view of the limited amount of available genetic information.

Sperry reformulated the theory proposing

an orderly cytochemical mapping in terms of two or more gradients of embryonic differentiation that spread across and through each other with their axes roughly perpendicular. These separate gradients successively superimposed on the retinal and tectal fields and surroundings would stamp each cell with its appropriate latitude and longitude expressed in a kind of chemical code with matching values between the retinal and tectal maps (Sperry, 1963, p. 707).

In the light of accumulating empirical data about retinotectal systems in all classes of vertebrates, Sperry's theory has been widely accepted and elaborated. Fraser and Perkel (1990) constructed a model that is centred around the chemoaffinity principle, but integrates several mechanisms: While selecting their targets, retinal growth cones are guided by mathematically defined multiple constraints. These conditions are (1) position-independent affinity for the tectum, (2) competition for synaptic space, and (3) position-dependent affinities of the optic fibers to appropriate tectal targets. The latter position-dependent adhesion is assumed to be coded in two gradients, one along the dorsoventral axis and one in anterior–posterior direction. Computer simulations allowed to generate normal retinotopy and experimental results obtained in grafting and ablation experiments (Fraser and Perkel, 1990). The central issue in chemoaffinity remains, how the position specificity is encoded and by which molecular mechanisms axonal growth cones orient themselves in the target area. The program developed by Gierer (1981, 1987) assumes that axons respond to spatially graded concentrations of guiding substances. Gradients are required for both dimensions of the tectal surface, and along each axis two countergraded effects are necessary to create target positions *inside* the fields for each fiber terminal. These antagonistic effects depend quantitatively on molecular components of the axonal growth cones like receptor concentrations or modulated receptor affinities. To designate different specific locations along the gradients for individual axons by this system, the biochemical outfit of different growth cones themselves must be graded according to their retinal origin (Gierer, 1987; Fraser and Perkel, 1990). The physical mechanism for axonal guidance may be a force of maximal adhesion to the substrate (Letourneau, 1975) or, as it is most often assumed, chemoattractive and repulsive influences (Bonhoeffer and Gierer, 1984; Gierer, 1987; Walter et al., 1990). In this case, the problem arises, how relatively small growth cones can detect slight spatial gradients.

One possibility is a temporal detection of the gradient, as used in bacterial chemotaxis. As another solution, an adaptation of growth cone sensitivity to repulsive influences has been suggested (Bonhoeffer and Gierer, 1984). In analogy to the cAMP-chemotropism of cellular slime molds, Gierer conceived of a mechanism that enhances a slight external gradient within the growth cone. The amplification might result form receptor-mediated short-range autocatalytic reactions in combination with lateral inhibition or depletion. Thus, a restricted focus of activity would be created at the growth cone leading to oriented fiber growth or even axonal branching. A computer model, based on these principles, simulated empirical growth cone pathways (Gierer, 1987). These theoretical considerations enjoy considerable experimental support.

Evidence for Signals Encoding Positional Information

Before documenting the chase for tectal gradients that evolved in the last decade, the strong but indirect evidence for the real existence of a chemoaffinity principle in the chick tectum should be noted: This support comes first from the *observed behavior of individual axons in vivo.* Thanos and Bonhoeffer (1983, 1987) and Thanos and Dütting (1987) employed anterograde labeling techniques to demonstrate axonal growth and branching patterns on the tectal surface: A majority of axons course along direct routes. Some apparently ectopic axons, which occur in normal development and after experimental disturbance, correct their path along the dorsoventral axis in a manner that is consistent with Gierer's model (figure 10.3). This is especially found in early arriving fibers (Thanos et al., 1984), which, additionally, display more complex growth cones than the later arriving ones (Thanos and Bonhoeffer, 1983). It is therefore likely that the first axons orient themselves in a field of positional cues, while following fibers fasciculate with preexisting axons that belong to neighboring ganglion cells (Thanos and Dütting, 1987). The close arrangement of ingrowing axons and radial glia led to the suggestion that positional cues are expressed on glial endfeet (Silver and Rutishauser, 1984; Vanselow et al., 1989).

The second line of evidence that lends support to the chemoaffinity hypothesis derives from *in vitro studies on retinotectal affinity.* Measuring cell–cell adhesion between dissociated retinal cells and tectal tissue in vitro, Barbera (1975) discovered that cells from dorsal retina adhered preferentially to ventral tectal halves and vice versa. In addition, the effect seemed to be developmentally matched with the time course of the process in vivo: Ventral retinal cells, for instance, expressed the preference for dorsal tectum only when dissociated after E6 (Barbera, 1975). A variety of other in vitro models on regional specificity have since then been developed. They examine retinal cell–cell adhesion (Gottlieb et al., 1976), tectal membrane attachment to retinal neurites (Halfter et al., 1981), retinal neurite growth on monolayers of tectal cells (Bonhoeffer and Huf, 1985), or membranes (Walter et al., 1987a), stimulation of neuritic growth by tectum extracts (Carri and Ebendal, 1987), and growth cone collapse induction by tectal membrane preparations (Cox et al., 1990). These systems often could detect some preference of

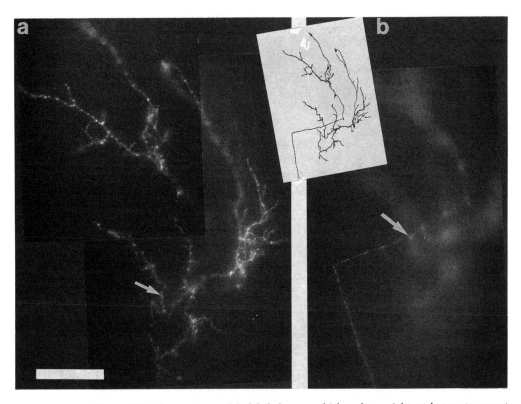

Figure 10.3 One anterogradely labeled axon, which makes a right-angle turn to correct its position in dorsal direction before terminating in the SGFS of the tectum. (a) Terminal arborization within the SGFS, the axon is out of focus. (b) Course of the axon in the SO; the site where it submerges into the deeper layer of the tectum is marked with arrows in a and b. Scale bar: 100 μm. (Insert) Combined drawing of the correcting axon and its terminal branches.

retinal neurites toward corresponding parts of the tectum. For example, the growth of (E6) nasal fibres is best stimulated by extracts from (E18) anterior tectal halves (Carri and Ebendal, 1987). The most convincing results are obtained with the assay developed by Bonhoeffer and co-workers (Walter et al., 1987a,b). Growing retinal neurites are offered membrane carpets from different tectal origin on alternating stripes. It turned out that temporal retinal axons avoid posterior tectal membranes when given a choice, but are still able to grow almost equally fast on tectal membranes of whatever origin (Walter et al., 1987a, 1989). This preference seems to be caused by a repellent substance rather than differential attraction, because prior treatment of posterior tectal membranes with heat or proteases converted them into an equally good growth substrate as anterior membranes (Walter et al., 1987b). Axons from nasal, dorsal, and ventral retina showed no preference. Recently, an avoidance reaction of temporal fibres could be reproduced in vitro: Neurites growing against an increasing gradient of posterior tectal mem-

Mey & Thanos: Anatomy of the Retinotectal Projection

branes stopped, when the slope of the gradient was steeper than 1% per 25μm (Baier and Bonhoeffer, 1992).

All previous in vitro experiments, however, failed to bring forth conclusive evidence for a gradient model, because (1) they were far to unspecific to detect any preference that could account for target specificity in the chemoaffinity model (Barbera, 1975; Gottlieb et al., 1976; Carri and Ebendal, 1987; Cox et al., 1990) or (2) they failed to reveal any *graded* characteristics along the tectal axes instead of a sharp transition (Halfter et al., 1981; Walter et al., 1987a,b, 1989; Baier and Bonhoeffer, 1992), and (3) often differences were detected along one axis only but not along the other (Halfter et al., 1981; Bonhoeffer and Huf, 1985; Walter et al., 1987a; Cox et al., 1990).

The most recent investigation of axon growth in the artificial gradient in vitro again showed a sharp discrimination between all nasal fibers, which lacked any response to the gradient, against all temporal fibers, which showed avoidance behavior (Baier and Bonhoeffer, 1992). This is precisely not to be expected if the gradient were to define spatial position along the entire rostrocaudal axis of the tectum. Problems to detect graded responses in vitro should not be taken as arguments against the chemoaffinity model, which is justified by fiber orientation in vivo. They may still be due to the technical constraints of the available assays.

Candidates for Guidance Molecules

The chemoaffinity postulate triggered research programs in several laboratories to find such guiding molecules. So far, these efforts, based on the technique of raising monoclonal antibodies, have revealed four possible candidates of guidance molecules in the chick retina (for review see: Stirling, 1991), and one tectal molecule that may guide growth cones by relative repulsion (Stahl et al., 1990).

Trisler and his colleagues were the first who discovered a molecule, called "TOP," that is continuously graded with respect to cell position in the retina. The expression of this cell surface molecule increases 35-fold from ventroanterior to the dorsoposterior pole (Trisler et al., 1981). Later, Trisler and Collins (1987) discovered an inverted distribution of TOP in the tectum, again rising in a graded fashion, here 10-fold from dorsal to ventral. Unfortunately, the expression of TOP drops continuously between E3 and E10. However, since it is still present at the time when first retinotectal axons arrive, and given the graded distributions, a homophilic binding mechanism has been suggested (Trisler and Collins, 1987). To our knowledge, no function could be assigned to TOP so far. Stirling (1991) argues that TOP rather plays a role in synaptic maturation than in axonal guidance, because its expression is highest in the retinal plexiform layers, is not temporally linked to fiber arrival on the tectum, and synapse formation can be affected with antibodies against TOP.

Two other monoclonal antibodies, "Julia" and "Dolce," bind preferentially to the developing dorsal retina of chicks, mice, rats and *Xenopus*. They recognize a 68-kDa and a 44-kDa protein. The 68-kDa protein and its mRNA are found throughout the whole retina, but the molecule seems to occur in a different configuration in the dorsal retina (Rabacchi et al., 1990). The protein is also involved in laminin binding. However, since the molecules are present on intracellular organelles, distributed in various other tissues, and under strong translational control, the hypothesis of its direct involvement in chemoaffinity has been substituted by the assumption of a role in differential control of protein synthesis (Stirling, 1991).

Recently, McLoon (1991) developed an antibody, "TRAP," that recognizes an asymmetric antigen expression along the nasal-temporal axis of the retina. The protein has an approximate molecular weight of 135 kDa, is present on the surface of axons and growth cones, and TRAP binding is most abundant on the temporal side. However, its distribution describes not a gradient, but a step function with a sharp transition in the vertical retinal midline (McLoon, 1991).

Further experiments in vitro specified the repulsive character of posterior tectal membranes to fibers from the temporal retina: the effect, tested with growth cone collapse and the stripe assay, was destroyed by treatment with proteases, heat, and phospholipase C, suggesting that the molecule is a protein, ankered with phosphatidylinositol to the membrane (Walter et al., 1987a,b, 1989; Cox et al., 1990). Antibodies were raised against purified tectal membrane extracts, and biochemical analysis led to the discovery of a 33-kDa glycoprotein that is expressed in higher concentration on the posterior surface of the tectum than anteriorly (Stahl et al., 1990). The gene of this molecule has been sequenced and its expression found to be developmentally regulated. A preliminary resumee of these results might be that not only a possible guidance molecule for retinal fibres has been found but that the avoidance of inappropriate targets appears as a central principle in CNS connectivity (Walter et al., 1989, Cox et al., 1990; Keynes and Cook, 1992).

Transplantation studies performed by Itasaki and others (Itasaki et al., 1991) provide evidence that the nuclear protein of the *engrailed* gene is expressed in chick and quail tecta in a graded fashion. The expression is highest at the caudal and lowest at the rostral pole of the mesencephalon. Heterotopic transplantations indicate that the gradient is controlled by a repressive influence from the junction between mes- and diencephalon, and that this determination takes place before the 25 somite stage is reached. Since the pattern of *engrailed* expression under normal and experimental conditions is a marker for the rostrocaudal polarity of cytoarchitectonic development and of the retinotectal projection map as well, it may be involved in the establishment of a rostrocaudal guidance gradient. The investigators also performed transplantations of half tecta after their determination and examined retinal fibre terminals following focal DiI labeling in the retina. In three cases, chick embryos with double rostral tecta (with respect to *engrailed* expression) were obtained and nasal fibers stained. They grew to their topographically correct caudal position on the graft, but degenerated later, indicating that their initial growth seemed to be independent of a presumed guidance gradient, whereas later termination and survival cannot be supported by rostral tectal tissue. In homotopic control operations or grafts before the 25 somite stage, the projections developed normally (Itasaki et al., 1991).

In a series of recent experiments, Dütting and Thanos resected the prospective temporal eye halves in 1.5-day-old chick embryos and investigated the ensuing retinotectal projection with retrograde labeling in juvenile birds. Experimental ablations at that early stage were compensated by complete regeneration with cells from the remaining nasal eye vesicle, thus giving rise to the development of eyes with normal size and morphology. Retrograde labeling revealed that the population of RGC in the regenerated temporal retinae projected in part to the anterior tecta (correct projection) and in part to the posterior tecta (corresponding to the target region of nasal ganglion cells). The RGC that lay in the temporal retina and were connected with the posterior tectum were aggregated in patches and surrounded by ganglion cells projecting to their correct anterior targets. This patchy distribution of RGC with respect to their central connection can be interpretated as evidence for very early determination of the positional specificity. Patches were interpreted as clones, descending from neuroblasts which invaded from the presumptive nasal eye half into the regenerating eye anlage (Dütting and Thanos, unpublished results). If this is correct, already neuroblasts at E1.5, the ancestors of may RGC and other neurons will be marked with some biochemical label for temporal or nasal position in the retina. In addition, this early determination of positional specificity would set limits to the topographical precision of the postulated biochemical markers.

ELIMINATION OF ECTOPIC CONNECTIONS

An elegant model that does not require specific recognition molecules or exact temporal sequences in development assumes that optic axons grow to the tectum in a diffuse manner, while interactions in the target field refine the projection into the ordered pattern of the adult (Rager, 1980; McLoon, 1982). Aberrant connections can be functionally identified and then be eliminated by cell death (Rager and Rager, 1978; Catsicas et al., 1987) or degeneration of axon terminals (Ehrlich and Mills, 1985; Williams and McLoon, 1991).

The conception of initially diffuse projection and random search for targets in the tectum is now refuted without doubt: Ingrowing axons are conclusively demonstrated to change their paths in correct directions to their targets (Thanos and Bonhoeffer, 1986; Nakamura and O'Leary, 1989); and computer simulations calculated growth paths for the random search proposal that were "in no way characteristic of actually observed axonal pathways" (Gierer, 1987). However, it is equally well established that many axons enter the tectum at erroneous positions (McLoon, 1982; Nakamura and O'Leary, 1989; Kobayashi et al., 1990), and that detection and elimination of ectopic connections take place a posteriori: The developing chick retinotectal system shows a linear decline in the percentage of fibres that overshoot their target in the tectum. This occurs between E14 and E18, after terminals are established. The refinement can partly be inhibited by treatment with tetrodotoxin and grayanotoxin I, which block and open sodium channels respectively. Therefore, neuronal activity is assigned a role in the reduction of overshooting axons. However, this was hardly seen in the correction of dorsoventrally aberrant fibers (Kobayashi et al., 1990).

Further evidence comes from projections of the chick visual system that are transiently formed and entirely disappear during development. One example is the ipsilateral retinotectal projection, which is eliminated between E12 and E16, but may partly persist, if the contralateral eye is removed during the first days of incubation (O'Leary et al., 1983). Other similarly transient systems include the efferent projections from the isthmooptic nucleus (ION) to the optic tectum and from the retina to the contralateral ION (Wizenmann and Thanos, 1990). Retrograde labeling of RGC shows that the elimination of the ipsilateral retinotectal connection is—to a large extent—not achieved by cell death (Williams and McLoon, 1991). Light dependent degeneration of retinotectal terminals has been detected earlier (Ehrlich and Mills, 1985). The projection from the retina to the ION is organized in a topographic manner with a number of connections made at ectopic positions. Here, nearly all ectopic terminals are eliminated between E12 and E14, and this refinement has been shown to occur by cell death of the respective RGC affecting 60% of the original population (Catsicas et al., 1987). All these findings support the notion that cell death, degeneration of axon collaterals, or degeneration of terminals are important processes for the establishment of the mature connectivity patterns. It is most likely that precise topographic projections as that of the visual system require subsidiary control processes, one of them being activity-dependent refinement.

CONCLUSIONS

1. Between E6 and E12, retinal axons spread over the tectal surface, forming a fiber front, which advances from the anterior ventral edge toward the posterior pole of the tectum. On E9, retinal fibers start to invade the outer layers in the central tectum, where simultaneously the

recipient laminae emerge from the neuroepithelium, and so create receptive structures for afferent fibers. The first synapses belonging to RGC that are situated in the central retina are also found in the central tectal area. Although some overshooting of fibers occurs, incoming axons appear to steer directly to their targets. Fibers can also correct their position along the dorsoventral axis before submerging beneath the surface and branching into terminal arborizations.

2. Several models have been proposed to account for the orderly connection between retinal fibers and central targets, resulting in the retinotopic map of the visual field on the tectal surface, which is so typical for primary sensory projections. Since observations of deflected axons conclusively show that early arriving retinal fibers recognize their position relative to a specific target, the chemoaffinity hypothesis, which postulates a molecular mechanism to encode positional information, has gained the widest support. However, despite considerable effort to find such guidance molecules, substances that are distributed in a spatial gradient in conformity with the theory *and* have functional significance with respect to fiber guidance *in vivo* have thus far eluded discovery. Moreover, the impression is that a crude positional information on the level of tectal quadrants (like dorsoventral plus anterior–posterior) may be determined by the substances tested in vitro, but no gradient emerges so far that would define each point on the tectal surface in interaction with retinal axons.

3. Since the precision of the retinotectal projection is physiologically important, more that the one process of fiber navigation in a gradient can be expected to ensure a correct development of the system. Much less will a single molecule solve the problem of preserving retinal topography in the central connections. Therefore, the concept of sequential fiber growth and cellular maturation, possibly supported by stabilizing fiber–fiber interaction, may still supply part of the answer. At least, it stresses the importance of spatiotemporal patterns of development, like transient receptivity for afferents at a given location on the tectum. After ingrowth of retinal fibers, ectopic connections are eliminated. Thus, function-dependent mechanisms for the finetuning of the system are very likely to occur, although physiological processes have, in this chapter, not been discussed in detail.

REFERENCES

Alvardo-Mallart, R.-M., and Sotelo, C. Homotopic and heterotopic transplantations of quail tectal primordia in chick embryos: organization of the retinotectal projections in the chimeric embryos. *Dev. Biol.* 103 (1984), 378–398.

Arees, E. A., and DeLong, G. R. Temporary contacts formed between developed optic fibers in the chick. *J. Embryol. Exp. Morphol.* 37 (1977), 211–216.

Baier, H., and Bonhoeffer, F. Axon guidance by gradients of a target-derived component. *Science* 255 (1992), 472–475.

Barbera, A. J. Adhesive recognition between developing retinal cells and the optic tecta of the chick embryo. *Dev. Biol.* 46 (1975), 167–191.

Bonhoeffer, F., and Gierer, A. How do retinal axons find their targets on the tectum? *Trends Neurosci.* 7 (1984), 378–381.

Bonhoeffer, F., and Huf, J. Position-dependent properties of retinal axons and their growth cones. *Nature (London)* 315 (1985), 409–410.

Cantino, D., and Sisto Daneo, L. Synaptic junctions in the developing chick optic tectum. *Experientia* 29 (1973), 85–87.

Carri, N. G., and Ebendal, T. Target-field specificity in the introduction of retinal neurite outgrowth. *Dev. Brain Res.* 31 (1987), 83–90.

Catsicas, S., Thanos, S., and Clarke, P. G. H. Major role for neuronal death during brain development: refinement of topographical connection. *Proc. Natl. Acad. Sci. U.S.A.* 84 (1987), 8165–8168.

Cowan, W. M., Adamson, L., and Powell, T. P. S. An experimental study of the avian visual system. *J. Anat.* 95 (1961), 545–562.

Cowan, W. M., Martin, A. H., and Wenger, E. Mitotic patterns in the optic tectum of the chick during normal development and after early removal of the optic vesicle. *J. Exp. Zool.* 169 (1968), 71–92.

Cox, E. C., Müller, B., and Bonhoeffer, F. Axonal guidance in the chick visual system: Posterior tectal membranes induce collapse of growth cones from the temporal retina. *Neuron* 4 (1990), 31–37.

Crossland, W. J., Cowan, W. M., Rogers, L. A., and Kelly, J. P. The specification of the retinotectal projection in the chick. *J. Comp. Neurol.* 155 (1974), 127–164.

Crossland, W. J., Cowan, W. M., and Rogers, L. A. Studies of the development of the chick optic tectum IV. An autoradiographic study of the development of retino-tectal connections. *Brain Res.* 91 (1975), 1–23.

DeLong, R. G., and Coulombre, A. J. Development of the retinotectal topographic projection in the chick embryo. *Exp. Neurol.* 13 (1965), 351–363.

DeLong, R. G., and Coulombre, A. J. The specificity of retinotectal connections studied by retinal grafts onto the optic tectum in chick embryos. *Dev. Biol.* 16 (1967), 513–531.

Ehrlich, D., and Mark, R. The course of axons of retinal ganglion cells within the optic nerve and tract of the chick (*Gallus gallus*). *J. Comp. Neurol.* 223 (1984), 583–591.

Ehrlich, D., and Mills, D. Evidence for self-absorption of terminals by developing axons of retinal ganglion cells in the chick. *Dev. Brain Res.* 17 (1985), 285–289.

Ehrlich, D., Keyser, K. T., and Karten, H. J. Distribution of Substance P-like immunoreactive retinal ganglion cells and their pattern of termination in the optic tectum of chick (*Gallus gallus*). *J. Comp. Neurol.* 266 (1987), 220–233.

Fraser, S. E., and Perkel, D. H. Competitive and positional cues in the patterning of nerve connections. *J. Neurobiol.* 21 (1990), 51–72.

Fujisawa, H., Thanos, S., and Schwarz, U. Mechanisms in the development of retinotectal projections in the chick embryo studied by surgical deflection of the retinal pathway. *Dev. Biol.* 102 (1984), 356–367.

Gierer, A. Development of projections between areas of the nervous system. *Biol. Cyb.* 42 (1981), 69–78.

Gierer, A. Directional cues for growing axons forming the retinotectal projection. *Development* 101 (1987), 479–489.

Goldberg, S. Studies on the mechanics of development of the visual pathways in the chick embryo. *Dev. Biol.* 36 (1974), 24–43.

Goldberg, S., and Coulombre, A. J. Topographical development of the ganglion cell fiber layer in the chick retina. A whole mount study. *J. Comp. Neurol.* 146 (1972), 507–518.

Gottlieb, D. I., Rock, K., and Glaser, L. A gradient of adhesive specificity in developing avian retina. *Proc. Natl. Acad. Sci. U.S.A.* 73 (1976), 410–414.

Gremo, F., Viglietti-Panzica, C., and Panzica, G. C. Development of neural connections in chick embryonic retino-tectal system: an overview. *Neurochem. Res.* 7 (1982), 243–259.

Halfter, W., and Deiss, S. Axon growth in embryonic chick and quail retinal whole mounts in vitro. *Dev. Biol.* 102 (1984), 344–355.

Halfter, W., and Deiss, S. Axonal pathfinding in organ-cultured embryonic avian retinae. *Dev. Biol.* 114 (1986), 296–310.

Halfter, W., Claviez, M., and Schwarz, U. Preferential adhesion of tectal membranes to anterior embryonic chick retina neurites. *Nature (London)* 292 (1981), 67–70.

Hamdi, F. A., and Whitteridge, D. The representation of the retina on the optic lobe of the pigeon. *Quart. J. Exp. Physiol.* 39 (1954), 111–119.

Horder, T. J., and Mashkas, A. The developmental programme for retinal embryogenesis with special reference to the chick. *Biblthca. Anat.* 23 (1982), 103–123.

Itasaki, N., Ichijo, H., Hama, C., Matsuno, T., and Nakamura, H. Establishment of rostrocaudal polarity in tectal primordium: *Engrailed* expression and subsequent tectal polarity. *Development* 113 (1991), 1133–1144.

Kahn, A. J. Ganglion cell formation in the chick neural retina. *Brain Res.* 63 (1973), 285–290.

Kahn, A. J. An autoradiographic analysis of the time of appearance of neurons in the developing chick neural retina. *Dev. Biol.* 38 (1974), 30–40.

Keynes, R. J., and Cook, G. M. W. Repellent cues in axon guidance. *Curr. Opin. Neurobiol.* 2 (1992), 55–59.

Kobayashi, T., Nakamura, H., and Yasuda, M. Disturbance of refinement of retinotectal projection in chick embryos by tetrodotoxin and grayanotoxin. *Dev. Brain Res.* 57 (1990), 29–35.

LaVail, J. H., and Cowan, W. M. The development of the chick optic tectum I. Normal morphology and cytoarchitectonic development. *Brain Res.* 28 (1971), 391–419.

Letourneau, P. C. Cell-to-substratum adhesion and guidance of axonal elongation. *Dev. Biol.* 44 (1975), 92–101.

McGill, J. I., Powell, T. P. S., and Cowan, W. M. The retinal representation upon the optic tectum and isthmo-optic nucleus in the pigeon. *J. Anat.* 100 (1966), 5–33.

McGraw, C. F., and McLaughlin, B. J. Fine structural studies of synaptogenesis in the superficial layers of the chick optic tectum. *J. Neurocytol.* 9 (1980), 79–93.

McLoon, S. Alterations in precision of the crossed retinotectal projection during chick development. *Science* 215 (1982), 1418–1419.

McLoon, S. Evidence for shifting connections during development of the chick retinotectal projection. *J. Neurosci.* 5 (1985), 2570–2580.

Development of the Avian Visual System

McLoon, S. A monoclonal antibody that distinguishes between temporal and nasal retinal axons. *J. Neurosci.* 11 (1991), 1470–1477.

Nakamura, H., and O'Leary, D. D. M. Inaccuracies in initial growth and arborization of chick retinotectal axons followed by course corrections and axon remodeling to develop topographic order. *J. Neurosci.* 9 (1989), 3776–3795.

Navascués, J., Rodríguez-Gallardo, L., Martín-Partido, G., and Alvarez, I. S. Proliferation of glial precursors during the early development of the chick optic nerve. *Anat. Embryol.* 172 (1985), 365–373.

Navascués, J. Martín-Partido, G., Alvárez, I. S., Rodríguez-Gallardo, L. and García-Martínez V., Glioblast migration in the optic stalk of the chick embryo. *Anat. Embryol.* 176 (1987a), 79–85.

Navascués, J., Rodríguez-Gallardo, L., García-Martínez, V., Alvárez, I. S., and Martín-Partido, G. Extra-axonal environment and fibre directionality in the early development of the chick embryo optic chiasm: a light and scanning electron microscopic study. *J. Neurocytol.* 16 (1987b), 299–310.

O'Leary, D. D. M., Gerfen, R., and Cowan, W. M. The development and restriction of the ipsilateral retinofugal projection in the chick. *Dev. Brain Res.* 10 (1973), 93–109.

Panzica, G. C., and Viglietti-Panzica, C. V. Electron microscopy of synaptic structures in the optic tectum of developing chick embryos. *Biblthca. Anat.* 19 (1981), 167–173.

Patten, B. M. *Early Embryology of the Chick*, 5th ed. McGraw-Hill, New York, 1971.

Puelles, L., and Bendala, M. C. Differentiation of Neuroblasts in the chick optic tectum up to eight days of incubation: A Golgi study. *Neuroscience* 3 (1978), 307–325.

Rabacchi, S. A., Nerve, R. L., and Drager, U. C. A positional marker for the dorsal embryonic retina is homologous to the high-affinity laminin receptor. *Development* 109 (1990), 521–531.

Rager, G. Morphogenesis and physiogenesis of the retino-tectal connection in the chicken II. The retino-tectal synapses. *Proc. R. Soc. London B.* 192 (1976), 353–370.

Rager, G. Die Ontogenese der retinotopen Porjektion. *Naturwissenschaften* 67 (1980), 280–287.

Rager, G., and v. Oeynhausen, B. Ingrowth and ramification of retinal fibers in the developing optic tectum of the chick embryo. *Exp. Brain Res.* 35 (1979), 213–227.

Rager, G., and Rager, U. Systems-matching by degeneration. I A quantitative electron microscopic study of the generation and degeneration of retinal ganglion cells in the chicken. *Exp. Brain Res.* 33 (1978), 65–78.

Rager, U., Rager, G., and Kabiersch, A. Transformations of the retinal topography along the visual pathway of the chicken. *Anat. Embryol.* 179 (1988).

Ramón y Cajal, S. *Histologie du systéme nerveux de l'homme et des verébrés*, Vol. II, Madrid, 1911, segudna reimpresion, 1972. Le lobe optique des vertébrés inférieurs, toit optique des oiseaux, pp. 196–212.

Senut, M. C., and Alvardao-Mallart, R. M. Development of the retinotectal system in normal quail embryos: cytoarchitectonic development and optic fiber innervation. *Dev. Brain Res.* 29 (1986), 123–140.

Silver, J., and Rutishauser, U. Guidance of optic axons *in vivo* by a preformed adhesive pathway on neuroepithelial endfeet. *Dev. Biol.*, 106 (1984), 485–499.

Sperry, R. W. Chemoaffinity in the orderly growth of nerve fiber patterns and connections. *Proc. Natl. Acad. Sci. U.S.A.* 50 (1963), 703–790.

Stahl, B., Müller, B., v.Boxberg, Y., Cox, E. C., and Bonhoeffer, F. Biochemical characterization of a putative axonal guidance molecule of the chick visual system. *Neuron* 5 (1990), 735–743.

Stieda. Studien über das centrale Nervensystem der Vögel und Säugenthiere, Z. *Wiss. Zool.*, XIX (1868), reference from Ramón y Cajal, 1911.

Stirling, V. Molecules, maps and gradients in the retinotectal projection. *Trends Neurosci.* 14 (1991), 509–512.

Thanos, S., and Bonhoeffer, F. Investigations on development and topographic order of retinotectal axons: Anterograde and retrograde staining of axons and their perikarya with Rhodamine in vivo. *J. Comp. Neurol.* 219 (1983), 420–430.

Thanos, S., and Bonhoeffer, F. Course corrections of deflected retinal axons on the tectum of the chick embryo. *Neurosci. Lett.* 72 (1986), 31–36.

Thanos, S., and Bonhoeffer, F. Axonal arborization in the developing chick retinotectal system. *J. Comp. Neurol.* 261 (1987), 155–164.

Thanos, and Dütting, D. Outgrowth and directional specificity of fibers from embryonic retinal transplants in the chick optic tectum. *Dev. Brain Res.* 32 (1987), 161–179.

Thanos, S., Bonhoeffer, F., and Rutishauser, U. Fiber-fiber interaction and tectal cues influence the development of the chick retinotectal system. *Proc. Natl. Acad. Sci. U.S.A.* 81 (1984), 1906–1910.

Thanos, S., Vanselow, J., and Mey, J. Ganglion cells in the juvenile chick retina and their ability to regenerate axons in vitro. *Exp. Eye Res.* 54 (1992), 377–391.

Trisler, G. D., and Collins, F. Corresponding spatial gradients of TOP molecules in the developing retina and optic tectum. *Science* 237 (1987), 1208–1209.

Trisler, G. D., Schneider, M. D., and Nirenberg, M. A topographic gradient of molecules in retina can be used to identify neuron position. *Proc. Natl. Acad. Sci. U.S.A.* 78 (1981), 2145–2149.

Vanselow, J., Thanos, S., Godement, P., Henke-Fahle, S., and Bonhoeffer, F. Spatial arrangement of radial glia and ingrowing of retinal axons in the chick optic tectum during development. *Dev. Brain Res.* 45 (1989), 15–27.

Walter, J., Kern-Veits, B., Huf, J., Stolze, B., and Bonhoeffer, F. Recognition of position-specific properties of tectal cell membranes by retinal axons in vitro. *Development* 101 (1987a), 685–696.

Walter, J., Henke-Fahle, S., and Bonhoeffer. Avoidance of posterior tectal membranes by temporal retinal axons. *Development* 101 (1987b), 909–913.

Walter J., Müller, B., and Bonhoeffer, F. Axonal guidance by an avoidance mechanism. *J. Physiol. (Paris)* 83 (1989), 1988–1989.

Walter, J., Allsopp, T. E., and Bonhoeffer, F. A common denominator of growth cone guidance and collapse? *Trends Neurosci.* 13 (1990), 447–452.

Watanabe, M., Rutishauser, U., and Silver, J. Formation of the retinal ganglion cell and optic fiber layers. *J. Neurobiol.* 22 (1991), 85–95.

Williams, C. V., and McLoon, S. C. Elimination of the transient ipsilateral retinotectal projection is not solely achieved by cell death in the developing chick. *J. Neurosci.* 11 (1991), 445–453.

Wizenmann, A., and Thanos, S. The developing chick isthmo-optic nucleus forms a transient efferent projection to the tectum. *Neurosci. Lett.* 113 (1990), 241–246.

11 Development, Plasticity, and Differential Organization of Parallel Processing of Visual Information in Birds

G. Fontanesi, G. Casini, A. Ciocchetti,
and P. Bagnoli

The vertebrate visual system has long been regarded as a suitable model for the studies of the development, plasticity, and organization of neural networks. While most of this work has been carried out with mammals, comparative studies on the avian visual system may make useful contributions. There are, of course, some differences between the visual systems of birds and mammals: (1) the presence in birds of a completely crossed retinofugal projection, (2) the partial recrossing of the thalamofugal fibers, which allows binocular interactions to take place in telencephalic visual centers, (3) the nuclear organization of the avian equivalents of the mammalian neocortical laminae, and (4) the greater development of the tectofugal as compared to the geniculocortical system.

Despite these differences, birds are capable of comparable and in some cases superior performance in acuity, discrimination, and binocular processing (see chapters 1 and 9). It is now clear that there are a number of parallels between the organization of the visual pathways in birds and in mammals (see chapter 6). Moreover, experimental manipulations, such as monocular deprivation and retina removal during critical periods in development, produce similar changes in the structural and functional organization of visual pathways in birds and mammals. Such similarities increase the utility of the avian visual system for studies of development. This chapter reviews recent studies on the maturation, plasticity, and organization patterns of central visual pathways in birds. Special attention will be paid to maturational changes mediating the use of visual processing strategies unique to birds.

DEVELOPMENT OF VISUAL PATHWAYS

The development of the avian retinotectal system has been studied primarily in chicks and pigeons: the first a precocial and the second an altricial species. Not surprisingly, the two species differ with respect to the time course of maturational events. In chickens, they are confined primarily to the embryonic periods (Mathers and Ostrach, 1979; Mc-

Graw and McLaughlin 1980), while in pigeons they are delayed until the first 10 days after hatching. Pigeons therefore offer the advantage of a continuing susceptibility to experimental manipulations during early posthatching periods.

The organization of the visual system displays the same immature characteristics in newly hatched pigeons and embryonic chicks. At the retinal level, the maturation of synapses and photoreceptors shows a progression from center to periphery, with numerous synapses present in the inner plexiform layer (IPL) at a time when photoreceptor lamellae have yet to appear. By the time photoreceptor disks first appear, only a few synapses are present in the outer plexiform layer (OPL). They increase in number as the lamellar structures complete their maturation. This developmental pattern is correlated with a gradual increase in the amplitude of the flash-evoked electroretinogram (FERG). Simultaneous with the appearance of FERG responses, pattern-evoked ERGs (PERGs) can be recorded from the pigeon eye and their amplitude increases over the first posthatching month. During the first 10 days of this period, the cloudiness of the optical media progressively disappears and retinal acuity improves. The pigeon's eyelids open between days 6 and 9, at which time the maturation of its retina is almost complete, and is paralleled by the structural and functional development of the retino-fugal pathways (Porciatti et al., 1985; Bagnoli al., 1985, 1987).

Although ipsilateral, retinofugal fibers reaching the thalamus and the optic tectum (TeO) are present at hatching, they disappear almost completely during the following week. During the same period, retinal afferents that, at hatching, are confined to the central tectal quadrant, progressively invade the superficial layers of TeO. The time course of retinal invasion is characterized by the late innervation of the ventro-medial tectal quadrant, which may reflect a delayed origin of ganglion cells in the corresponding retinal region. The lamination of the super-ficial TeO takes place within this same period. The development of the retinotectal projection in chicks and pigeons is illustrated schematically in figure 11.1.

The time course of tectal development, as indicated by responses to flash- and pattern-evoked stimuli, parallels that of retinal FERG and PERG responses, and their amplitude increases, as does tectal acuity, over the first month of life. Thus the development of the avian retino-tectal system is characterized by a temporal correlation among eyelid opening, the appearance of photoreceptor disks, the specification of retinotectal connections, and the maturation of tectal neurons. These data suggest that the organization of retinotectal connections may be a product of developmental processes occurring during the early pos-thatching period. Comparable developmental patterns are observed in other nonmammalian vertebrates, as well as in some mammals (McLoon and Lund, 1982; Williams and Chalupa, 1982; Thanos and Bonhoeffer, 1984; Insausti et al., 1985). The initial presence and subsequent disap-

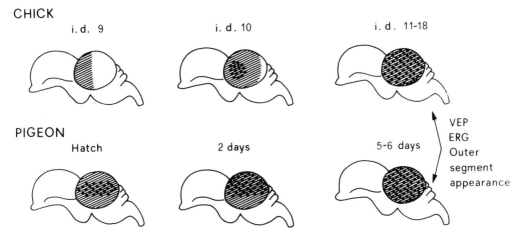

Figure 11.1 Development of the retinotectal system in chicks and pigeons. Note that the organizational pattern is almost comparable in the two species, but with a different time course. Retinal axons overlying the tectal surface are indicated by lines whereas fibers entering the superficial tectal layers are indicated by dots. In chicks, the adult pattern is reached between 11 and 18 days of incubation whereas in pigeons the final organization is obtained at the end of the first week after hatching. i.d., incubation day; ERG, electroretinogram; VEP, visually evoked potential (see text for details).

pearance of an ipsilateral retinofugal pathway parallel similar events in mammals, where there is also a reduction (although not a complete disappearance) of the initially present ipsilateral component. This may provide a mechanism for the segregation of ipsilateral and contralateral retinal terminals within the primary visual targets (Rakic, 1986; Sretavan and Shatz, 1986). These comparative observations suggest that birds and mammals use similar developmental strategies for the organization of central visual connections.

PLASTIC CHANGES INDUCED BY VISUAL DEAFFERENTATION AND DEPRIVATION

Visual inputs appear to play a critical role in the development of the visual pathways in birds. For example, unilateral retina removal, if performed immediately after hatching, results in a marked shrinkage of the main contralateral primary and secondary visual regions, with associated alterations in their cytoarchitecture, which are maintained in the adult. Similarly, after early removal of one retina, the ipsilateral retinofugal projection, which normally disappears during development, is retained into adulthood, and the lamination of the superficial TeO is prevented (Bagnoli et al., 1989a). Unilateral retina removal also induces a drastic reorganization of thalamofugal connections (figure 11.2), altering the relative contribution of thalamic afferents to the Wulst, and producing an enlargement of the crossed thalamofugal component originating from the visual thalamus on the side innervated by the intact

Fontanesi et al.: Parallel Processing of Visual Information

A

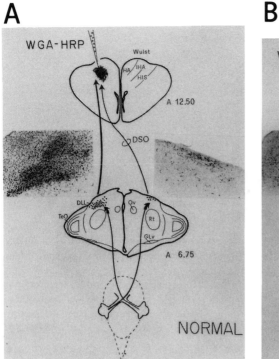

B

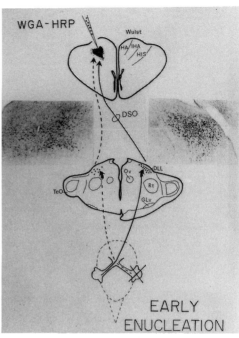

Figure 11.2 Schematic representation of the relative contribution of ipsilateral and contralateral thalamo-Wulst projections in normal adult pigeons and in adults with unilateral retina removal at hatching. Photomicrographs of frontal sections through the diencephalon show retrogradely labeled neurons in the dorsolateral thalamus following WGA-HRP injection into the visual Wulst. DLL, nucleus dorsolateralis anterior thalami, pars lateralis; DSO, decussatio supraoptica; GLv, nucleus geniculatus lateralis, pars ventralis; HA, hyperstriatum accessorium; HD, hyperstriatym dorsale; HIS, hyperstriatum intercalatus superior; IHA, nucleus intercalatus hyperstriati accessorii; Ipc, nucleus isthmi, pars parvocellularis; nBOR, nucleus of the basal optic root (l, d, and p, lateralis, dorsalis, and proper, respectively); Ov, nucleus ovoidalis; PT, nucleus pretectalis; Rt, nucleus rotundus; TeO, optic tectum; TrO, tractus opticus. Anatomical nomenclature after the stereotaxic atlas of Karten and Hodos (1967).

eye. The deafferented visual thalamus establishes reduced connections with the ipsilateral Wulst, while the crossed pathway originating in the remaining, (normally innervated) thalamus appears increased. Therefore, visual information reaching the dorsolateral thalamus must play a key role in establishing the normal balance of thalamic inputs to the Wulst. These findings are consistent with the hypothesis, derived from studies in mammals, that competitive processes involving thalamic neurons driven by the two eyes have an important role in determining the organization of the thalamocortical pathway (Rakic, 1981; Jeffery, 1984; Shook et al., 1985). Thus, despite some important differences in the organization of visual pathways in birds and mammals, competitive interactions represent a basic mechanism for normal maturation of thalamocortical connections in both classes (see also Engelage and Bischof, this volume).

The "competition" hypothesis, based on visual deafferentation studies, is further supported by 2-[^{14}C]deoxyglucose studies of functional visual deprivation (e.g., monocular occlusion) in pigeons. In such birds, marked functional asymmetries in the response to illumination are present at the level of the visual Wulst, with higher incorporation of the tracer on the brain side contralateral to the deprived eye. This effect is likely to be due to enhanced functional activity in the crossed thalamo-Wulst pathway carrying information from the nondeprived eye (Bagnoli et al., 1982; Burkhalter et al., 1982).

DEVELOPMENT OF SPECIFIC TRANSMITTER PHENOTYPES IN NEURONS OF THE CENTRAL VISUAL RELAYS

The transmitter phenotype of a neuron is generally determined by multiple factors, including genetic program, afferent influences, hormones, efferent innervation, etc. Among these factors, afferent innervation plays an important role during brain maturation (see Huntley et al., 1988). The role of such innervation in the development of the avian visual system has been examined, by comparing the distribution of neurotransmitter types in normal and visually deprived pigeons. Using immunocytochemical methods, the development of cell populations expressing either classical transmitters, e.g., γ-aminobutyric acid (GABA), acetylcholine (Ach), norepinephrine (NA), and serotonin (5HT) or neuropeptides, e.g., substance P (SP), neuropeptide Y (NPY), and somatostatin (SS) has been investigated (Bagnoli et al., 1989b, 1991, 1992; Fontanesi et al., 1993). Quantitative evaluations have been made at different developmental stages, using computer-assisted image analysis techniques.

These studies demonstrate that the anatomical and functional maturation of the pigeon visual system is paralleled by changes in neurotransmitter distribution in the developing visual neurons. Normal transmitter maturation is likely to depend on retinal input at critical times during development, since the adult distribution of transmitters is generally reached when the morphological and functional maturation of visual connectivities is completed. Except for Ach, NPY, and SS, which are generally expressed in the embryo, expression of the other investigated neurotransmitters can first be detected at hatching. Changes in the pattern of transmitter expression during maturation generally include a progressive decrease in the density of transmitter-identified cells, with a parallel increase in neuropilar processes. Some identified cell populations are also found to transiently express specific transmitters only at early developmental stages. Loss of immunopositive cell bodies can be attributed to numerous factors, including cell death, secondary migration, morphological transformation, variation in transmitter level, change in phenotype expression, etc. Experiments with visually deaf-ferented pigeons can help to elucidate the mechanisms underlying transmitter expression during development by clarifying the possible role of incoming retinal afferents in regulating the final distribution of transmitters.

Early retinal deafferentation generally affects transmitter distribution in the pigeon visual system. Unilateral deafferentation, performed at hatching, produces marked effects upon TeO and related pretectal nuclei. The thalamic visual relays are almost unaffected, except for cholinergic cell populations of the dorsolateral thalamus, which appear drastically reduced on the brain side contralateral to the removed retina. In the telencephalon, most transmitter systems of the visual Wulst are unaffected by unilateral deafferentation, except for a drastic decrease in the density of cholinergic fibers originating from Ach-positive cells of the visual thalamus. In contrast, marked but quite different effects of early bilateral deafferentation on the distribution of peptidergic transmitters are seen in the telencephalic targets of the thalamofugal and tectofugal systems. In the visual Wulst, the distribution of SS-positive cells retains an immature pattern since their total number does not increase during development. In contrast, bilateral deafferentation results in a significant increase of SS-positive cells in the ectostriatum. Comparable effects, e.g., loss of transmitter-identified cells after retina removal have been reported in mammals (Nakagawa et al., 1988; Miguel-Hidalgo et al., 1990). Numerous phenomena might explain such cell loss, including (1) the lack of adequate innervation, (2) the trans-synaptically induced loss of intrinsic cells, (3) possible changes in the rate of transmitter biosynthesis, and (4) the lack of trophic molecules originating in retinal afferents. Similarly, the number of SS-positive cells of the mammalian visual cortex increases following retinal removal, suggesting an inhibitory role for developing thalamocortical connections on SS expression (Jeffery and Parnavelas, 1987). Figures 11.3 and 11.4 summarize qualitative and quantitative data on neurotransmitter distribution during normal development, and in adults subjected to unilateral or bilateral retina removal posthatching.

CONCLUSION

Maturational changes of neural structures have been reported at different levels of the visual system of lateral-eyed birds. The posthatching remodeling of visual regions suggests that visual inputs play a role in their development. As shown in this review and previous papers, substantial rearrangements occur in either the thalamofugal or tectofugal pathway (Adret and Rogers, 1989; Rogers and Bell, 1989; ref in Bischof et al., 1991). The present results also demonstrate that retinofugal axons influence the development of neurotransmitter systems in the pigeon visual areas since drastic modifications are induced by early deafferen-

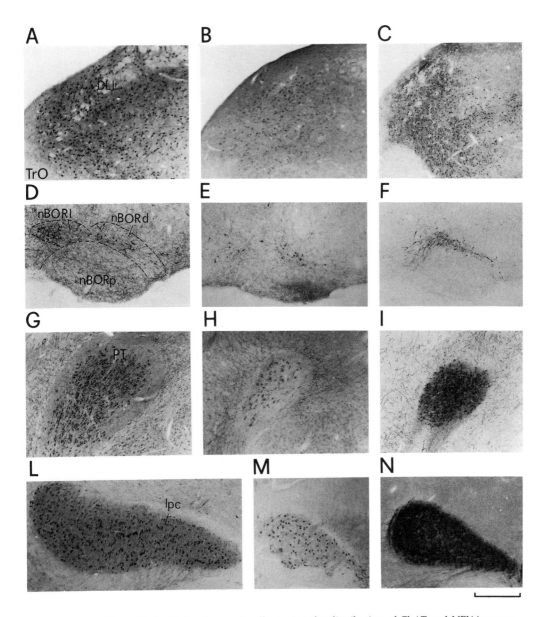

Figure 11.3 Photomicrographs illustrating the distribution of ChAT and NPY immuno-reactivity in some visual regions of adult (A, D, G, and L), unilaterally retina ablated (B, E, H, and M), and newly hatched pigeons (C, F, I, and N). ChAT-positive cells and processes are present in the nucleus dorsolateralis anterior thalami, pars lateralis (DLL), and in the nucleus isthmi, pars parvocellularis (Ipc) (A–C and L–N, respectively). NPY immunoreactivity is present in the nucleus of the basal optic root (nBOR) and in the nucleus pretectalis (PT) (D–F and G–I, respectively). Note the loss of immunoreactive cell bodies as a result of early retina ablation. From hatching to adulthood, there is an increase of ChAT immunopositive cells in the DLL. Over the same period, a drastic decrease in the density of NPY and ChAT immunopositive cell bodies is observed in PT and Ipc, respectively. In contrast, no changes are detected in the density of NPY immunopositive cells of the nBOR. Modified from Bagnoli et al. (1992). Calibration bar: 390 μm, A–C and L–N; 310 μm, D–F; 340 μm, G–I.

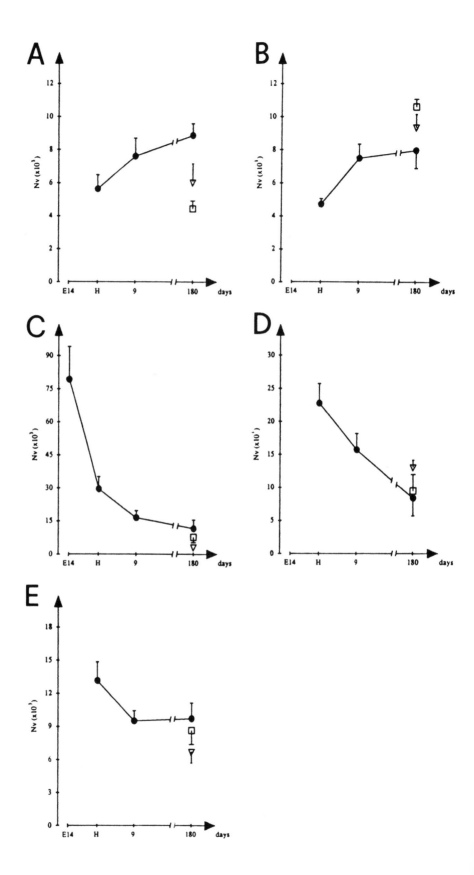

Development of the Avian Visual System

Figure 11.4 Example of computer-assisted image analysis from immunohistochemically processed sections of the pigeon visual system. The diagrams show changes in the number of SS-positive cells per cubic millimeter of tissue (Nv) over maturation and in adults with early retina removal. Filled circles refer to different stages (H, hatching). Open squares and open triangles refer to pigeons that have had one or both retinas removed at hatching. In unilaterally deafferented animals, quantitative data are obtained from visual regions contralateral to the removed retina. In pigeons with bilateral deafferentation, measurements are obtained from both brain sides. Maturative changes result in cell density increase at the level of the optic tectum (layer 7 and 10 shown in A and B, respectively), whereas a drastic decrease in the density of labeled cells is shown by the nucleus of the basal optic root (C), the ectostriatum (D), and the visual Wulst (E). Unilateral retina removal has significant effects on the immunolabeled cell populations in the optic tectum and the nucleus of the basal optic root, while no effects are observed in the visual Wulst and ectostriatum. In contrast, bilateral deafferentation induces a decrease of immunostained cell density in the visual Wulst and an increase in the ectostriatum. Modified from Fontanesi et al. (1993).

tation. These effects are, however, difficult to explain in terms of simple interactions between incoming visual afferents and neurotransmitter expression during maturation. Several interacting factors, either intrinsic (e.g., genetic) or extrinsic (e.g., environmental) appear to be necessary for the correct development of the visual pathways as well a their neurochemical characteristics.

ACKNOWLEDGMENTS

Immunohistochemical results, except for GABA, 5HT, and SS were obtained in collaboration with Dr. J. T. Erichsen (SUNY at Stony Brook). Supported by the C. N. R. Target Project on Biotechnology and Bioinstrumentation (Ct 92.01167. PF70 to P. Bagnoli).

REFERENCES

Adret, P. and L. J. Rogers. (1989). Sex difference in the visual projection of young chicks: A quantitative study of the thalamofugal pathway. *Brain Res.* 478:59–73.

Bagnoli, P., A. Burkhalter, A. Vischer, H. Henke, and M. Cuenod. (1982). Effects of early monocular deprivation on choline acetyltransferase and glutamic acid decarboxylase in pigeon visual Wulst. *Brain Res.* 247:289–302.

Bagnoli, P., V. Porciatti, A. Lanfranchi, and C. Bedini. (1985). Developing pigeon retina: light-evoked responses and ultrastructure of outer segments and synapses. *J. Comp. Neurol.* 235:384–394.

Bagnoli, P., V. Porciatti, G. Fontanesi, and L. Sebastiani. (1987). Morphological and functional changes in the retinotectal system of the pigeon during the early posthatching period. *J. Comp. Neurol.* 256:400–411.

Bagnoli, P., G. Casini, G. Fontanesi, and L. Sebastiani. (1989a). Reorganization of visual pathways following posthatching removal of one retina in pigeons. *J. Comp. Neurol.* 288:512–527.

Bagnoli, P., G. Fontanesi, P. Streit, L. Domenici, and R. Alesci. (1989b). Changing distribution of GABA-like immunoreactivity in pigeon visual areas during the early posthatching period and effects of retinal removal on tectal GABAergic systems. *Visual Neurosci.* 3:491–508.

Bagnoli, P., S. Di Gregorio, M. Molnar, C. Romei, and G. Fontanesi. (1991). Maturation and plasticity of neuropeptides in the visual system. In P. Bagnoli and W. Hodos (Eds.), *The Changing Visual System.* Plenum Press, New York, pp. 114–128.

Bagnoli, P., G. Fontanesi, R. Alesci, and J. R. Erichsen. (1992). Distribution of neuropeptide Y, substance P and choline acetyltransferase in the developing visual system of the pigeon and effects of unilateral retina removal. *J. Comp. Neurol.* 318:392–414.

Bischof, H. J., K. Herrmann, and J. Engelage. (1991). Development and plasticity of the tectofugal visual pathway in the zebra finch. In P. Bagnoli and W. Hodos (Eds.), *The Changing Visual System.* Plenum Press, New York, pp. 199–208.

Burkhalter, A., P. Streit, P. Bagnoli, A. Vischer, H. Henke, and M. Cuenod. (1982). Deprivation-induced functional modifications in the pigeon visual system. In C. Ajmone Marsan and H. Matthies (Eds.), *Neuronal Plasticity and Memory Formation.* Raven Press, New York, pp. 477–485.

Fontanesi, G., G. Traina, and P. Bagnoli. (1993). Somatostatin-like immunoreactivity in the pigeon visual system: developmental expression and effects of retina removal. *Visual Neurosci.* 10:1–15.

Huntley, G. W., S. H. C. Hendry, H. P. Killacrey, L. M. Chalupa, and E. G. Jones. (1988). Temporal sequence of neurotransmitter expression by developing neurons of fetal monkey visual cortex. *Dev. Brain Res.* 43:69–96.

Insausti R., C. Blakemore, and W. C. Cowan. (1985). Postnatal development of the ipsilateral retinocollicular projections and effects of unilateral enucleation in the golden hamster. *J. Comp. Neurol.* 234:393–409.

Jeffery, G. (1984). Transneuronal effects of early eye removal on geniculo-cortical projection cells. *Dev. Brain Res.* 13:257–263.

Jeffery, G., and J. G. Parnavelas. (1987). Early visual deafferentation of the cortex results in an asymmetry of somatostatin labeled cells. *Exp. Brain Res.* 67:651–655.

Karten, H. J., and W. Hodos. (1967). *A Stereotaxic Atlas of the Brain of the Pigeon Columba livia.* Baltimore: J. Hopkins University Press.

Mathers, L. H., and L. H. Ostrach. (1979). Mechanisms controlling axonal misrouting in the visual system of the chick embryo. *Anat. Rec.* 193:614–620.

McGraw, C. F., and McLaughlin. (1980). Fine structural studies of synaptogenesis in the superficial layers of the chick optic tectum. *J. Neurocytol.* 9:79–93.

McLoon, S. C., and R. D. Lund. (1982). Transient retinofugal pathways in the developing chick. *Exp. Brain Res.* 45:277–284.

Miguel-Hidalgo, J. J., E. Semba, K. Takatsuji, and M. Tohyama. (1990). Substance P and enkephalins in the superficial layers of the rat superior colliculus: differential plastic effects of retinal deafferentation. *J. Comp. Neurol.* 299:389–404.

Nagakawa, S., Y. Hasegawa, T. Kubozono, and K. Takuni. (1988). Substance P-like immunoreactive retinal terminals found in two retinorecipient areas of the Japanese monkey. *Neurosci. Lett.* 93:32–37.

Porciatti, V., P. Bagnoli, A. Lanfranchi, and C. Bedini. (1985). Interactions between photoreceptors and pigmented epithelium in developing pigeon retina: an electrophysiological and ultrastructural study. *Doc. Ophthalmol.* 60:413–419.

Rakic, P. (1981). Development of visual centers in the primate brain depends on binocular competition before birth. *Science* 214:928–931.

Rakic, P. (1986). Mechanisms of ocular dominance segregation in the lateral geniculate nucleus: competitive elimination hypothesis. *Trends Neurosci.* 9:11–15.

Rogers, L. J., and G. A. Bell. (1989). Different rates of functional development in the two visual systems of the chicken revealed by 14C 2-deoxyglucose. *Dev. Brain Res.* 49:161–172.

Shook, B. L., L. Maffei, and L. M. Chalupa. (1985). Functional organization of the cat's visual cortex after prenatal interruption of binocular interactions. *Proc. Natl. Acad. Sci. U. S. A.* 82:3901–3905.

Sretavan, D. W., and C. Shatz. (1986). Prenatal development of retinal ganglion cell axons: segregation into eye-specific layers within the cat's lateral geniculate nucleus. *J. Neurosci.* 6:234–251.

Thanos, S., and F. Bonhoeffer. (1984). Development of the transient ipsilateral retinotectal projection in the chick embryo: A numerical fluorescence microscopic analysis. *J. Comp. Neurol.* 224:407–414.

Williams, R. W., and L. M. Chalupa. (1982). Prenatal development of retinocollicular projections in the cat: an anterograde tracer transport study. *J. Neurosci.* 2:604–622.

12 Development of the Tectofugal Visual System of Normal and Deprived Zebra Finches

Kathrin Herrmann and Hans-Joachim Bischof

Extensive studies in the mammalian visual system have demonstrated that the specificity of connections that characterizes the adult nervous system results from a complicated interplay between genetic and environmental influences early in an animal's life. Important insights into the problem of visual system development came from the studies of Hubel and Wiesel, who demonstrated that monocular deprivation and other manipulations of the rearing conditions during early infancy profoundly influence the morphological and physiological development of the geniculocortical pathway of mammals (review in Wiesel, 1982). To determine whether similar processes played a role in the development of the avian visual system, we examined the effects of monocular and binocular deprivation on the normal development of the visual system of zebra finches.

We chose the zebra finch (*Taeniopygia guttata castanotis*) because it is an altricial species, born very immature with closed eyes, after an in ovo period of only 13 days, so that most of its visual system development takes place posthatching. An ethological study of the ontogeny of visual function suggested that young birds do not react to visual stimuli before day 10, which is 4 or 5 days after eye opening (Bischof and Lassek, 1985).

In zebra finches, as in many other avian species (e.g., chickens, pigeons), the eyes are situated laterally, so that the binocular visual field is rather narrow ($\pm$ 15°, Bischof, 1988), relative to the monocular field (about 150°). These size differences of the binocular and monocular visual fields are correlated with differences in the relative size of the tectofugal and thalamofugal visual systems, which have been thought to process information about the unilateral and bilateral visual fields, respectively (but see chapter 8). The thalamofugal system has been homologized with the geniculostriate system of mammals; the tectofugal system has been assumed to correspond to the mammalian extrageniculostriate system (Nauta and Karten, 1970). Our studies focused on the development of the tectofugal system because of its extensive size in this lateral-eyed species.

Previous anatomical studies have shown that the tectofugal system conveys information from the retina via the tectum opticum to the nucleus rotundus of the thalamus and thence to a telencephalic nucleus, the ectostriatum (Benowitz and Karten, 1976; Nixdorf and Bischof, 1982). Because the optic nerve crosses completely in the optic chiasm, it was originally assumed that the tectofugal pathway processes information exclusively from the contralateral eye (figure 12.1). However, there is evidence suggesting that tectofugal nuclei (rotundus, ectostriatum) may also process information from the ipsilateral retina. Physiological data demonstrate that the ectostriatum can be driven by stimulation of either eye (Engelage and Bischof, 1988, 1990; this volume), although up to now there are no reports of truly binocular neurons in any tectofugal nucleus. There are at least three sources for such input: the projection from the visual wulst back to the tectum opticum (Bagnoli et al., 1980), the tectotectal projection (Robert and Cuenod,

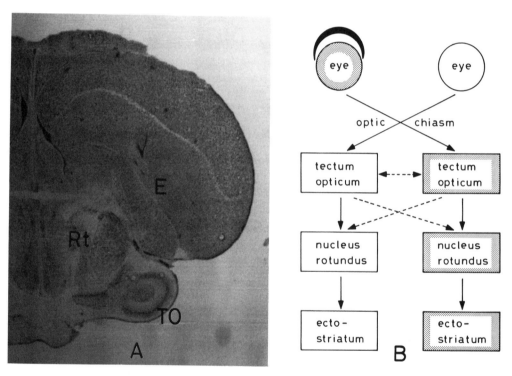

Figure 12.1 (A) Nissl-stained cross section through the right hemisphere of a zebra finch brain, showing the main stations of the tectofugal visual pathway: retinal axons (Ret) enter superficial layers of the contralateral tectum opticum (TO). Visual information is then processed to deeper tectal layers. From there, visual information in transferred via the nucleus rotundus in the thalamus (Rt) to the telencephalic way-station of this pathway, the ectostriatum (E). (B) Due to the complete crossing of the optic nerve in the optic chiasm, monocular deprivation in birds creates a "deprived" hemisphere contralateral to the closed eye (graphically depicted by shading). The stippled lines, however, show interhemispheric projections that seem to be of much greater importance than previously expected. From Herrmann and Bischof (1986b).

1969; Bischof and Niemann, 1990), and the projection from the tectum opticum to the contralateral nucleus rotundus (Benowitz and Karten, 1976; Bischof and Niemann, 1990, figure 12.1B). A transient ipsilateral retinotectal connection, which has been demonstrated in chicks (O'Leary et al., 1983) and in pigeons (Bagnoli et al., 1983) is not detectable in adult birds and thus cannot be a source for the input from the ipsilateral eye.

It is, therefore, not improbable that binocular interactions are possible in all three relays of the tectofugal pathway. This is an important possibility, since, in mammals, deprivation-induced changes in visual system development have been attributed almost exclusively to unbalanced binocular competition (e.g., Wiesel and Hubel, 1965; Hubel et al., 1988; Guillery, 1972). The data presented in this chapter demonstrate that, as in mammals, monocular deprivation does effect the anatomical development of tectofugal nuclei, and that most of these effects are best interpreted as effects of a crosstalk of the tectofugal systems of both sides of the brain.

NORMAL DEVELOPMENT OF THE NUCLEUS ROTUNDUS AND THE ECTOSTRIATUM

Nucleus Rotundus

The nucleus rotundus is the largest thalamic area in adult zebra finches, with a volume of about 0.4 mm^3. At birth, however, its volume comprises only one-fifth of the adult volume. Nucleus rotundus quadruples in size between birth and day 10, and by day 20 it is significantly (ca. 20%) larger than in adults.

The development of individual rotundal neurons shows a similar pattern, i.e., an increase in size between birth and day 20 followed by a reduction until adulthood (figure 12.2a). Myelination of axons within the nucleus starts between days 5 and 10, and the adult pattern is achieved between days 20 and 40 (Herrmann and Bischof, 1986a). Electron microscopic data indicate that the density of synapses, as well as the size of the presynaptic terminals, increase steadily between hatching and day 20, the largest increase in synapse density occurring between days 5 and 10, around the time of eye opening (Nixdorf and Bischof, 1986).

Ectostriatum

The development of zebra finch ectostriatum (figure 12.2a) follows a time course similar to that of rotundus. Cell size increases between birth and day 20 and decreases thereafter. The myelination process of ectostriatal axons starts slightly later than in rotundus, between days 10

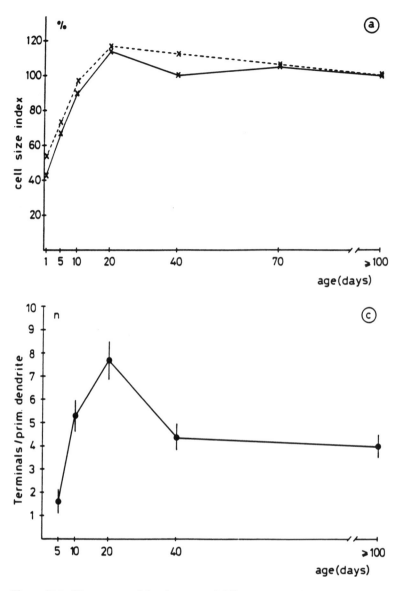

Figure 12.2 Time course of development of different neuronal elements. (a) Neuron size (% of adult values). Stippled line, ectostriatum; full line, n. rotundus. After Herrmann and Bischof (1986a). (b–d) Ectostriatal measurements. (b) Average radius of dendritic field. (c) Branching index: number of terminal dendritic segments per primary dendrite.

Development of the Avian Visual System

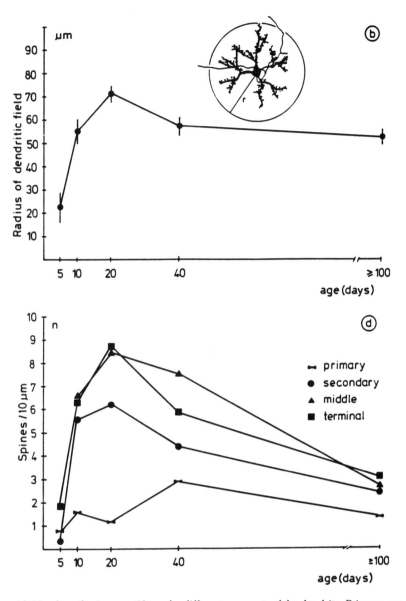

(d) Number of spines per 10 μm for different segments of the dendrite. Primary, segments directly adjacent to the cell body; secondary, segments following the primary ones; terminal, end segments of each dendrite; medial, segments that were not primary or terminal. After Herrmann and Bischof (1988a).

and 20, adult myelin density being achieved by 40 days (Herrmann and Bischof, 1986a).

Using the Golgi-impregnation technique, which stains not only cell bodies but also their axons and dendrites, we have followed the morphological development of ectostriatal neurons. The major neuron type in this structure resembles the spiny stellate cell of mammalian neocortex, with a soma diameter of about 15 μm and three to five radially oriented primary dendrites. Each dendrite branches three or four times and bears a significant number of dendritic spines of different morphology. The dendrites extend about 55 μm from the soma but never leave the ectostriatum. Axons could be traced in some preparations as far as 100 μm. They sometimes arborize, and single axon collaterals could be traced into the paleostriatum or the neostriatum (Herrmann and Bischof, 1988b). The same neuron type has been reported for the ectostriatum of chicken (Tömböl et al., 1988) and quail (Watanabe et al., 1988).

Figure 12.3 illustrates selected examples of the development of the main ectostriatal neuron type. The most rapid development occurs between days 5 and 10, at the time of eye opening. Neurons of 5-day-old finches are typically undifferentiated cells, with irregularly thickened, short dendrites bearing growth cones and filopodia. Between days 5 and 10 there is a tremendous growth spurt, reflected in increasing soma diameter, the growth and bifurcation of dendrites, and the occurrence of numerous thin dendritic spines. Between days 10 and 20 there is a further increase in dendritic length and branching frequency. After day 20, a substantial reduction in dendritic length, branching frequency, and the number of spines can be detected.

A quantitative analysis of these parameters was carried out and the results are plotted in figure 12.2b–d. Taken together there seems to be a good correlation between cell size, nucleus volume, dendritic field size, number of branch points, and number of dendritic spines. All these parameters show an increase between birth and day 20, followed by a decrease to adulthood. Thus early neuronal development in the zebra finch, as in other birds and mammals, is characterized by both proliferative and regressive phenomena (see, e.g., Changeux and Danchin, 1976; Herrmann and Bischof, 1986a).

The transient overproduction of neuronal elements is often interpreted as providing conditions under which selection processes can eliminate nonfunctional synapses while stabilizing functional ones. The model, however, implies the existence of competitive processes that have not been thus far demonstrated directly for the tectofugal system. Indirect evidence, however, indicates that binocular competition may be possible in the ectostriatum. Engelage and Bischof (1988) have recently shown that ipsilaterally evoked visual potentials could be recorded as acutely enucleated zebra finches, suggesting that there may

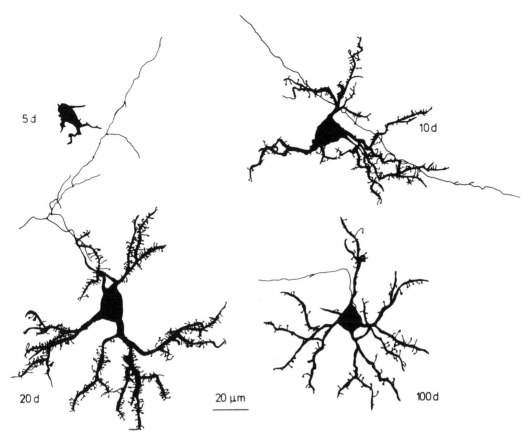

Figure 12.3 Typical examples of ectostriatal neurons at postnatal days 5, 10, 20, and 100. The most pronounced growth spurt occurs between days 5 and 10, right around the time of eye opening. From Herrmann and Bischof (1988b).

indeed be binocular interaction, which is difficult to detect under normal conditions (see chapter 8).

Against this background, then, the remainder of the chapter examines the effects of monocular deprivation on the retina and the tectofugal pathway.

EFFECTS OF MONOCULAR DEPRIVATION

Retina

It is now well established that monocular deprivation in birds, as in mammals, causes a substantial elongation in the anterior-posterior length of the eyeball accompanied by a major myopia (Bagnoli et al., 1985; Wiesel and Raviola, 1977; Yinon et al., 1982, 1983). Surprisingly, however, in pigeons, the only avian species studies thus far, electroretinograms (ERGs) evoked by presentation of alternating gratings to the deprived and nondeprived eyes were not different in amplitude (Bagnoli et al., 1985).

The ERG is generated by sources other than retinal ganglion cells and probably reflects the activity of cells in the inner nuclear layer of the retina (Bagnoli et al., 1984). To see whether and to what extent retinal ganglion cells were affected by monocular deprivation, we deprived zebra finches from birth to 20, 40, or 100 days. We examined retinal ganglion cells in two locations: in the fovea, where they are known to be small and densely packed, and in the far periphery, where they are larger and loosely packed (figure 12.4). The results show that retinal ganglion cells in both the fovea and the periphery are only marginally affected by monocular deprivation. If changes were seen, they were in the direction opposite from what might be predicted, i.e., retinal ganglion cells were lightly larger in the *deprived* eye. While more detailed morphological data and physiological studies are needed, the evidence

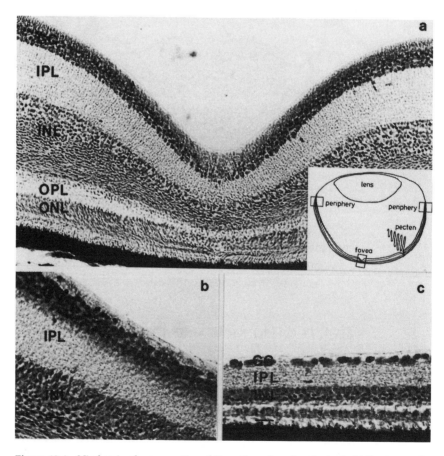

Figure 12.4 Nissl-stained cross section of the retina of a zebra finch. (a, b) Sections right through the fovea centralis; (c) a section through the periphery, as shown in the inset of (a). Note the difference in the size and density of retinal ganglion cells in (b, fovea) and (c, periphery).

Development of the Avian Visual System

to date suggests that retinal ganglion cells are more or less unaffected by deprivation. Thus the more central changes seen after monocular deprivation are not due to the effects of peripheral atrophy but reflect effects on central processes.

Thalamofugal System

While much known about the mechanisms mediating monocular deprivation effects on the mammalian geniculocortical pathway, surprisingly little is known about deprivation effects on the visual Wulst, the avian homologue of area 17. Pettigrew and Konishi (1976) were the first to demonstrate that neurons in the owl Wulst respond to monocular deprivation in a manner similar to that of neurons in mammalian visual cortex. Almost all neurons recorded from had lost their binocularity and could be driven only monocularly by the nondeprived eye. Correlated with this loss of binocularity was a morphological change. Whereas ocular dominance columns are not seen in normal owls, they seem to appear after monocular deprivation, forming stripes running orthogonal to the vertical meridian as in mammals (Pettigrew and Gynther, 1990).

Bagnoli and co-workers demonstrated that monocular visual deprivation produced changes in the neurotransmitter phenotypes of neurons in visual Wulst. These included a loss of GAD activity and an increase in ChAT activity in the dorsolateral Wulst contralateral to the deprived eye, as well as a decrease in the endogenous level of norepinephrine in the ipsilateral hemisphere (Bagnoli et al., 1982, 1983).

Nucleus Rotundus and Ectostriatum: Anatomical Effects

In these experiments deprivation began on the first or second day of life (when the eyes were still closed) by covering one eye (left or right) with an eye cap, just like for the measurements of retinal ganglion cells. The deprivation was maintained until the day of sacrifice on day 20, 40, or 100 (adulthood), so that the birds actually never saw with the occluded eye. Cell size and volume of the nucleus rotundus and ectostriatum were measured in Nissl-stained sections and compared to normally reared birds of the same age (Herrmann and Bischof 1986b,c).

Deprivation during the first 20 days of life did not result in morphological differences between the deprived and the nondeprived rotundus or ectostriatum. In contrast, following eye closure for a longer period (40 or >100 days), neurons in the deprived hemisphere were about 15% smaller than in the contralateral, nondeprived hemisphere. However, when the data of the deprived birds were compared to age-matched normally reared zebra finches, there were several unexpected findings.

As figure 12.5 shows, both rotundal and ectostriatal cell sizes of 20-day-old deprived birds are about 10% larger than those of normal birds.

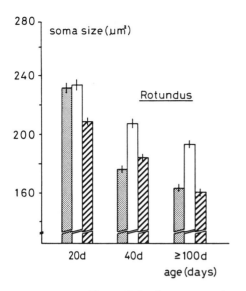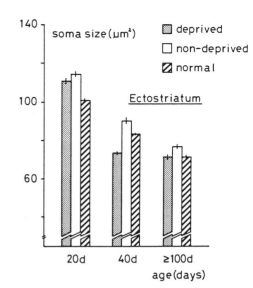

Figure 12.5 Comparison of the mean cross-sectional areas of neurons in the nucleus rotundus (a) and ectostriatum (b) of normal and monocularly deprived zebra finches of different ages. Gray bars, cell size in the deprived hemisphere (i.e., contralateral to the deprived eye); open bars, cell size in the nondeprived hemisphere (contralateral to the open eye); hatched bars, cell size of normal control birds (from Herrmann and Bischof, 1986b,c).

Also, the observed left-right asymmetry after 40 or 100 days of monocular deprivation must be attributed to a hypertrophy of neurons in the nondeprived rotundus, not to a shrinkage in the deprived hemisphere: neurons in n. rotundus and ectostriatum contralateral to the deprived eye are not statistically different from normal controls, while the neurons of n. rotundus and ectostriatum driven by the nondeprived eye are larger than those in controls. Thus, the effects of monocular deprivation are biphasic. Short-term deprivation leads to an "unselective" growth of neurons in both hemispheres. A longer deprivation period, however, causes the neurons driven by the deprived eye to shrink to a size that is also observed in normal animals. In contrast, the neurons driven by the nondeprived eye remain hypertrophied as they were with 20 days of deprivation. These effects of monocular deprivation can be shown not only for the neuron size within n. rotundus and ectostriatum, but also for the total volume of nucleus rotundus.

Our data indicate that there must be some crosstalk between the tectofugal system of both sides of the brain: the hemisphere driven by the nondeprived eye obviously also responds to deprivation and must therefore gain the information that the other hemisphere is deprived. Likely sources of this interhemispheric transfer are the tectotectal, the tectocontralateral rotundal, or the Wulst-tectum projections (see Engelage and Bischof, this volume). By these connections information from both eyes could meet in both sides of the brain.

Guillery and Stelzner (1970) and Guillery (1972) found in the cat that cell size of neurons in the monocular segment of the LGN is less affected by monocular deprivation compared to that of neurons of the binocular lamina. This can be interpreted as to show that cell size changes occur only if there is competitive interaction between the inputs from both eyes. Our results can be interpreted accordingly: Cell size changes due to monucular deprivation can be observed in areas where, by connections between the two brain sides, binocular interaction (and competition) is possible. The retina and the outer layers of the tectum, which do not have input from the nondeprived ipsilateral hemisphere, do not show effects.

Monocular deprivation also affects ultrastructural parameters in nucleus rotundus. The size of the presynaptic terminals is significantly reduced in both hemispheres after deprivation from birth to day 20 and stays low in the deprived hemisphere, if deprivation is maintained into adulthood. In addition, synapse density was much higher in the deprived hemisphere (Nixdorf and Bischof, 1987). These changes in ultrastructural parameters should be reflected in dendritic parameters like dendritic length or branching frequency. To our surprise, this was not the case for the ectostriatum. However, monocular deprivation did not have an effect on either dendritic length or branching frequency of the main ectostriatal neuron type. Both parameters paralleled the normal development, were at a maximum at 20 days, and declined until adulthood. We found, however, that monocular deprivation interfered with the development of dendritic spines. In zebra finches deprived for at least 40 days, neurons in the deprived hemisphere bear significantly fewer spines than those in the nondeprived hemisphere. This interhemispheric difference is mainly due to a lack of the normally occurring spine reduction in the nondeprived hemisphere, rather than to spine loss in the deprived hemisphere. We can conclude this because in comparison with normally reared birds, spine density is not lower in the deprived hemisphere, but rather is higher in the nondeprived brain side (figure 12.6). The excess of spines can be interpreted as a retention of a juvenile status, and might reflect a longer susceptibility to environmental changes. Another speculation might be that the amount of processed stimuli positively correlates with the number of spines. It could be argued that the nondeprived hemisphere has to compensate the lack of information in the hemisphere driven by the deprived eye and therefore retains more spines. These two hypotheses must not be mutually exclusive but rather the cause and consequence of the same process.

In any case, these results again point directly to interhemispheric interactions. As mentioned earlier, in contrast to the thalamofugal system, neither binocular neurons nor competitive interactions have been described before. Tectotectal as well as tectorotundal interhemispheric projections, however, indicate that such interactions between the two brain sides are possible. It can also not be excluded that then normally

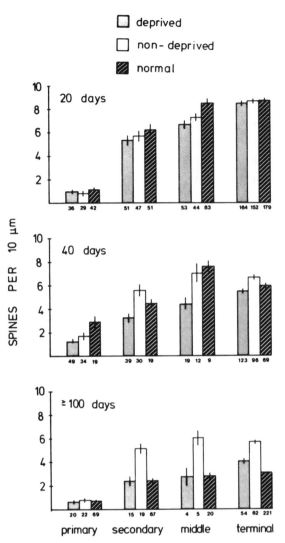

Figure 12.6 Spine density of neurons in the ectostriatum of zebra finches deprived from birth to day 20 (upper), 40 (middle), and >100 days of age (bottom). Bars represent median values + SEM for various dendritic segments (primary, secondary, middle, terminal). Gray bars, spine density in the deprived hemisphere (i.e., contralateral to the deprived eye); open bars, spine density in the nondeprived hemisphere (contralateral to the open eye); hatched bars, spine density of normally reared birds. Differences in spine density between deprived and nondeprived hemisphere occur only after 40 days of deprivation and manifest themselves basically in an excess of spines in the nondeprived hemisphere. Spine density in the deprived hemisphere appears to be normal (see data in bottom row; from Herrmann and Bischof, 1988b).

transient ipsilateral retinotectal projection might be maintained as a result of monocular deprivation, as it was demonstrated in enucleation studies in chickens (O'Leary et al., 1983). However, our preliminary findings that cell size is not altered by monocular deprivation in the outer tectal layers indicate that this is not a likely explanation.

Nucleus Rotundus and Ectostriatum: Functional Effects

To determine whether the deprivation-induced morphological changes discussed above might have functional correlates, we used the 2-deoxy-glucose (2DG) method. This technique identifies differential activity in various brain areas by measuring the accumulation of a radioactively tagged glucose marker as an index of the energy utilization, and hence the functional involvement, of these areas.

For this study, zebra finches were monocularly deprived from birth to adulthood. The day before the 2DG experiment the eyecaps were taken off, and the birds were allowed to see with both eyes while being exposed to the 2DG. The results were not surprising: despite the fact that the birds were now seeing binocularly, both the nucleus rotundus and the ectostriatum showed a tremendous asymmetry in the optical density: in the hemisphere contralateral to the deprived eye, the glucose consumption and therefore the activity was drastically lower than in the nondeprived hemisphere (Herrmann and Bischof, 1986b, figure 12.7). Nonvisual areas like the telencephalic auditory field were symmetrically labeled. It is likely that the asymmetry in the nucleus rotundus and the ectostriatum is due to a decrease of activity in the deprived

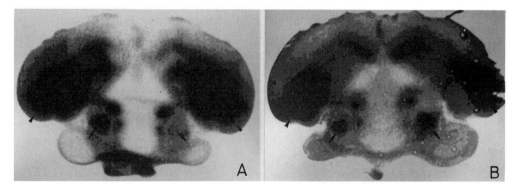

Figure 12.7 Computer-generated densitometric plot of 2-deoxyglucose autoradiography. (A) Cross section of the brain of a zebra finch that was monocularly deprived from birth to day 100, and stimulated binocularly during the 2DG experiment. Nucleus rotundus (arrow) and ectostriatum (arrowhead) are asymmetrically labeled. The deprived (right) hemisphere shows weaker labeling in both areas. In contrast, (B) shows a cross section of the brain of a bird that was deprived for the same length of time but as adult. 2DG labeling of both nucleus rotundus and ectostriatum is symmetrical in both hemispheres, indicating that monocular deprivation in adult birds does not lead to metabolic changes in these tectofugal areas.

hemisphere, because we know from experiments with intact birds that nucleus rotundus and ectostriatum are usually heavily labeled and stand out in 2DG experiments. This was not he case in the deprived hemisphere of our experimental animals.

In contrast to these results, however, Burkhalter et al., (1982) reported no asymmetries in 2DG activity in the tectofugal pathway of pigeons after monocular deprivation. While there are a number of methodological differences between the studies that might explain the discrepancy, it may also reflect species differences between pigeons and zebra finches. Güntürkün and Böhringer (1987) found that the tectum opticum of normally reared pigeons shows hemispheric differences (see also chapter 13), a phenomenon that is absent in zebra finches (Herrmann, unpublished observations). This asymmetry in normal pigeons might of course interfere with structural changes arising after monocular deprivation. At present we do not know whether the pigeons studied by Burkhalter et al., (1982) were consistently deprived on either the left or the right eye, but it is possible that the morphological asymmetry in pigeons might explain the absence of effects in the 2DG study of these animals.

THE SENSITIVE PERIOD FOR THE DEPRIVATION EFFECTS

In recent years a large body of literature has accumulated showing that the nervous system is susceptible to manipulations only during a brief time early in an animal's life, the so-called sensitive or critical period (Blakemore and VanSluyters, 1974; Hubel and Wiesel, 1970; Knudsen and Knudsen, 1986; Olsen and Freeman, 1980). We therefore wanted to establish whether such a sensitive period also existed for the effects of monocular deprivation in zebra finches. Using the 2DG method we deprived adult zebra finches for the same length of time as the neonates in the experiment mentioned above (for 100 days) and found that this late deprivation did not result in any asymmetric labeling of nucleus rotundus and ectostriatum as seen in developing animals (Herrmann and Bischof, 1986b, figure 7b). This suggests that during a critical period of development, birds were susceptible to deprivation manipulations to which adults, with fully differentiated nervous systems, are immune.

To explore the time course of this sensitive period for the effects of monocular deprivation, we measured cell size and volume changes in zebra finches subjected to a period of 40 days of unilateral eye closure (the time, when all deprivation effects seem to be stable) starting at ages spaced regularly throughout the first 70 days of life, i.e., we deprived birds from days 1 to 40, 10 to 50, etc. until days 70 to 110.

The result of this study (Herrmann and Bischof, 1988a) shows that monocular deprivation markedly affects cell size of nucleus rotundus and ectostriatum if the treatment starts at 1 or 10 days post hatching. The differences between deprived and nondeprived hemisphere decreased with increasing visual experience prior to deprivation. Surprisingly to us, however, was that deprivation onset at day 40 caused again as severe effects as early monocular closure. Deprivation starting at day 50 or later, on the other hand, did no longer lead to abnormalities.

The measurements of the rotundus volume parallel the cell size results, with the exception that the second increase in sensitivity occurred at day 50 instead of day 40 (figure 12.8). Taken together, these results indicate that the sensitive period for the effects of monocular deprivation may be double-peaked: the sensitivity to external stimuli declines from hatch until day 30, but has another peak at 40—50 days of life. Therefore we can conclude that a period of normal vision prior to deprivation reduces the sensitivity to anatomical and functional changes caused by deprivation. It is worth noticing that the first peak of sensitivity occurs at a time early in ontogeny, when both ectostriatum and nucleus rotundus are not fully developed: between hatching and day

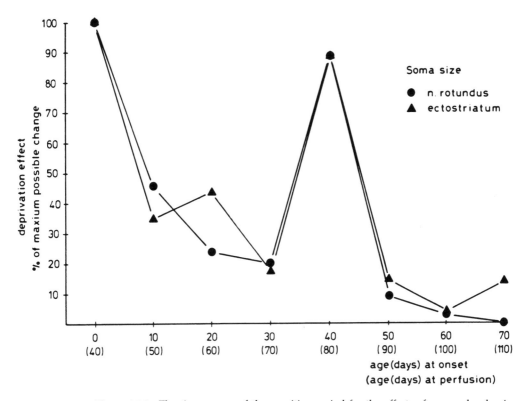

Figure 12.8 The time course of the sensitive period for the effects of monocular deprivation as derived from cell size measurements of rotundal and ectostriatal neurons. Birds were monocularly deprived for a constant period of 40 days starting at days 0, 10, 20, 30, 40, 50, 60, and 70, and sacrificed immediately after the deprivation period. The absolute difference between the soma size in the deprived and nondeprived hemisphere following neonatal eye closure for 40 days was set 100% (maximal possible change). The left–right differences in cell size following later deprivation onset were calculated with respect to this value.

Herrmann & Bischof: Development of the Tectofugal System

20 neurons grow, dendritic arbors increase in length and complexity, dendritic spines are being added, and synaptic contacts are still weak and probably modifiable. The peak of sensitivity seems to occur *before* the transient overshoot in all these parameters can be observed, and it would be interesting to find out whether the presence of redundant and superfluous neuronal elements allows plastic changes to occur.

At present we have no good explanation for the second rise in susceptibility at day 40, a time when the anatomical development of both nucleus rotundus and ectostriatum was thought to be completed. A study by Engelage and Bischof (1990) clearly demonstrated, however, that the physiological response pattern of neurons in the ectostriatum is not adultlike by day 30. Probably the second rise in susceptibility may be explained by late occurring projections, which weaken the previously established connections by competitive interactions. Interestingly, such a second rise in sensitivity after the end of the originally presumed sensitive period was also demonstrated in the LGN of primates (Headon et al., 1985). These authors, however, also did not provide an explanation. Thus further experiments will be needed to clarify the nature of this second peak.

BINOCULAR DEPRIVATION

Most effects of monocular deprivation in the tectofugal system arise in the hemisphere driven by the nondeprived eye, and these effects manifest themselves in a hypertrophy of cell size and volume, and an increased spine density. How would these parameters be affected if we deprived both eyes of vision? There are two arguments to suppose that binocular deprivation would not have any effect at all: first, if deprivation effects are due to an imbalance of the inputs from the two eyes to the competitive sites, one should not see an effect because both eyes are reduced in activity. Second, if the absence of effects in the deprived hemisphere, as demonstrated above, could be interpreted as to show that patterned visual input is not necessary for the establishment of these anatomical features, one could predict that binocular deprivation should have no effect at all. To test this hypothesis, we deprived zebra finches binocularly from birth until day 20 or 40, the age when deprivation effects were stable in monocularly deprived birds. As a first attempt, we measured cell size and volume of the nucleus rotundus and ectostriatum and compared those to normally reared birds of the same age.

As we predicted, the data of this study clearly demonstrated that binocular deprivation does not arrest neuron growth in the nucleus rotundus and the ectostriatum of zebra finches (figure 12.9). These results suggest that at least the anatomical development of tectofugal system can proceed in the total absence of patterned vision, although the possible physiological changes induced by binocular deprivation

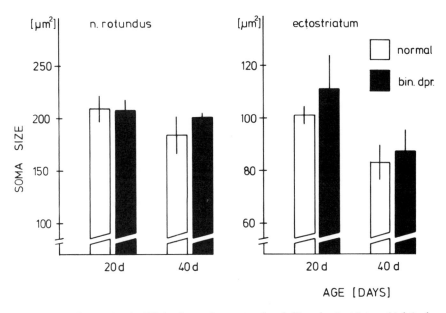

Figure 12.9 Soma size (+ SE) in the nucleus rotundus (left) and ectostriatum (right) of zebra finches that were binocularly deprived from birth until day 20 or 40, compared to age-matched normally reared control birds. Binocular deprivation does not lead to significant changes in neuron size of either area.

remain to be determined. It is also possible that in birds the exposure to light in ovo is sufficient to induce the normal course of development. A study in dark-reared primates has shown that even short periods of light are sufficient to trigger the normal cell differentiation process (Chow, 1955). The importance of light in ovo was established by Rogers and co-workers and will be reviewed in another chapter of this volume.

CONCLUSIONS

In this chapter we provided extensive evidence that both the tectofugal and the thalamofugal system of birds are susceptible to visual deprivation. We have shown that monocular deprivation affects cell size, volume, and spine density in the nucleus rotundus and the ectostriatum, and these effects are mainly due to a hypertrophy (or failure to decline) of these neuronal elements on the nondeprived hemisphere, whereas the hemisphere driven by the deprived eye seems more or less unaffected. We are far away from understanding the underlying cellular mechanisms that lead to these changes. We believe, however, that the morphological and physiological abnormalities in the tectofugal pathway, traditionally thought to be strictly monocular, have to be interpreted as a result of an imbalance of binocular interactions, and we speculate on the anatomical substrate for these interhemispheric interactions.

REFERENCES

Bagnoli, P., Grassi, S. and Magni, F. A direct connection between the visual wulst and the tectum opticum in the pigeon (*Columbia livia*) demonstrated by horseradish peroxidase. *Arch. Ital. Biol.* 118 (1980), 72–80.

Bagnoli, P., Burkhalter, A., Visher, A., Henke, H., and Cuenod, M. Effects of monocular deprivation in choline acetyltransferase and glutamic acid decarboxylase in the pigeon visual wulst. *Brain Res.* 247 (1982), 289–302.

Bagnoli, P. Barselotti, R., Pelegrini, M. and Alesci, R. Norepinephrine levels in developing pigeon brain: Effect of monocular deprivation on the wulst noradrenergic system. *Dev. Brain Res.* 10 (1983), 243–250.

Bagnoli, P., Porciatti, V., Francesconi, W., and Barsellotti, R. Pigeon pattern electroretinogram: A response unaffected by chronic section of the optic nerve. *Exp. Brain Res.* 55 (1984), 253–262.

Bagnoli, P., Porciatti, V., and Francesconi, W. Retinal and tectal responses to alternate gratings are unaffected by monocular deprivation in pigeons. *Brain Res.* 338 (1985), 341–345.

Benowitz, L., and Karten, H. J. Organization of the tectofugal pathway in the pigeon: A retrograde transport study. *J. Comp. Neurol.* 167 (1976), 503–520.

Bischof, H. J. The visual field and visually guided behavior in the zebra finch. *J. Comp. Physiol. A* 163 91988), 329–337.

Bischof, H. J., and Lassek, R. The gaping reaction and the development of fear in young zebra finches (*Taeniopygia guttata castanotis*). *Z. Tierphysiol.* 69 (1985), 55–65.

Bischof, H. J., and Niemann, J. Contralateral projections of the tectum opticum in the zebra finch (*Taeniopygia guttata castanotis*). *Cell Tissue Res.* 262 (1990), 307–313.

Blakemore, C., and VanSluyters, R. C. Reversal of the physiological effects of monocular deprivation in kittens: Further evidence for a sensitive period. *J. Physiol.* 237 (1974), 195–216.

Burkhalter, A., Streit, P., Bagnoli., Visher, A., Henke, H., and Cuenod, M. Deprivation induced functional modification in the pigeon visual system. In C. Ajmone Marsan, and H. Matthies, (Eds.), *Neuronal Plasticity and Memory Formation.* Raven Press, New York, 1982, pp. 477–485.

Changeux, J. P., and Danchin, A. Selective stabilization of developing synapses as a mechanism for the specification of neuronal networks. *Nature (London)* 264 (1976), 705–712.

Chow, K. L. Failure to demonstrate changes in the visual system of monkeys kept in darkness or in coloured lights. *J. Comp. Neurol.* 102 (1955), 597–606.

Engelage, J., and Bischof, H. J. Enucleation enhances ipsilateral flash evoked potentials in the ectostriatum of the zebra finch (*Taeniopygia guttata castanotis* Gould). *Exp. Brain Res.* 70 (1988), 79–89.

Engelage, J., and Bischof, H. J. Development of flash evoked responses in the ectostriatum of the zebra finch: An evoked potential and current source density analysis. *Vis. Neurosci.* 5 (1990), 241–248.

Guillery, R. W. Binocular competition in the control of geniculate cell growth. *J. Comp. Neurol.* 144 (1972), 117–127.

Guillery, R. W., and Stelzner, D. J. The differential effects of unilateral lid closure upon the monocular and binocular segments in the dorsal geniculate nucleus in the cat. *J. Comp. Neurol.* 139 (1970), 413–422.

Güntürkün, O., and Böhringer, P. Lateralization reversal after intertectal comissurectomy in the pigeon. *Brain Res.* 408 (1987), 1–5.

Headon, M. P., Sloper, J. J., Hirons, R. W., and Powell, R. P. S. Effect of monocular closure at different ages on deprived and undeprived cells in the primate lateral geniculate. *Dev. Brain Res.* 18 (1985), 57–68.

Herrmann, K., and Bischof, H. J. Delayed development of song control nuclei in the zebra finch is related to behavioral development. *J. Comp. Neurol.* 245 (1986a), 167–175.

Herrmann, K., and Bischof, H. J. Effects of monocular deprivation in the nucleus rotundus of zebra finches: A Nissl and deoxyglucose study. *Exp. Brain Res.* 64 (1986b), 119–126.

Herrmann, K., and Bischof, H. J. Monocular deprivation affects neuron size in the ectostriatum of the zebra finch brain. *Brain Res.* 379 (1986c), 143–146.

Herrmann, K., and Bischof, H. J. The sensitive period for the morphological effects of monocular deprivation in two nuclei of the tectofugal pathway of zebra finches. *Brain Res.* 451 (1988a), 43–53.

Herrmann, K.,and Bischof, H. J. Development of neurons in the ectostriatum of normal and monocularly deprived zebra finches: A quantitative Golgi study. *J. Comp. Neurol.* 277 (1988b), 141–154.

Hubel, D. H., and Wiesel, T. N. The period of susceptibility to the physiological effects of unilateral eye closure in kittens. *J. Physiol. (London)* 208 (1970), 419–436.

Hubel, D. H., Wiesel, T. N., and Levay, S. Plasticity of ocular dominance columns in monkey striate cortex. *Phil. Trans. R. Soc. London B.* 278 (1977), 377–409.

Knudsen E. I., and Knudsen, P. F. The sensitive period for auditory localization in barn owls limited by age, not by experience. *J. Neurosci.* 6 (1986), 1918–1924.

Nauta, W. J. H., and Karten, H. J. A generale profile of the vertebrate brain with sidelights of an ancestry of the cerebral cortex. In F. O. Schmitt (Ed.), *The Neuroscience Second Study Program.* Rockefeller University Press, New York, 1970, pp. 7–26.

Nixdorf, B. E., and Bischof, H. J. Afferent connections of the ectostriatum and the visual wulst in the zebra finch (*Taeniopygia guttata castanotis* Gould): an HRP-study. *Brain Res.* 248 (1982), 9–17.

Nixdorf, B., and Bischof, H. J. Posthatching development of synapses in the neuropil of nucleus rotundus of the zebra finch: A quantitative electron microscopic study. *J. Comp. Neurol.* 250 (1986), 133–139.

Nixdorf, B., and Bischof, H. J. Ultrastructural effects of monocular deprivation in the neuropil of nucleus rotundus in the zebra finch: A quantitative electron microscopic study. *Brain Res.* 405 (1987), 326–336.

O'Leary, D. D. M., Gerten, C. R., and Cowan, C. M. The development and restriction of the ipsilateral retinotectal projection in the chick. *Dev. Brain Res.* 10 (1983), 93–109.

Olsen, C. R., and Freeman, R. D. Profile of the sensitive period for monocular deprivation in kittens. *Exp. Brain Res.* 39 (1980), 17–21.

Pettigrew, J. D., and Gynther, I. C. Dendritic changes in granule cells of owl visual cortex following visual deprivation. *Soc. Neurosci. Abs.* (1990), 474.

Pettigrew, J., and Konishi, M. Effects of monocular deprivation on binocular neurons in the owl's visual wulst. *Nature (London)* 264 (1976), 753–754.

Robert, F., and Cuenod, M. Electrophysiology of the intertectal commissures in the pigeon. I. Analysis of the pathway. *Exp. Brain Res.* 9 (1969), 116–122.

Tömböl, T., Magloczky, Z., Steward, M. G., and Czillag, A. The structure of chicken ectostriatum. I. Golgi study, *J. Hirnforsch.* 29 (1988), 525–546.

Watanabe, M., Ito, H., and Ikushima, M. Cytoarchitecture and ultrastructure of the avian ectostriatum: afferent terminals from the dorsal telencephalon and some nuclei in the thalamus. *J. Comp. Neurol.* 236 (1985), 241–257.

Wiesel, T. N. Postnatal development of the visual cortex and the influence of environment. *Nature (London)* 299 (1982), 582–591.

Wiesel, T. N., and Hubel, D. H. Comparison of the effects of unilateral and bilateral closure on cortical unit responses in kittens. *J. Neurophysiol.* 28 (1965), 1029–1040.

Wiesel, T. N., and Raviola, E. Myopia and eye enlargement after neonatal lid fusion in monkeys. *Nature (London)* 266 (1977), 66–68.

Yinon, U., Koslowe, K. C., Lobel, D., Landshman, N., and Barishak, Y. R. Lid suture myopia in developing chicks: Optical and structural considerations. *Current Eye Res.* 2 (1982/83), 877–882.

13 Developmental Mechanisms of Lateralization

Lesley J. Rogers and Patrice Adret

Lateralization of function in the brain was first described for humans. It originally referred to specialization of one of the hemispheres to perform a particular function (e.g., control of speech by the left hemisphere), and to the consistency of this specialization across the majority of individuals. Lateralization is now known to be a well-developed characteristic of both mammalian and avian species (Bradshaw and Rogers, 1992). The earliest example of lateralization in the avian brain was for control of singing in songbirds (Nottebohm, 1977). Because the lateralization for control of song is consistent across all or most members of the same species, it can be considered as present at the species or population level. Other forms of lateralization in animals, for example, preferential paw use in mice (Collins, 1985), are present in individuals but without a consistent bias of direction in the population. Most examples of lateralization in birds have been found to occur at both the individual and population levels. Many of them involve the processing of visual inputs, and much of the data comes from studies using the chicken, *Gallus gallus domesticus*.

LATERALIZATION OF VISUALLY CONTROLLED BEHAVIOR IN BIRDS

Evidence from a variety of tasks suggests that the left and right hemispheres of the chicken forebrain are specialized to control different functions and that they undergo different time-courses of development. For example, administration of cycloheximide or glutamate to the left hemisphere of male or female chicks on day 2 post hatching results in slower learning to discriminate grains from a background of small pebbles, and an increase in the frequency of attack and copulation behavior, but similar treatment of the right hemisphere does not affect these behaviors (Rogers, 1986). These behavioral changes are long-lasting (possibly permanent), which suggests that the drugs disrupt development of the left hemisphere during a critical stage of its differentiation (for mode of action see Hambley and Rogers, 1979). The right and left hemispheres have also been shown to play different roles during the consolidation of imprinting memory (Cipolla-Neto et al., 1982) and during memory formation of a passive avoidance task (Rose, 1991). These instances of behavioral lateralization are correlated with lateralized changes at subcellular and neurochemical levels (e.g., McCabe et al., 1988; Stewart, 1991). In male chicks, functional lateralization of the hemispheres, as manifested by superior monocular performance with the right eye, has been demonstrated for several types of visual discrimination tasks (e.g., Gaston and Gaston, 1984; Mench and Andrew, 1986; see also Andrew and Dharmaretnam, 1991, and chapter 18). Comparable effects have been demonstrated in adult pigeons, including lateralization of visual discrimination performance and pecking rate during feeding (von Fersen and Güntürkün, 1990; Güntürkün, 1985; Güntürkün and Kesch, 1987).

Because there is virtually complete decussation of the optic tracts in most birds, the reported superiority of the right eye for acquisition and retention of visual discrimination tasks has often been interpreted as implying left hemisphere specialization for this type of learning. However, this interpretation should be made with caution, since the organization of the avian visual system provides ample opportunities for binocular processing of ipsilateral visual inputs (see chapters 8 and 11). Moreover, while the lateralization of discrimination learning and retention in pigeons closely parallels that of the young chick, left–right eye differences are no longer present in male chicks tested at 3 weeks of age (Rogers, 1991), and so it apparently does not persist into adulthood, as it does in the pigeon. Nevertheless, the ubiquity of lateralization for visual discrimination and other behaviors (for details see Bradshaw and Rogers, 1993, chapter 2) in the chick is striking, and this chapter reviews what is known about its ontogeny and neural correlates.

EFFECT OF LIGHT INPUT PRIOR TO HATCHING ON LATERALIZATION OF BRAIN FUNCTION

The chick embryo is oriented in the egg such that, during the later stages of incubation, it occludes its left eye with its body leaving the right eye positioned to receive light input entering the egg through the shell and penetrating its translucent eyelids. In addition, during the later stages of incubation the right eye is frequently opened, particularly in response to auditory and tactile stimulation (Gottlieb, 1968; Vince and Toosey, 1980), and during this period the hen frequently stands up to inspect the eggs or leaves the nest temporarily. Both behaviors would expose the embryos to light. It is during this same period that the visual connections to the forebrain become functional (Freeman and Vince, 1974). Thus, exposure of embryos in the egg to light will differentially stimulate visual structures connected to the right and left eyes, and could lead to advanced development of the neural circuits connected to the right eye.

A series of experiments from our laboratory has demonstrated that the functional lateralization of visual discrimination learning, attack and copulation in the chick brain are, at least in part, determined by this differential exposure of the left and right eyes to light prior to hatching (Rogers, 1982, 1990; Zappia and Rogers, 1983). Chicks hatched from eggs incubated in darkness for the last 3 days lack the lateralization of those behaviors normally unmasked by unilateral treatment of either the left or right hemisphere with cycloheximide. This effect on lateralization occurs irrespective of whether or not the embryos have been exposed to light prior to the last three days of incubation. Thus, in this precocial species, the last 3 days of embryonic development represent a sensitive period for development of lateralization in response to visual stimulation. Recently, Güntürkün (1990) demonstrated a role for light in establishing lateralization in pigeons, an altricial species.

It is possible to reverse the direction of functional lateralization by withdrawing the embryo's head from the egg on day 19/20 of incubation, occluding the right eye with black tape and allowing the left eye to receive light exposure (figure 13.1). However, while as little as 2

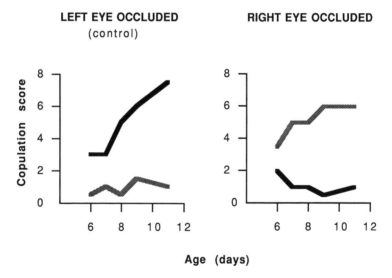

Figure 13.1 Lateralized light exposure and behavioral lateralization in chicks. Both groups had their heads withdrawn from the egg on day 19/20 of incubation; patches were applied to the left eye of controls and to the right eye of the experimentals, exposing the unoccluded eye to light. Following administration of glutamate into the left (black lines) or right (gray, dotted lines) hemisphere on day 2 post hatching, lateralization of copulation was scored according to a ranking scale from 1 to 10 in a standard hand-thrust test. In the control group the level of copulation was elevated following injection into the left hemisphere, and not the right. In the experimental group copulation was elevated following injection of glutamate into the right hemisphere, and not the left. Thus occlusion of the right eye on day 19/20 reversed the direction of lateralization. From Zappia and Rogers (1983).

Rogers & Adret: Developmental Mechanisms of Lateralization

hours of monocular light stimulation during the sensitive period is sufficient to organise the direction of lateralization, at least 6 hours of such stimulation is necessary to render it irreversible (Rogers, 1990).

An unexpected offshoot of these experiments was the finding of sex differences in lateralization. The lateralization effects of cycloheximide treatment on post-hatching day 2 was seen in both males and females, and reversal of its direction was equally possible in both sexes. Yet, males tested in their second week of life show lateralization of performance on the visual discrimination task when tested monocularly while females do not (Zappia and Rogers, 1987). Females tested monocularly in the visual discrimination task learn equally well with the left or right eye, and as well as they do when tested binocularly. This was the first indication that, although young females have lateralization at higher levels of brain organization, they may differ from males in the organization of the visual input pathways to these levels. These results led us to examine the development of visual structures of the chick's forebrain to determine whether the development of behavioral lateralization was paralleled by structural differences in the organization of the right and left hemispheres of the two sexes.

STRUCTURAL ASYMMETRY IN THE THALAMOFUGAL VISUAL PROJECTIONS

Using the fluorescent retrograde tracer True Blue (TB), we made injections into the telencephalic hyperstriatal areas that receive the thalamofugal visual projections, and compared the numbers of retrogradely labeled neurons in the ipsilateral and contralateral thalamic relay nuclei. Because it is impossible to control precisely the size of the injection, we could not compare absolute cell counts across subjects. We therefore used the ratio of the number of cells labeled contralaterally to the injection site to the number labeled ipsilaterally (C/I ratio), which was independent of the amount of dye injected (figure 13.2).

In both a domestic and a feral strain of male chicks, TB injections into the left hyperstriatum on day 2 post hatching resulted in lower C/I ratios than did injections into the right hyperstriatum (Rogers and Sink, 1988; Adret and Rogers; 1989). The use of C/I ratios, rather than absolute cell counts, precludes us from knowing whether this asymmetry in the thalamofugal visual projections of young males reflects a property of the ipsilateral or the contralateral projections, or indeed whether it is present in both projections. Nevertheless, higher C/I ratios following injection of the right side clearly indicate a more extensive projection from the left thalamic nuclei. As figure 13.3 illustrates, more ipsilateral and contralateral projections from the left side of the thalamus compared to the right would both lower the C/I ratio resulting from injection of the left side and raise the C/I ratio resulting from injection of the right. Using HRP labeling and absolute cell counts, Boxer and Stanford

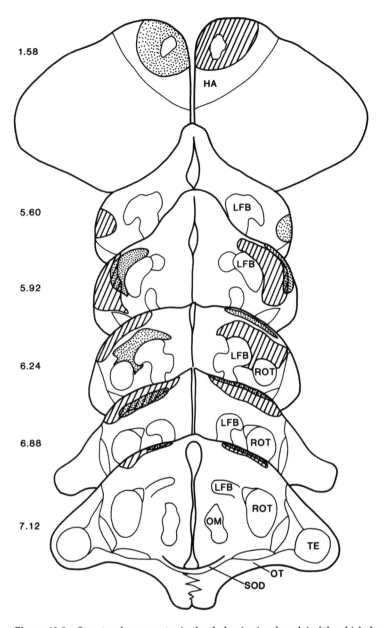

Figure 13.2 Structural asymmetry in the thalamic visual nuclei of the chick demonstrated by hyperstriatal injections of True Blue (dotted, left) and Fluoro-Gold (hatched, right). Transverse sections (40 μm) through the hyperstriatal region and the diencephalon at indicated distances (mm) from the rostral pole, illustrating the injection site (1.58) and the distribution of labeled cell bodies in the thalamus (5.60–7.12). Ipsilaterally projecting cell bodies (dotted on left and hatched on right) are more medial, skirting the lateral forebrain bundle and the nucleus rotundus and lying in the nucleus dorsolateralis anterior thalami, DLA. Contralaterally projecting cell bodies (hatched on left and dotted on right) are more superficially placed, within the dorsolateral thalamus (DLA). The area containing FG-labeled cells on the left side of the thalamus (contralateral to the FG injection site) is larger than that for the TB-labeled cells on the right side of the thalamus (contralateral to the TB injection site). HA, hyperstriatum accessorium; LFB, lateral forebrain bundle: ROT, nucleus rotundus; OM, occipito-mesencephalic tract; TE, tectum; OT, optic tract; SOD, supraoptic decussation.

Rogers & Adret: Developmental Mechanisms of Lateralization

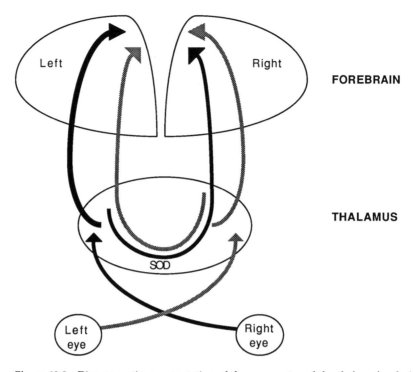

Figure 13.3 Diagrammatic representation of the asymmetry of the thalamofugal visual system in the young male chick. C/I = the ratio of the number of cell bodies in the thalamus labeled contralaterally (C) to the injection site to the number labeled ipsilaterally (I) to the same site. A lower left C/I ratio could reflect increased numbers of ipsilaterally projecting neurons from the left side of the thalamus to the forebrain (black line, left side), or more contralateral projections from this side of the thalamus to the right side of the forebrain (black line). Lateralization resulting from exposure to light prior to hatching could be due either to increased growth of the C and/or I projections from the left side, or to a reduction or the loss of some of these projections during development (see text for details). SOD, supraoptic decussation.

(1985) reported that the asymmetry is present in the contralateral projections. In our study, changes in the C/I ratios covaried significantly with the number of contralaterally labeled cells but not with the ipsilateral ones, which also suggests an asymmetry of the contralateral projections (see also, Rogers and Bolden, 1991). The most striking demonstration of structural asymmetry comes from a double labeling experiment with True Blue injections into the hyperstriatum on one side of the forebrain and Fluoro-Gold into the other. This permits measurement, within the same subject, of the contralateral and ipsilateral projections from each side of the thalamus to the hyperstriata on both sides of the forebrain. Significant asymmetry of the C/I ratios was found in male chicks of both domestic and feral strains injected with the dyes on day 2 post hatching.

As the models presented in figure 13.4 indicate, such asymmetries could reflect either differences in the actual numbers of thalamic pro-

MODEL A

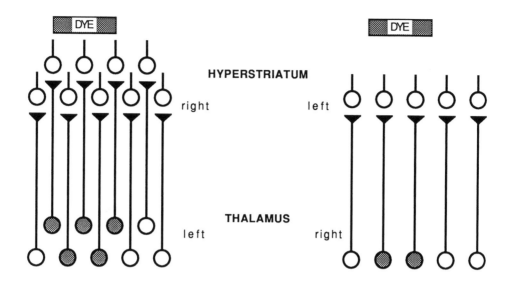

MODEL B

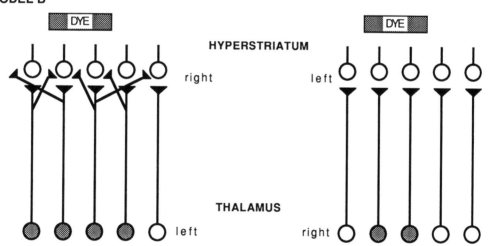

Figure 13.4 Two models of processes leading to asymmetry in the C/I ratios of thalamic visual projection neurons following lateralized exposure to light. Projections from each side of the thalamus to the hyperstriatum of the opposite telencephalon are illustrated. Dye is retrogradely transported to label thalamic cell bodies, and more cells are labeled on the left side of the thalamus. In model A there are more cell bodies that project their axons from thalamus to contralateral (right) hyperstriatum. On the right side of the thalamus there are fewer cells that project to the contralateral (left) hyperstriatum and so fewer cells are labeled. In model B, increased arborization of the axon terminals of these cells produces labeling of more cell bodies in the left side of the thalamus.

Rogers & Adret: Developmental Mechanisms of Lateralization

jection neurons or in the extent of their terminal arborization with in the hyperstriata, or both. That is, sensory information may be processed in a lateralized manner either at the level of the thalamus (figure 13.4A), or at the level of the visual hyperstriatum (figure 13.4B). Model A implies either a larger population of thalamorecipient target neurons in the right hyperstriatum, or that the number of target neurons in the hyperstriatum is the same on both sides but more convergence of inputs occurs on the right side. Model B postulates a greater divergence of visual input to the right hyperstriatum and consequently more integration of information on this side. Interestingly, the synaptic density per unit volume is significantly higher in the right than in the left hyperstriatum accessorium (HA) of 2-day-old male chicks (Stewart et al., 1992). While HA does not receive a direct thalamofugal projection, such inputs could originate in the known projections from adjacent hyperstriatal regions (Dubbeldam, 1991). Thus, an increased density of synapses in right HA may reflect either an increased number of thalamic projection neurons or more arborization of the end terminals of existing projections from the left thalamus to right visual telencephalon.

The enhanced development of projections from the left side of the thalamus (right eye) to the forebrain may account or the superior monocular visual (pebble/grain) discrimination performance by males using their right eye. Unfortunately, there is no independent evidence that the thalamofugal visual system is involved in this discrimination task. On the other hand, the possibility of light-dependant developmental asymmetry in the tectofugal visual system of the chick remains to be explored. An asymmetry with respect to cell size has been reported in the different layers of the pigeon tectum, and has been shown to depend on light stimulation of the embryo (Melsbach et al., 1991; Güntürkün, 1990).

SEX DIFFERENCE IN ASYMMETRY OF THE THALAMOFUGAL VISUAL PROJECTIONS

In contrast to the asymmetry characteristic of males, female chicks of the feral strain, treated in a similar manner, proved to have symmetry of these visual projections (Adret and Rogers, 1989). A recent study, which applied the more precise double-labeling technique to a larger sample of domestic females, has revealed asymmetry (the right C/I ratio being significantly higher than the left), but to a much lesser degree than in males (Rajendra and Rogers, 1993). The C/I ratios of the left and right sides of the females approximate the C/I ratios determined following injection of the right side of the male. This suggests that in females both sides of the thalamus (and thus both eyes) have well-developed visual projections to the hyperstriata, equivalent to those of the left side of the thalamus (right eye) of the male. The finding could potentially explain why females learn equally well with either eye when they are tested for visual discrimination learning and why both eyes of the female learn the visual discrimination task as well as does the right eye of the male.

EFFECT OF LIGHT INPUT PRIOR TO HATCHING ON ASYMMETRY OF THE THALAMOFUGAL VISUAL PROJECTIONS

We have shown that the direction of functional lateralization in the male chick is determined by differential exposure of the embryo to light, and that lateralization is correlated with structural asymmetry. Moreover, these effects occur at the stage of embryonic development when visual connections to the forebrain are becoming functional (Freeman and Vince, 1974). We therefore proceeded to examine the effects of light exposure on the symmetry/asymmetry of thalamofugal visual projections (figure 13.5).

Embryos were exposed to various lighting conditions during the last stages of incubation, and then injected with fluorescent tracers on day 2 post hatching (Rogers and Sink, 1988; Rogers and Bolden, 1991). As in our previous experiments, the direction of the effect was manipulated by withdrawing the embryo's head from the egg on day 19/20 of incubation, applying a patch of black tape to the right eye and exposing the left eye to light for 24 hours before removing the eye-patch. In contrast to controls, which had a patch placed on the left eye, this manipulation reversed the normal direction of structural asymmetry. Thus, monocular light input determines the asymmetrical development of the visual projections from thalamus to telencephalon. The sensitive period to light stimulation is over by the time of hatching, since the asymmetry persists into the third week post hatching despite the fact that the chicks received light input to both eyes after hatching.

Another group of embryos was incubated in darkness and not exposed to light until after hatching, so that both eyes were simultaneously stimulated with light. Males treated in this way were found to have symmetrical organization of their thalamofugal visual projections, with high C/I ratios (ca. 50% for each side). They resembled females in having well-developed sets of contralateral projections (relative to the ipsilateral ones) from both sides of the thalamus to the telencephalon. A third group of embryos was incubated in the dark, hatched in the dark, injected with dye under low lighting conditions on day 2 and raised in the dark. Males so treated also had symmetry of their thalamofugal visual projections, but with lower C/I ratios (ca. 25% for each side), than those whose eyes were exposed to light simultaneously after hatching.

Lack of light stimulation apparently prevents either full development of the contralateral thalamofugal projections (relative to the ipsilateral ones) or loss of the ipsilateral projections (relative to the contralateral ones). Structural symmetry is present in both dark-incubated groups,

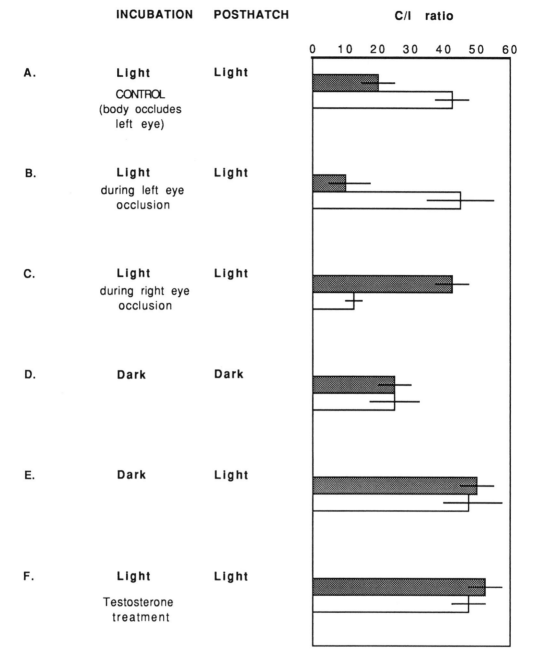

Figure 13.5 Light exposure and structural changes in developing chicks. C/I ratios have been determined after injecting fluorescent markers into the left (black bars) and the right (white bars) sides of the hyperstriatum of 2-day-old chicks exposed to various conditions of light and darkness during the last days of incubation. Data for males only. The C/I ratios are plotted as mean values with standard errors. (A) Controls, hatched from eggs that received exposure to light during the last 3 to 4 days of incubation and also after hatching (*n* = 10); (B) the left eye of each embryo was occluded for 24 hours on day 19/20 of incubation and the right eye exposed to light, both eyes were exposed to light after

irrespective of posthatching light exposure, but the C/I ratios are higher in those which do receive light after hatching. These findings suggest that, if the eggs receive no light exposure prior to hatching, the sensitive period for light can extend into the immediate post-hatching period. Moreover, since male embryos exposed to lateralized light input prior to hatching retain asymmetry despite binocular stimulation of the eyes with light after hatching, the light exposure prior to hatching must close the sensitive period before hatching occurs. In this respect, the development of structural asymmetry and functional lateralization in chicks is similar to the way in which the sensitive period of imprinting in chicks is closed by exposure to the imprinting stimulus, but remains open for an extended period if the chick is held in the dark (Horn, 1985). However, in emphasizing the role of light stimulation during development, it is important to remember that most chicks used in imprinting studies have hatched from eggs incubated in darkness; yet, they have lateralization of memory processes. Thus lateralized light stimulation is clearly not the sole determinant of brain lateralization in this species.

AGE-DEPENDENT CHANGES IN THE ASYMMETRY OF THE THALAMOFUGAL VISUAL PROJECTIONS

Since in a precocial species like the chick, much development takes place over the embryonic period, we examined the organization of the thalomofugal visual projections in the late embryonic stage. Embryos were injected with fluorescent tracers on day 19 of incubation—the "tucking" stage of Hamburger and Oppenheim (1967)—and then put back into its normal position within the egg (Rogers et al., 1993) and kept there until day 2 post hatching. Half of the embryos received light exposure from day 18 of incubation on, while the other half were held in the dark. The resulting C/I ratios are presented in figure 13.6. No left/right differences in the C/I ratios were present in any of the groups. Comparison of the dark-and light-exposed males reveals some effect of light in elevating the mean C/I ratio, as determined by injecting the right side. Apparently this indicates a trend that becomes significant in the early post-hatching period. We have also investigated the organization of the thalamofugal visual projections in males aged 12 to 16 days and 21–25 days post hatching (Rogers and Sink, 1988). Structural asymmetry is present between approximately days 2 and 16, but by the

hatching ($n = 7$); (C) as for group B but with right, instead of left, eye occlusion before hatching ($n = 6$); (D) a group incubated and reared in the dark ($n = 6$); (E) a group incubated in the dark and exposed to light after hatching so that both eyes were simultaneously stimulated with light ($n = 8$); (F) a group injected with testosterone on day 16 of incubation (25 mg of testosterone oenanthate injected into the egg) and exposed to the same lighting conditions as group A ($n = 9$). Significant asymmetry is present in the C/I ratios of groups A, B, and C. Note the reversed direction of asymmetry in group C.

Rogers & Adret: Developmental Mechanisms of Lateralization

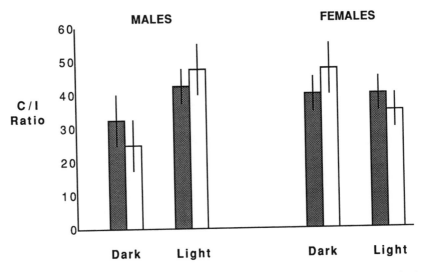

Figure 13.6 The C/I ratios for male and female embryos following injection (incubation day 19/20; 4 day survival) of one fluorescent dye into the left hyperstriatum (black bars) and the other into the right hyperstriatum (white bars). Half the embryos were incubated, injected, hatched, and raised in the dark, and the other half were exposed to light from day 18 of incubation on. Means and standard errors are plotted. No significant asymmetry was present in any of these groups (*n* = 6 to 8 per group). Note that the male embryos exposed to light tend to have higher C/I ratios than those held in the dark (details in text).

third week of life it is no longer present. Even in males, therefore, structural asymmetry of the thalamofgual visual projections is transient. This does not detract from its importance, occurring as it does through-out those stages of development when the chicks are undergoing im-portant forms of learning which have permanent or long-lasting consequences for later behavior. Some lateralities in the chicken brain are independent of asymmetry in the visual projections, but possibly others may be determined by the left/right bias in visual projections which occurs during early life. The latter may well persist after asym-metry in the visual projections is no longer present. Thus, while asym-metry may not be evident in the thalamofugal visual projections of adult chickens or pigeons, functional lateralities determined by the early asymmetry of these projections may exist in adult birds.

SEX HORMONES AND LIGHT-DEPENDENT DEVELOPMENT OF THE THALAMOFUGAL VISUAL PROJECTIONS

Although both male and female embryos are oriented in the egg in the same way, and both receive lateralized light stimulation prior to hatch-ing, females have less asymmetry of their thalamofugal visual projec-tions. The development of these projections in females must therefore be less sensitive to light, or the sensitive period for females must extend into the post-hatching period, so that an initial asymmetry in the pro-

Development of the Avian Visual System

jections is removed by exposure of both eyes to light after hatching. Since we failed to detect asymmetry in females even at the embryo stage, the latter explanation is unlikely. These data thus suggest that development of the thalamofugal visual projections in the female is almost completely independent of light stimulation. The sex difference in the sensitivity to light of the developing visual projections is likely to be dependent on the circulating levels of sex hormones during the later stages of embryonic development. Using a slow-release vehicle technique for testosterone delivery, Schwarz and Rogers (1992) have shown that high levels of this hormone in the male embryo prevent the normal development of structural asymmetry in the visual pathways. The males had a slight but significant reversal of asymmetry, and the females had no asymmetry.

Interestingly, in control male embryos the level of endogenously released testosterone rises until day 17 of incubation (Woods et al., 1975), and then falls to a trough during the last days of incubation, to rise again after hatching (Tanabe et al., 1979). Low levels of testosterone during the last few days of embryonic development appear to have a permissive effect on the development of asymmetry in the light-dependent thalamofugal projections. Administration of the hormone on day 16 of incubation would keep hormone levels high at a time when they are normally low.

EVIDENCE FOR LATERALITY OF MOTOR BEHAVIOR

In contrast to, for example, handedness in primates, the demonstration of functional lateralization for visual processing in birds involves discriminative processes and its "unmasking" requires specialized behavioral tests (e.g., monocular testing). However, "footedness" in parrots has been reported (Harris, 1989; Rogers, 1989), with most species being left-footed. Given their laterally placed eyes, this also means that the left eye is used to a greater extent to view the food object during feeding. The head is frequently titled to the left so that the food object is viewed by the left monocular field of vision. Some degree of footedness is also present in chickens (Rogers and Workman, 1992), which show a bias toward the use of the right foot to initiate ground scratching for food. Such behavior is directed toward the animal's right eye and foot, and is thus consistent with the already demonstrated superiority of the right eye in a visual search task. There is also some evidence for lateralized eye use during courtship display (Workman and Andrew, 1989) and in the control of vocal behavior (see chapter 18).

THE EVOLUTION OF BRAIN LATERALIZATION

In lateral-eyed species, processing of visual information from the two lateral, monocular fields may occur simultaneously and independently, at least at lower levels of brain organization. This could produce conflicting and potentially disruptive commands to the motor system, were it not for the presence of commissural structures, which permit interaction of such information at higher brain levels. The hemispheric dominance characteristic of brain lateralization may be viewed as an information processing mechanism that functions to minimize such conflict by biasing the direction of the motor response (see chapter 19). Andrew (1983) has suggested that brain lateralization or hemispheric specialization may have evolved as a consequence of having laterally placed eyes, and that lateralization of other functions (such as singing) may have followed. The discovery of lateralization in birds has made primatologists and human psychologists rethink the evolution of lateralization, which was once thought to be an uniquely human trait.

Whatever its evolutionary origin, the ubiquity of structural and behavioral lateralization suggests it has considerable functional significance. The developing chicken brain provides us with an excellent model system in which to study its ontogeny, the way in which environmental and hormonal factors interact to produce sex-related differences in lateralization, and the nature of the neural lateralities that correlate with the lateralized behaviors. Finally, comparative analyses of lateralization mechanisms in birds and mammals (e.g., Denenberg and Yutzey, 1985) should contribute to our understanding of structural and behavioral development.

REFERENCES

Adret, P., and Rogers, L. J. Sex difference in the visual projections of young chicks: A quantitative study of the thalamofugal pathway. *Brain Res.* 478 (1989), 59–73.

Andrew, R. J. Lateralization of emotional and cognitive function in higher vertebrates, with special reference to the domestic chick. In J-P. Ewert, R. R. Capranica, and D. Ingle, (Eds.), *Advances in Vertebrate Neuroethology*. Plenum Press, New York, 1983, pp. 477–509.

Andrew, R. J., and Dharmaretnam, M. A timetable of development. In R. J. Andrew (Ed.), *Neural and Behavioural Plasticity: The Use of the Domestic Chick as a Model*. Oxford University Press, Oxford, 1991, pp. 166–173.

Boxer, M. I., and Stanford, D. Projections to the posterior visual hyperstriatal region in the chick: An HRP study. *Exp. Brain Res.* 57 (1985), 494–498.

Bradshaw, J. L., and Rogers, L. J. *The Evolution of Lateral Asymmetries, Language, Tool Use and Intellect*. Academic Press, San Diego, 1993, in press.

Cipolla-Neto, J., Horn, G., and McCabe, B. J. Hemispheric asymmetry and imprinting: the effect of sequential lesions of the hyperstriatum ventrale. *Exp. Brain Res.* 48 (1982), 22–27.

Collins, R. L. On the inheritance of direction and degree of asymmetry. In S. D. Glick (Ed.), *Cerebral Lateralization in Nonhuman Species*. Academic Press, Orlando, 1985, pp. 41–71.

Denenberg, V. H., and Yutzey, D. A. Hemispheric laterality, behavioural asymmetry and the effects of early experience in rats. In S. D. Glick (Ed.), *Cerebral Lateralization in Nonhuman Species*. Academic Press, New York, 1985, pp. 109–133.

Dubbledam, J. L. The avian and mammalian forebrain: correspondences and differences. In R. J. Andrew (ed.), *Neural and Behavioural Plasticity: The Use of the Domestic Chick as a Model*. Oxford University Press, Oxford, 1991, pp. 65–91.

Fersen, L. von, and Güntürkün, O. Visual memory lateralization in pigeons. *Neuropsychologia* 28 (1990), 1–7.

Freeman, B. M., and Vince, M. A. *Development of the Avian Embryo*. Chapman and Hall, London, 1974.

Gaston, K. E., and Gaston, M. G. Unilateral memory after binocular discrimination training: Left hemisphere dominance in the chick? *Brain Res.* 303 (1984), 190–193.

Gottlieb, G. Prenatal behavior of birds, *Quart. Rev. Biol.* 43 (1968), 148–173.

Güntürkün, O. Lateralization of visually controlled behaviour in pigeons. *Physiol Behav.* 34 (1985), 575–577.

Güntürkün, O. Embryonale Orientierung als Ontogenetischer Auslöser für Visuelle Lateralisation. In D. Frey (Ed.), *Bericht über den 37. Kongress der Deutschen Gesellschaft für Psychologie in Kiel 1990*, Volume 1. Verlag für Psychologie, 1990, pp. 51–52.

Güntürkün. O. and Kesch, S. Visual lateralization during feeding in pigeons. *Behav. Neurosci.* 101 (1987), 433–435.

Hambley, J. W., and Rogers, L. J. Retarded learning induced by amino acids in the neonatal chick. *Neuroscience* 4 (1979), 677–684.

Hamburger, V., and Oppenheim, R. Prehatching motility and hatching behavior in the chick. *J. Exp. Zool.* 166 (1967), 171–204.

Harris, L. J. Footedness in parrots: Three centuries of research, theory, and mere surmise. *Canad. J. Psychol.* 43 (1989), 369–396.

Horn, G. *Memory Imprinting and the Brain*. Clarendon Press, Oxford, 1985.

McCabe, B. J., and Horn, G. Learning and memory: Regional changes in N-methyl-D-aspartate receptors in the chick brain after imprinting. *Proc. Natl. Acad. Sci. U. S. A.* 85 (1988), 2849–2853.

Melsbach, G., Hahmann, U., Waldmann, C., Wörtwein, G., and Güntürkün, O. Morphological asymmetries of the optic tectum of the pigeon. In N. Elsner and H. Penzlin (Eds.), *Synapse—Transmission and Modulation, Proc. 19th Göttingen Neurobiol Conf.* George Thieme Verlag, Stuttgart, 1991, p. 553.

Mench, J., and Andrew, R. J. Lateralization of a food search task in the domestic chick. *Behav. Neural Biol.* 46 (1986), 107–114.

Nottebohm, F. Asymmetries of neural control of vocalisation in the canary. In S. Harnard, R. W. Doty, L. Goldstein, and G. Krauthamer (Eds.), *Lateralisation in the Nervous System*. Academic Press, New York, 1977, pp. 23–44.

Rajendra, S., and Rogers, L. J. Asymmetry is present in the thalamofugal projections of female chicks. *Exp. Brain Res.* 92 (1993), 542–544.

Rogers, L. J. Light experience and asymmetry of brain function in chickens. *Nature* (*London*) 297 (1982), 223–225.

Rogers, L. J. Lateralization of learning in chicks. *Adv. Study Behav.* 16 (1986), 147–189.

Rogers, L. J. Laterality in animals. *Int. J. Comp. Psychol.* 3 (1989), 5–25.

Rogers, L. J. Light input and the reversal of functional lateralization in the chicken brain. *Behav. Brain Res.* 38 (1990), 211–221.

Rogers, L. J. Development of lateralization. In R. J. Andrew (Ed.), *Neural and Behavioural Plasticity: The Use of the Domestic Chick as a Model.* Oxford University Press, Oxford, 1991, pp. 507–535.

Rogers, L. J., and Bolden, S. W. Light-dependent development and asymmetry of visual projections. *Neurosci. Lett.* 121 (1991), 63–67.

Rogers, L. J., and Sink, H. S. Transient asymmetry in the projections of the rostral thalamus to the visual hyperstriatum of the chicken, and reversal of its direction by light exposure. *Exp. Brain Res.* 70 (1988), 378–384.

Rogers, L. J., and Workman, L. Footedness in birds. *Anim. Behav.* 45 (1993), 409–411.

Rogers, L. J., Bolden, S. W., and Adret, P. (1993). In preparation.

Rose, S. P. R. How chicks make memories; the cellular cascade from c-fos to dendritic modelling. *Trends Neurosci.* 14 (1991), 390–397.

Schwarz, I. M., and Rogers, L. J. Testosterone: A role in the development brain asymmetry in the chick. *Neurosci. Lett.* 146 (1992), 167–170.

Stewart, N. G. Changes in dendritic and synaptic structure in chick forebrain consequent on passive avoidance learning. In R. J. Andrew (Ed.), *Neural and Behavioural Plasticity; The Use of the Domestic Chick as a Model.* Oxford University Press, Oxford, 1991, pp. 305–328.

Stewart, M. G., Rogers, L. J., Davies, H. A., and Bolden, S. W. Structural asymmetry in the thalamofugal visual projections in 2-day old chicks is correlated with a hemispheric difference in synaptic number in the hyperstriatum accessorium. *Brain Res.* 585 (1992), 381–385.

Tanabe, Y., Nakamura, T., Fujioka, K., and Doi, O. Production and secretion of sex steroid hormones by the testes, the ovary and adrenal glands of embryonic and young chickens. *Gen. Comp. Endocrinol.* 39 (1979), 26–33.

Vince, M. A., and Toosey, F. M. Posthatching effects of repeated prehatching stimulation with an alien sound. *Behaviour* 72 (1980), 65–76.

Woods, J. E., Simpson, R. M., and Moore, P. L. Plasma testosterone levels in the chick embryo. *Gen. comp. Endocrinol.* 27 (1975), 543–547.

Workman, L., and Andrew, R. J. Population lateralization in zebra finch courtship: an unresolved issue? *Anim. Behav.* 41 (1989), 545–546.

Zappia, J. V., and Rogers, L. J. Light experience during development affects asymmetry of forebrain function in chickens. *Dev. Brain Res.* 11 (1983), 93–106.

Zappia, J. V., and Rogers, L. J. Sex differences and reversal of brain asymmetry by testosterone in chickens. *Behav. Brain Res.* 23 (1987), 261–267.

IV Visuomotor Mechanisms

Introduction

H. Philip Zeigler

The immensely sophisticated visual apparatus of birds is, ultimately, at the service of its motor systems. The chapters in this section examine the use of visual information in the control of a variety of motor patterns, from the relatively simple (eye movements) to the formidably complex (predator–prey interactions at an air–water interface).

Chapter 14, by Wallman and Letelier, will be of particular interest to anyone who has ever puzzled at the "head-bobbing" movements of a walking pigeon. It reviews what is known about the behaviors that stabilize the bird's visual world in the face of the perturbation of visual inputs, produced either by stimulus movement or the bird's own locomotor activities. Such stabilization involves the integration of signals from both the vestibular and visual systems and their use to control eye and head movements. The chapter corrects the misleading assumption that eye movements are lacking or minimal in birds, discusses their possible role in mediating binocular vision, and describes some of their unique properties.

In chapter 15, Zeigler, Jäger, and Palacios review studies of the response topography and visual control of pecking, probably the most exhaustively studied response in behavioral science. For the ethologist, pecking has all the earmarks of a "fixed action pattern," while for the psychologist, pecking has served primarily as an indicator response in studies of conditioning and learning. Both groups have viewed pecking as a unitary response, both elicited and directed by the food. The studies reviewed in this chapter show that pecking involves a sensorimotor chain, made up of head movement and jaw movement segments, which are linked by visual and tactile stimuli from the food object. Pecking behavior may be experimentally dissociated into localization, grasping, and manipulation components, each of which has its own sources of sensory control. Moreover, experiments involving a reversible "visual decerebration" demonstrate that the several response components are mediated by structures at different levels of the neuraxis.

An important feature of the pigeon's pecking behavior is its susceptibility to associative control by stimulus-reinforcer and response-reinforcer contingencies. Moreover, the conditioned key peck preserves the essential topographic features of the ingestive peck, including the saccade-like movements of the head and the variations in jaw movement with reinforcer type. Using both operant and classical conditioning paradigms, Allan (chapter 16) has taken advantage of these features to carry out an analysis of the behavioral control of the head movement and jaw movement components of pecking. He has shown that each of the components may be brought under control using either operant or classical conditioning paradigms. His work extends the analysis of conditioned response form and provides a preparation for experimental studies of sensorimotor control.

In nature, pecking functions primarily to transport a prehensile effector organ (the beak) toward objects precisely localized in space. In this respect, pecking may be considered a form of predation, with a stationary target as prey. Accurate peck localization and grasping behavior require the processing of visual information as to the size of the target and its egocentric distance and direction. This is a complex enough task when the target is stationary. Its complexity increases considerably when the target is moving, since target distance and direction are continually changing. Information processing by avian predators such as hawks and falcons must involve the continual updating of information on the orientation and distance to the prey and on its relative motion. The task becomes truly daunting when—as is the case for many piscivorous water birds—both the predator and prey are moving, and when the processing involves compensation for visual distortions produced at an air-water interface. The task faced by a diving gannet or kingfisher also involves accurate estimations of the time to contact, split-second decisions as to when to dive, and moment-to-moment control of wing position in relation to the predicted collision time. The visuomotor mechanisms involved in such behaviors are discussed in chapter 17 by Katzir, and his studies help to remind us of some of the ecological factors that have constrained the evolution of the visual system in birds.

14 Eye Movements, Head Movements, and Gaze Stabilization in Birds

Josh Wallman and Juan-Carlos Letelier

Television commercials to the contrary, the visual system functions poorly with momentarily presented images of random parts of our visual surroundings. Rather, the brain requires both stable views of its surroundings and self-directed changes of gaze. The oculomotor system accomplishes these tasks with only a few behaviors, each of which is quite stereotyped with respect both to its form and its eliciting stimuli. Thus, in contrast to one's ability to move one's hand with any speed, acceleration, or direction, following any aspect of the target motion, the eyes are constrained to a small number of behaviors each of which is guided by highly restricted stimuli. In these respects, the behaviors of the eyes possess the stereotypy that the early ethologists sought in more conspicuous courtship and parental behaviors. In this chapter, we will first introduce these several behaviors and the stimuli that control them, relying mostly on research on primates; then we will review the modest amount of research on the eye movements of birds, with emphasis on the work of our laboratory.

GAZE-CHANGING BEHAVIORS

Eye movement behaviors can be divided into two broad classes: gaze-changing behaviors and gaze-holding behaviors. Two of the behaviors that change the direction of gaze are *pursuit movements,* unstudied in birds, which move the eye smoothly to track moving targets, and *saccades,* which abruptly shift gaze from one target to another. The two behaviors are quite distinct in that pursuit movements in general attempt to match the target velocity, regardless of the target position, whereas saccadic eye movements ignore target velocity and attempt to match target position.

This functional difference can be used to illustrate the distinctness of these two types of oculomotor behavior. In a classic experiment in humans, a target is made to jump to the left of where the eye is looking and then slowly move to the right. In this situation the pursuit eye movements are to the right—the direction of the velocity vector of the target—even though they take the eye away from the target. The saccades, on the other hand, are to the left—the direction of the position error—and compensate for the "wrong-way" pursuits (Rashbass, 1961). These results resemble the stimulus specificity shown by food-begging in young thrushes in which the full behavior is elicited by rather arbitrary shapes, with the release and orientation of the behavior being dependent on different parameters of the visual stimuli (Tinbergen and Kuenen, 1939). In the case of the eye movements the different stimulus specificities reflect the existence of two rather independent behaviors that track targets concurrently but are driven by different stimulus components.

A similar experimental paradigm illustrates another aspect of oculomotor behavior: If, after jumping left, the target jumps back to its starting position before the eye makes a saccade, the eye often makes a saccade to the left (where the target is not) and then makes a second saccade back to the starting position, where the target has been throughout these saccades (Westheimer, 1954). This is somewhat similar to the observation of Lorenz and Tinbergen (1938) that incubating geese, using their bills to retrieve eggs that have rolled out of the nest, will continue this egg-rolling movement until the bill reaches the nest even if the egg has meanwhile gone out of reach. In contrast with the mysteriousness of the stereotypy of the egg-rolling behavior, the "fixed action patterns" of the oculomotor system offer one a reasonable prospect of working out both their formal and neurophysiological determinants. For example, in the saccade example the reason for the "pointless" saccades has been studied in terms of the interactions among the decision to make a saccade, the programming of its amplitude and direction, and attentional factors (reviewed by Becker, 1989). In general, because much is known about how and where oculomotor programming takes place, and what its dynamic constraints are, it is possible to design models that permit clear and testable predictions of the properties of neurons at different levels of the oculomotor system (reviewed by Van Gisbergen and Van Opstal, 1989).

Vergence movements are a third type of gaze changing behavior. If objects are to be viewed with both eyes simultaneously, the eyes must change their angle to each other depending on the distance of the object. In animals with obligatory binocular vision, like ourselves, this is accomplished mostly by a distinct slow eye movement behavior—vergence—driven either by the disparate location of an image on the two retinas (retinal disparity vergence) or by changes in the distance at which the eyes are focused (accommodative vergence) (Carpenter, 1988). In addition to these slow vergence movements, unequal saccades in the two eyes can also change the vergence state. In birds, these saccadic vergence changes are the principal and perhaps the only vergence mechanism. In species that keep the eyes unaligned most of the time, large oppositely directed saccades are used to position the eyes for binocular vision (Bloch et al., 1984, 1987; Wallman and Pettigrew, 1985).

GAZE-HOLDING BEHAVIORS

Gaze-holding movements maintain the visual surroundings stationary on the retina despite locomotion by the animal or movements of the head. Two behaviors—optokinetic and vestibulo-ocular reflexes—stabilize the eyes, and two others—optomotor and vestibulocollic reflexes—stabilize the head. Critical differences among these four behaviors lie in the nature of their eliciting stimuli and the relation of the response to the stimuli. In optokinetic and optomotor behaviors, a specialized part of the visual system (including dedicated retinal ganglion cells and nuclei in the accessory optic system and pretectum) responds to visual motion over a large part of the retina and produces an eye or head movement that reduces the velocity of the retinal image. In the vestibulocollic reflex, the head moves to reduce the stimulation from the semicircular canals. Thus these three reflexes all operate as negative feedback loops. In contrast, in the fourth behavior, the vestibulo-ocular reflex, the eye movements produced that compensate for the head motion stimulating the semicircular canals do not affect the input to the semicircular canals, and so the vestibulo-ocular reflex is not a negative feedback loop.

Although these four gaze-stabilizing reflexes may be experimentally isolated in the laboratory, under normal conditions they do not exist independently, since every head movement produces both vestibular and visual stimulation. One indication of the intimate intermingling of visual and vestibular sensation is that circularvection—the perception that one is rotating—can be elicited indistinguishably by rotating either the person or the visual surroundings as long as the velocities and accelerations are within the range of the optokinetic system (Flandrin et al., 1990).

AVIAN EYE MOVEMENTS

The several types of eye-movement behaviors just discussed probably occur in all animals. Why then have a chapter on the eye movements of birds? For one, avian saccades have mysterious peculiarities that warrant study. For another, head-stabilizing behaviors are especially prominent in birds and especially relevant to their visual behaviors. Although at one time head movements would have been viewed as quite different behaviors from eye movements, it is becoming clear that gaze-related behaviors are organized principally in terms of outcomes—

the effect on gaze—with the particular effector system involved—eye or head—being of lesser importance.

HEAD-STABILIZING AND HEAD-BOBBING

One freedom of morphological evolution that birds, unlike mammals, enjoy is that they are not constrained to have only seven neck vertebrae or massive skulls anchoring powerful jaws. As a consequence there are many birds with small heads on long, flexible necks. These attributes confer an additional freedom: Such birds can not only stabilize their visual surroundings when they are standing still, as can all visual animals, but they can keep the visual world quite stationary even during locomotion. Thus a pigeon or chicken walking does not suffer the visual streaming of the image of the surroundings (optic flow) as mammals do, but keeps its head stationary with respect to the surroundings most of the time, while the legs move the body forward; when the legs have overtaken the head, the bird thrusts its head forward (a head saccade, really), putting the head again in front of the body and then again stabilizing it with respect to the surroundings. (Any changes the bird wishes to make in where the eyes are looking are saved up to the next head thrust, the only time when eye saccades are made, thereby further reducing interruptions of stable gaze [Pratt, 1982].)

The ability of birds to stabilize their heads in space can be appreciated by holding a long-necked bird in one's hand and twisting or translating its body; the degree of stabilization is so good that it almost seems as if the head is fixed in space with the neck passively joining it to the moving body. In this situation, as in the walking one, many cues—proprioceptive, vestibular, and visual—help stabilize the head. A variety of experiments have demonstrated that visual signals are by far the most important, generally overruling conflicting signals from other sources.

This visual predominance has been shown by several clever experiments on the head-bobbing during locomotion described just above. Friedman (1975) showed that when the visual environment is made to move with the head, walking pigeons do not bob their heads. Similarly, if the birds do not move with respect to the surroundings, either because they are on a treadmill (Frost, 1978) or because the visual surroundings move with their body (Friedman, 1975), head-bobbing also ceases. Even more convincing, if one arranges to have a bird on a stationary perch surrounded by an oscillating visual environment, the head moves with the visual surroundings, even though this visual stabilizing behavior perturbs the vestibular stabilization mechanism. In these laboratory situations we are provoking the bird to move its head to stabilize its visual surroundings, whereas in normal circumstances movements of the whole visual field would usually result from perturbations of head position, and the responses to them would be part of head-stabilizing behavior.

LABORATORY MANIFESTATIONS OF GAZE-STABILIZING BEHAVIORS

If a bird or its visual surroundings are sinusoidally oscillated at modest amplitude and frequency, the eyes generally follow the stimulus with high gain (that is, the responses mostly compensate for the stimulus motion). If the stimulus motion is unidirectional, the responses of the eye or head became nystagmic, that is, alternating between a slow phase, during which gaze is stabilized, and quick phases, saccadic in form, in the opposite direction. Thus, optokinetic nystagmus (OKN) or vestibular nystagmus can be seen as made up of two competing behaviors: The slow phases minimize gaze velocity with respect to the surroundings and the quick phases keep gaze centered.

The slow phase of OKN is itself made up of two rather independent behaviors: an early component present only during stimulation, and a delayed component that takes seconds to build up in speed ("velocity storage") and persists in darkness after stimulation ceases (afternystagmus). Velocity storage is thought to compensate for the decaying response of the semicircular canals to unidirectional stimulation. One theory holds that the delayed responses are part of a rotational compensatory system, while the early responses are part of a translational one (Miles, 1993).

When OKN is elicited by visual stimuli seen by only one eye, strong asymmetries are seen: stimulus motion from back to front (temporal to nasal motion) results in stronger responses than the reverse. Prominent in animals with lateral eyes, this asymmetry is commonly thought to be an adaptation to prevent optokinetic stimulation during forward locomotion, while preserving rotational sensitivity (left eye driving left turns and right eye driving right turns).

Finally, although head and eye movements stabilize gaze by different motor pathways, their stimulus characteristics are quite similar. They show the same response curves both as a function of stimulus speed, when the drum is rotating at a constant speed, and as a function of either temporal frequency or velocity, when the drum is oscillating (Gioanni, 1988), suggesting that one sensory pathway drives both behaviors.

Although stabilization of gaze has been in general viewed as a simple reflexive response to movements of the animal or its surroundings, one experiment with pigeons shows how important the behavioral context can be. If the visual surroundings are rotated about a restrained pigeon, as in the usual laboratory situation, its head will follow the movements with a high fidelity up to 30°/sec. If the same experiment is carried out with a bird in tethered flight, the head will follow the surroundings up to 200°/sec (Bilo, 1992).

INTEGRATION OF VISUAL AND VESTIBULAR SIGNALS

As suggested above ("Gaze-Holding Behaviors"), the identification of the VOR and OKN as separate behaviors is a bit of a laboratory artifact, because normally both are simultaneously elicited during head turns; that is, both visual and vestibular indications of head movements are summed to elicit stabilizing head and eye movements. This summation presents no particular problem when confined to horizontal head rotation and visual motion in the central retina, as both motion signals are approximately horizontal. Problems arise, however, when one considers the nonhorizontal motion directions produced by head rotations about a horizontal axis. For a simple head rotation that stimulates one of the vertical semicircular canals (the left anterior for example), the motion seen by the right eye ranges from upward in the left part of the visual field to downward in the right, with the central visual field seeing a mostly cyclorotational (torsional) motion (arrows in figure 14.1A).

How can retinal directional signals, which code linear motion, be added to the canal signals, which code rotational motion, to give a measure of head rotation whether sensed by the eyes or the canals? One solution, advocated by several investigators, is that from the signals carried by retinal neurons with linear directional selectivities the accessory optic system synthesizes a visual signal that approximates the optic flow experienced during rotation about the axis of one of the semicircular canals (Simpson and Hess, 1977; Burns and Wallman, 1981; McKenna and Wallman, 1985).

The evidence for a linkage of the purely visual optokinetic responses to the semicircular canals is somewhat indirect. If one measures the gain of optokinetic nystagmus in chickens to visual motion about a variety of horizontal axes, the highest gain is to the pattern of optic flow approximating that which would be experienced if the animal were rotated about an axis coinciding with that which optimally excites the contralateral anterior semicircular canal (figure 14.1A "4-week-old"; Wallman and Velez, 1985). According to this view, each eye signals principally two directions of whole-field optic flow: temporal-to-nasal horizontal optic flow, which corresponds to excitation of one of the horizontal canals, and the combination of vertical and torsional signals described in the preceding paragraph, which corresponds to excitation of the contralateral anterior canal.

More direct evidence that the brain computes the rotational components of the optic flow is the finding of neurons in the pigeon vestibulocerebellum that respond selectively to visual rotations about the same two axes just described (Wylie and Frost, 1991).

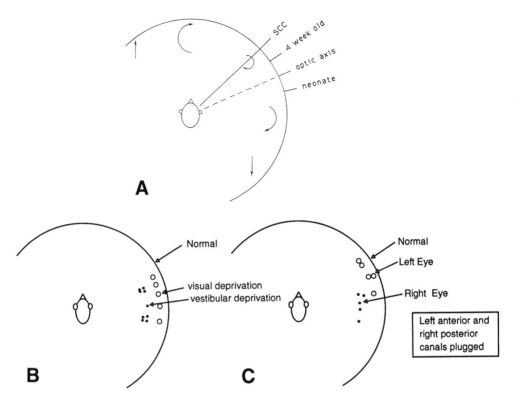

Figure 14.1 Optic flow and optokinetic nystagmus about various horizontal axes. (A) Diagrammatic top view of optic flow experienced (arrows) during head rotation (down and leftward) optimally stimulating the left anterior semicircular canal (SCC). Also shown are the median axes of highest optokinetic nystagmus gain for right eye of normal 4-week-old chicks and of newly hatched chicks. (B) Effect on best OKN axis of visual deprivation (only diffuse diurnal light permitted) or vestibular deprivation (daily streptomycin injections) from hatching. Note that both deprivations prevent the normal development change in OKN axis. Data points are best Fourier fit to data of individual animals. Arrows are medians of each group. "Normal" is same axis as "4 week old" in A. (C) Effect of neonatal plugging of one pair of semicircular canals. Note that the right eye is much more developmentally retarded than the left eye, suggesting an association of each eye with one canal pair.

Recent evidence from developmental studies (Rojas et al., 1985 and unpublished) suggests that inputs from the canals play a developmental role in the organization of the optokinetic system in chicks. First, after hatching the horizontal axis of highest optokinetic gain shifts toward the axis of the contralateral anterior canal mentioned above (figure 14.1A, compare "neonate" and "4-week-old"). Second, this shift in the axis of highest optokinetic gain does not take place if the animals are denied either visual motion experience (by diffusers over the eyes) or vestibular experience (by killing the vestibular hair cells with streptomycin injections) (figure 14.1B). Third, plugging one pair of vertical canals (the left anterior and the right posterior) prevented this shift in the optokinetic axis in the right eye (the one that would normally be associated with high gain in the motion direction of the plugged anterior canal), but not in the other eye (figure 14.1C).

These results suggest that during development the vestibular system affects the connectivity of visual system neurons so as to create a visual analog of each of the semicircular canals. This may occur by altering the synapses from the accessory optic system, which responds to optic flow, to the vestibular nuclei, by selecting or strengthening those visual synapses well correlated with the canal-related activity of the vestibular nuclear neurons. We presume that this developmental matching facilitates the addition of visual and vestibular motion signals to yield a head velocity signal that is reliable whether the input modality is visual or vestibular.

INTEGRATION OF ROTATION AND TRANSLATION

The stability of vision can be affected both by rotational perturbations, which change the angles of the head to the surroundings, and translational perturbations, which change the distances to the surroundings. Most studies of gaze stabilization have concerned stabilization against rotations, either of the head or of the surroundings. However, for the eye to be stable in space, the translational perturbations must also be compensated for. This generally is done by head movements (especially in birds) or by whole-body movements, because the eyes can only rotate. As in the case of the rotation, translation can be detected by the vestibular and visual systems and can be described as separate behaviors (translational VOR, translational OKN). In pigeons there are separate zones of the cerebellum for rotational and translational optic flow (Wylie and Frost, 1991).

For humans, there is a very clear perceptual distinction between rotational and translational visual motion. Thus, the illusion of translation, produced, for example, when an adjacent vehicle begins to move past the stationary vehicle in which you are seated, is never mistaken for rotation. Conversely, rotating visual surroundings can induce the illusion that one is rotating (circularvection), but never that one is translating. One exception, however, is that in chickens and pigeons rotations of the visual surroundings can induce strong side-to-side translations of the head when the frequency of the oscillatory stimulus motion is high (Nalbach, 1993; Marin and Wallman, unpublished). Nalbach suggests that this demonstrates that the visual system cannot, in this artificial stimulus situation, perfectly decompose optic flow into its rotational and translational components; it relies on integration of the vectors of local visual motion across the visual field, with the frontal vectors being more potent. We suggest that this translation occurs because at high frequencies the more effective head rotation would cause the vestibular stabilizing mechanism (the vestibulocollic reflex) to oppose the visual stabilization and clamp the head. This leaves the bird with only head translation, which can at best stabilize the region in front of it. This interpretation, different from, but not incompatible with that of Nalbach, is supported by our finding that if the horizontal semicircular canals are plugged, the birds do not translate their heads even at high frequencies. The presence of this dysfunctional translation behavior emphasizes how tightly linked are eye and head responses; otherwise the bird could use optokinetic eye rotations to achieve optimal stabilization.

SPONTANEOUS EYE MOVEMENTS AND PRIMARY GAZE POSITIONS

Because we humans enjoy the illusion that nearly all of our behaviors are purposive, we tend to assume that our eye movements are purposive, with position of our eyes at any moment being controlled by the position of an object of interest, and that most saccades—the primary voluntary gaze-changing movements—are carried out to look at particular objects. These assumptions cannot be entirely true because we make saccades nearly as frequently in darkness as when there is a scene to view. Furthermore, in those few species studied, the eyes tend to remain within a few degrees of a particular position, the so-called primary position of gaze, most of the time, suggesting that some process influences the probability of saccades in different directions to return the inquisitive eye to its home position. (Collewijn, 1977; Wallman and Pettigrew, 1985). In the Little Eagle and Tawny Frogmouth, the eyes are kept near the primary gaze position by having saccades toward the primary position becoming more probable with increasing distance away from the primary position, and by having those saccades toward the primary position occur after a shorter intersaccadic interval than those away from it (Wallman and Pettigrew, 1985).

Keeping the eye in one region could have several adaptive functions, including minimizing of muscle effort, and simplification of oculomotor or perceptual calibration. Whatever its function, the existence of a primary gaze position has several consequences for birds.

First, it causes the retinas generally to view the world from the vicinity of a particular eye position. Because the head as well is generally held in a particular posture (Duijm, 1951, 1958; Erichsen et al., 1989; see chapter 2), particular regions of the retina tend to view particular parts of the visual world. As a result appropriate specializations of retina and eye are possible. Thus one region of the dorsal retina of pigeons, called the red field because of the abundance of red oil droplets, views the ground in front of the bird. Similarly, some birds have two foveae or areas specialized for acute vision, one located near the optic axis, thereby looking somewhat laterally, and the other in the temporal retina, which looks frontally and tends to align with the corresponding region of the other eye when the eyes are near the primary gaze position; this fovea is presumably used for binocular vision.

Furthermore, in many terrestrial species, both avian and nonavian, the density of retinal neurons is greatest along a horizontal streak that aligns with the horizon and compensates for the foreshortening of perspective—that is, that the closer to the ground one is, the more of one's world is crammed into a small visual angle around the horizon (Hughes, 1977, 1981).

A similar specialization has been suggested with respect to moving objects (Maldonado et al., 1988). When a slow (or static) object is presented to a pigeon it keeps it in front of the head. When a rapidly moving object is presented, it keeps it in its lateral visual field. Such observations suggest that in addition to retinal specializations devoted to acuity (foveae and streaks) and to color vision or contrast (red field), some birds have retinal regions (or corresponding brain regions) specialized for processing different velocity ranges.

Second, if the eye and head are consistently maintained in a particular position, the optics of the eye can be specialized for this position. In a number of species of birds the refractive state of the eye changes with vertical angle below the horizon, such that the entire retina can view the ground in focus at once, as long as the bird is at a typical height above the ground (Fitzke et al., 1985; see chapters 1 and 2).

Third, the range of positions that the eye frequents may reflect, not some hypothetical morphological constraint, but rather the strength of the tendency to restore the eye to its primary gaze position. This tendency probably accounts for early reports that birds have negligible eye movements, especially species with small heads and large eyes, which generally move the head more than the eyes.

In at least one group of birds, however, the impression of ocular near immobility is veridical: Owls have large tubular eyes that appear to fill the orbit and that move only a few degrees in each direction, with most gaze-changing and gaze-holding being carried out by means of head movements. Nonetheless, owls raised without binocular vision develop strabismus of up to 11° (Knudsen, 1989), suggesting that, as in humans, the binocular eye alignment is actively achieved with visual mediation. What function might this restricted effective oculomotor range serve? In animals with two eyes, the disparity of images on the two retinas yields information about relative depth (stereopsis), but functions poorly in perception of absolute depth because disparity depends on the degree of convergence of the eyes, as well as on depth. With relatively immobile eyes the animal can use the two eyes as a range-finder, as does the toad (Collett and Harkness, 1982). Perhaps owls do as well.

CONJUGATE VS. INDEPENDENT EYE MOVEMENTS

We primates are constrained to make movements of the two eyes that are conjugate, that is, in which both eyes go right or left by nearly the same amount. This may be an adaptation to facilitate stereopsis or other aspects of binocular vision, or simply to ease the task of knitting together the views seen by the two eyes into a single percept. Many birds lack this constraint, and can move the two eyes independently, although when saccades occur, they occur synchronously (Lemeignan et al., 1992). One consequence of this freedom from conjugacy is that the brain is presented moment to moment with two often quite different views of the world, lacking even overlapping features. One wonders whether these two views are processed independently in parallel or whether only one is attended to at a time.

If visual attention is unitary as in humans, might the views provided by the two eyes or even by different parts of the visual field of one eye be made more or less salient at the level of the retina by the centrifugal projection from the brain? This projection is especially large in granivourous birds, which might have a particular need to time-share their visual attention between potential food on the ground and potential predators in the sky. The centrifugal projection is smaller in birds of prey and said to be even smaller in swans, a pattern consistent with this conjecture. Another line of evidence perhaps bearing on the centrifugal fibers playing a role in oculomotor attention is the finding that activity of centrifugal neurons is modulated by saccadic eye movements even in darkness (Marin et al., 1990). Although saccadic modulation of retinal activity would not be surprising, its occurrence in darkness suggests an oculomotor role for the centrifugal projection.

The occurrence of independent movements of the two eyes raises the issue of how stereopsis, which is clearly present in pigeons (McFadden, 1987 and chapter 3) and kestrels (Fox, 1978), is achieved. One possibility is that the birds can establish a correspondence between the two retinal images, regardless of their degree of overlap and angle of alignment, rather as though we could push one eyeball in any direction and still have the images from the two eyes remain fused. More plausibly, birds could have a particular position of gaze that the two eyes adopt when they wish to use binocular vision. Evidence of this is that some birds of prey have foveas in the temporal retina presumably used for stereopsis and that pigeons converge the two eyes before pecking (Bloch et al., 1984, 1987). Both groups of birds probably achieve stereopsis by aligning the receptive fields of retinal afferents in both eyes that project to binocular neurons in either the optic tectum or the Wulst (McFadden, 1988; Pettigrew and Konishi, 1976)).

TORSIONAL EYE POSITION

Birds, unlike primates, do not have frontally placed eyes. That is, in no avian species are the optic axes of the two eyes parallel in the primary gaze position. In pigeons and chickens this angle is 65–70° (Wallman and Velez, 1985; Nalbach et al. 1990), and in ducks it is nearly 90°. As a result, if a bird wishes to track an object moving vertically in front of it, it must make torsional (cyclorotational) eye movements. In chickens, the range of torsional eye positions is approximately as great as of vertical or horizontal positions. This contrasts dramatically with us primates, in whom torsional movements are small and occur mostly to fuse images in the two eyes. More formally, one says that primate eye positions are constrained by their neural organization to being two-dimensional, meaning that there is only one eye position from which one can regard a particular object (Donder's law). This is clearly not the case in birds, in which it appears that any combination of vertical, horizontal, and torsional positions within the effective oculomotor range can occur. (If binocular fusion can be achieved at more than one eye position, the brain must deal not only with differences in horizontal and vertical alignment, but also in torsion.)

PANORAMIC VISION VS. BINOCULAR FUSION: CAN ONE BIRD HAVE BOTH?

The advantages of panoramic vision and independent eye movements are obvious: maximal visual field, perhaps the ability to track two targets at once, and having different states of accommodation and pupillary contraction in the two eyes. Similarly obvious are the advantages are of moving the two eyes conjugately to view objects binocularly: stereopsis, increases in both acuity and sensitivity through probability summation, and use of the convergence angle of the eyes as a cue for depth and accommodation. Might it be that some birds (or other animals) gain all these advantages by switching between two oculomotor modes—a panoramic mode in which the eyes have the optic axes far apart (little binocular overlap) and the eyes move rather independently, and a frontal mode in which the eyes are more aligned (substantial binocular overlap) and move conjugately? The Frogmouth might be one such animal. In contrast to the eagle, which seems somewhat specialized for binocular vision (eyes stay in binocular field, most saccades are in the same direction in both eyes, many saccades are conjugate, and the primary gaze position nearly aligns the two temporal foveas), the Frogmouth has the eyes quite divergent at the primary gaze position, and most saccades are in opposite directions, but it frequently makes large convergent saccades (not seen in the eagle) that briefly center the eyes in the frontal visual field (Wallman and Pettigrew, 1985). The pigeon

(Bloch et al., 1987) and other species may also be able to switch between a panoramic and a frontal mode.

SACCADIC OSCILLATIONS

One oculomotor behavior is unique to birds. During saccades, the eye in several species studied does not proceed directly to the target in a straight line, but executes a series of spiraling oscillations, often much larger than the saccade of which they are a part (figure 14.2) (owls: Steinbach and Money, 1973; Pettigrew et al., 1990; chickens: Turkel and Wallman, 1977; Tawny Frogmouth and Little Eagle, Bush Thick-knee, Kookaburra: Pettigrew et al., 1990). In chickens, these oscillations are mostly torsional, consisting of 2–6 cycles with an almost invariant frequency of 28 Hz, an amplitude of 10–12° and a mean duration of 180 msec. In chickens and pigeons it is clear that all saccades involve oscillations.

The presence of saccadic oscillations is correlated with an unusual organization of the extraocular motor pools. In mammals, all ocular motoneurons carry signals related to both the position and velocity of the eye. In the chicken, there are two distinct classes of motoneurons: position-velocity motoneurons fire continuously at a rate proportional to the eye position and velocity. These neurons hold the eye during fixations and move it slowly from one position to another. They cease firing for most of each saccade, leaving the eye relatively free from muscular restraints on its motion (figure 14.3A). At this time, the second type of motoneuron, the saccade-related ones, becomes active, firing a

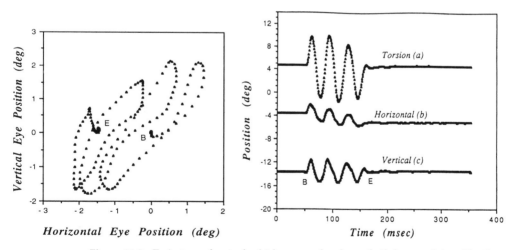

Figure 14.2 Trajectory of a single chicken saccade, shown both by x–y plot and by time course of three orthogonal components (upward deflection means intorsion, temporalward horizontal movement, and upward vertical movement; B, beginning of saccade; E end of saccade). Eye movements were rcorded by 3-D magnetic search coil method and are presented in Fick's coordinates.

Wallman & Letelier: Eye and Head Movements, Gaze Stabilization

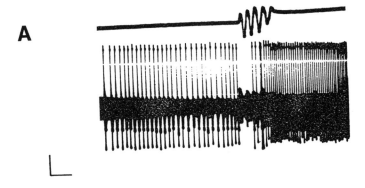

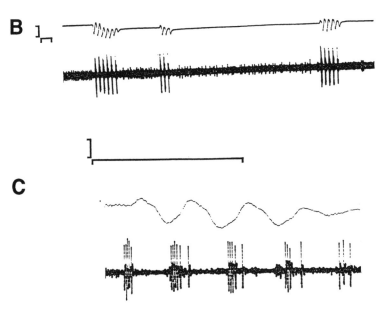

Figure 14.3 Characteristic firing pattern during saccades of the two classes of motoneu-rons in the trochlear nucleus. (A) Position-velocity neuron. Note that the saccade has an intorsional (upward on page) component, which is associated with increased spike fre-quency, but during much of the saccade, unit is silent. (B, C) . Saccade-related neuron. Note that unit is silent between saccades, but fires with each intorsional phase of the eye movement. In all three parts of this figure, calibrations are 100 msec and 5°.

short burst for each oscillatory cycle, thereby producing the saccadic oscillations (figure 14.3B; Letelier, 1992).

A curious feature of the timing of the activity of the saccade-related motoneurons is that although the first burst precedes the first intor-sional phase, subsequent ones occur after the eye has started its intor-sional motion, as though the eye were a pendulum, in the sense that, once in oscillation, the eye reverses its direction of motion passively, with the motoneurons only accelerating it (figure 14.3C).

Because disconnection of one muscle does not change the pattern of contraction of its antagonist, oscillations are not likely to be due to proprioceptive interactions. Instead, the complementary responses of these two types of motoneurons probably reflect their different inputs. Intracellular recordings from axons projecting to the motor nuclei show that some have the general pattern of the position-velocity motoneurons, while others have the regular 28 Hz bursts of the saccade-related type. Thus it appears that birds must have a central pattern generator, above the level of the motoneurons, that generates these highly regular oscillations and sends them to both eyes at once, producing conjugate oscillations during saccades. Avian oculomotor neurons thus appear to be an exception to the general principle of motor organization that all the motoneurons to a muscle generally share common inputs. We speculate that this difference reflects an adaptation to maximize the eye speed during the oscillations.

Two advantages accrue to having separate saccade-related and position-velocity motoneurons, with the position-velocity ones inhibited during much of the saccade. First, because contracting muscles are stiffer (require more force per mm of contraction) than those at rest, if a contracting muscle must stretch a contracting antagonist, the eye will move more slowly. Since an eye muscle twitch (in cats) lasts 19 msec, the only way to avoid stretching a contracting antagonist while oscillating the eye with a period of 36 msec is to stimulate each muscle only during a brief burst at the start of its contraction. This is possible in birds but not in mammals, because each mammalian motoneuron fires with a rate proportional to eye position, and thus would continue its firing throughout its half-cycle of activity. Consequently, during the next half-cycle, the muscle would still be contracting and hence stiff. A second possible advantage of the avian mode is that it permits the eye to act like a pendulum, reversing its direction of motion passively, with the motoneurons firing afterward. This too could not occur in mammals, because the continuous motoneuron activity would not leave the eye free to oscillate.

Whatever the reasons for the motor mechanism of saccadic oscillations, an astonishing consequence of the saccadic oscillations is that they stir the vitreous humor. If the small fluorescent molecule fluorescein is injected into the blood and allowed to leak out from the pecten, the saccadic oscillations cause spectacular fluorescent plumes to shoot across the liquid part of the vitreous near the retina (Pettigrew et al., 1990). These plumes had been observed earlier (Bellhorn and Bellhorn, 1975), but their relation to the saccadic oscillations not discerned.

What function might avian oscillations serve? Early researchers imagined that the movements helped to polish the cornea against the nictitating membrane (third eyelid), or assumed that the heavy eyes of birds could not move fast enough to provide the blurring necessary to suppress vision during saccades without this additional twirling (Nye, 1969;

Brooks and Holden, 1973). However, the oscillations are not very tightly related to the movements of the nictitating membrane and the chicken eye moves just about as fast as a human one during saccades.

We suggest that the oscillations play a role in retinal nutrition. The large avascular avian retina may well need some mechanical assistance in obtaining nutrients and oxygen from the pecten, which, in large birds, can be a centimeter from parts of the retina. Oscillating the eye would stir the vitreous humor, especially as the pecten is shaped rather like the agitator in a washing machine. Our consistent finding in several species that fluorescein moves across the retina during saccades supports this hypothesis and suggests that four avian features may have evolved together: saccadic oscillations, fan-shaped pectens, large eyes, and thick avascular retinas. Variations in each of these characteristics may be related to variations in the other; for example, birds with thicker retinas may have longer saccadic oscillations or larger pectens. Birds, therefore, may utilize a strategy giving them much higher acuity at all eccentricities than would be possible if retinal vascularization were used for retinal nourishment.

Saccadic oscillations may have more than a single function. It seems odd that birds avoid interruptions of vision during locomotion, and yet make extremely long oscillating saccades which obscure vision for more than 10% of the time. We speculate that these long oscillatory saccades may have some visual function, perhaps aiding in the detection of some kinds of motion. In chickens, brief movements of the visual surround during saccades are followed by shortening of the saccade (or at least of its oscillations), suggesting that birds can detect visual motion during saccades. Obtaining evidence in favor of this hypothesis remains a challenge.

CONCLUSIONS

Birds, like other animals, have distinct behaviors that change and stabilize gaze. Although reflex-like in that normal behavior is produced in highly reduced stimulus situations, each behavior is coming to be seen as part of several complex subsystems. Thus the VOR, long a paradigm of a simple three-neuron reflex arc, now turns out be modulated by the distance at which the eyes are looking even in darkness. Similarly OKN, long thought to respond only to the gross optic flow, responds better to background than foreground motion. Thus, despite their stereotypy, these behaviors may possess a complexity of inputs and serve a multiplicity of functions like the behaviors associated with higher cortical processing.

One could say that birds fascinate us because they combine a weirdness of form and behavior with a familiarity of inferred perceptual and mental processes. Perhaps with oculomotor processes as well, the weird behaviors of birds will illuminate the physiology of the familiar.

REFERENCES

Becker, W., Metrics. In R. H. Wurtz and M. E. Goldberg (Eds.), *The Neurobiology of Saccadic Eye Movements* (Vol. 3 of *Reviews of Oculomotor Research*). Elsevier, Amsterdam, 1989, pp. 13–61.

Bellhorn, R. W., and Bellhorn, M. S. The avian pecten. I. Fluorescein permeability. *Ophthal. Res.* 7 (1975), 1–7.

Bilo, D. Visual reflexes and neck flexion-related activity of flight control muscles in the airflow-stimulated pigeon. In A. Berthoz, P. P. Vidal, and W. Graf (Eds.), *The Head-Neck Sensory Motor System*. Oxford University Press, Oxford, 1992, pp. 96–100.

Bloch, S., Rivaud, S., and Martinoya, C. Comparing frontal and lateral viewing in the pigeon. III. Different patterns of eye movements for binocular and monocular fixation. *Behav. Brain Res.* 13 (1984), 173–182.

Bloch, S., Lemeignan, M., and Martinoya, C. Coordinated vergence for frontal fixation, but independent eye movements for lateral viewing, in the pigeon. In J. K. O'Regan and A. Levy-Schoen (Eds.), *Eye Movements: From Physiology to Cognition*. Elsevier, Amsterdam, 1987, pp. 47–56.

Brooks, B., and Holden, A. L. Suppression of visual signals by rapid image displacement in the pigeon retina: a possible mechanism for "saccadic" suppression. *Vision Res.* 13 (1973), 1387–1390.

Burns, S., and Wallman, J. Relation of single unit properties to the oculomotor function of the nucleus of the basal optic root (accessory optic system) in chickens. *Exp. Brain Res.* 42 (1981), 171–180.

Carpenter, R. H. S. *Movements of the Eyes*, 2nd ed. Pion, London, 1988.

Collett, T. S., and Harkness, L. I. K. Depth vision in animals. In D. I. Ingle, M. A. Goodale, and R. J. W. Mansfield (Eds.), *Analysis of Visual Behavior*. MIT Press, Cambridge, MA, 1982.

Collewijn, H. Eye and head movements in freely moving rabbits. *J. Physiol.* 266 (1977), 471–498.

Duijm, M. On the head posture in birds and its relation to some anatomical features. *Proc. Kon. Med. Akad. Wet. C.* 54 (1951), 202–211; 260–271.

Duijm, M. On the position of a ribbon-like central area in the eyes of some birds. *Arch. Neerl. Zool.* 13 (1958), 128–145.

Erichsen, J. T., Hodos, W., Evinger, C., Bessette, B. B., and Phillips, S. J. Head orientation in pigeons: Postural, locomotor and visual determinants. *Brain Behav. Evol.* 33 (1989), 268–278.

Fitzke, F. W., Hayes, B. P., Hodos, W., Holden, A. L., and Low, J. C. Refractive sectors in the visual field of the pigeon eye. *J. Physiol.* 369 (1985), 33–45.

Flandrin, J. M., Courjon, J. H., Magnin, M., and Arzi, M. Horizontal optokinetic responses under stroboscopic illumination in monkey and man. *Exp. Brain Res.* 81 (1990), 59–69.

Fox, R. Binocular vision and stereopsis. In S. J. Cool, E. L. Smith, and D. L. MacAdam (Eds.), *Frontiers in Visual Science*. Springer-Verlag, New York, 1978, pp. 316–327.

Friedman, M. B. Visual control of head movements during avian locomotion. *Nature (London)* 255 (1975), 67–69.

Frost, B. J. The optokinetic basis of head-bobbing in the pigeon. *J. Exp. Biol.* 74 (1978), 187–195.

Gioanni, H. Stabilizing gaze reflexes in the pigeon (*Columba livia*) I. Horizontal and vertical optokinetic eye (OKN) and head (OCR) reflexes. *Exp. Brain Res.* 69 (1988), 567–582.

Hughes, A. The topography of vision in mammals of contrasting life style: Comparative optics and retinal organisation. In F. Crescitelli (Ed.), *Handbook of Sensory Physiology*. Springer, New York, 1977.

Hughes, A. One brush tailed possum can browse as much pasture as 0.06 sheep which may indicate why this "arboreal" animal has a visual streak: Some comments on the "terrain" theory. *Vision Res.* 21 (1981), 957–958.

Knudsen, E. I. Fused binocular vision is required for development of proper eye alignment in barn owls. *Visual Neurosci.* 2 (1989), 35–40.

Lemeignan, M., Sansonetti, A., and Gioanni, H. Spontaneous saccades under different visual conditions in the pigeon. *NeuroReport* 3 (1992), 17–20.

Letelier, J. C. Neuroethology of saccadic eye movements in chickens. Ph. D. Dissertation, City University of New York, 1992.

Lorenz, K., and Tinbergen, N. Taxis und Instinkthandlung in der Eirollbewegung der Graugans. *Z. Tierpsychol.* 2 (1938), 1–29. [In C. H. Schiller (trans.), *Instinctive Behavior. The Development of a Modern Concept*. International Universities Press, New York, 1957.]

Maldonado, P. E., Maturana, H., and Varela, F. J. Frontal and lateral visual system in birds: Frontal and lateral gaze. *Brain Behav. Evol.* 32 (1988), 57–62.

Marin, G., Letelier, J. C., and Wallman, J. Saccade-related responses of centrifugal neurons projecting to the chicken retina. *Exp. Brain Res.* 82 (1990), 263–270.

McFadden, S. A. The binocular depth stereoacuity of the pigeon and its relation to the anatomical resolving power of the eye. *Vision Res.* 27 (1987), 1967–1980.

McFadden, S. A. Eye design for depth and distance perception in the pigeon. An observer oriented perspective. *J. Comp. Psychol.* 3 (1991), 1–22.

McKenna, O. C., and Wallman, J. Accessory optic system and pretectum of birds: comparisons with those of other vertebrates. *Brain Behav. Evol.* 26 (1985), 91–116.

Miles, F. A. The sensing of rotational and translational optic flow by the primate optokinetic system. In F. A. Miles and J. Wallman (Eds.), *Visual Motion and its Role in the Stabilization of Gaze* (Vol. 5 of *Reviews of Oculomotor Research*). Elsevier, Amsterdam, 1993.

Nalbach, H. O. Translational head movements of pigeons in response to a rotating pattern: Characteristics and tools to analyse mechanisms underlying detection of rotational and translational optical flow. *Exp. Brain Res.* (1993), in press.

Nalbach, H. O., Wolf-Oberhollenzer, F., and Kirschfeld, K. The pigeon's eye viewed through an ophthalmoscopic microscope: Orientation of retinal landmarks and significance of eye movements. *Vision Res.* 30 (1990), 529–540.

Nye, P. W. The monocular eye movements of the pigeon. *Vision Res.* 9 (1969), 133–144.

Pettigrew, J. D., and Konishi, M. Neurons selective for orientation and binocular disparity in the visual Wulst of the barn owl (*Tyto alba*). *Science* 193 (1976), 675–678.

Pettigrew, J. D., Wallman, J., and Wildsoet, C. F. Saccadic oscillations facilitate ocular perfusion from the avian pecten. *Nature (London)* 343 (1990), 362–363.

Pratt, D. W. Saccadic eye movements are coordinated with head movements in walking chickens. *J. Exp. Biol.* 97 (1982), 217–223.

Rashbass, C. The relationship between saccadic and smooth tracking eye movements. *J. Physiol.* 159 (1961), 326–338.

Rojas, X., McKenna, O. C., and Wallman, J. Functional parcellation of the accessory optic system requires visual experience. *Soc. Neurosci. Abstr.* 11 (1985), 1014.

Simpson, J. I., and Hess, R. Complex and simple visual messages in the flocculus. In R. Baker and A. Berthoz (Eds.), *Control of Gaze by Brain Stem Neurons*. Elsevier North-Holland, New York, 1977, pp. 351–360.

Steinbach, M. J., and Money, K. E. Eye movements of the owl. *Vision Res.* 13 (1973), 889–891.

Tinbergen, N., and Kuenen, D. J. Über die auslösenden und die richtunggebenden Reizsituationen der Sperrbewegung von jungen Drosseln (*Turdus m. merula* L. and *T. e. ericetorum* Turton). *Z. Tierpsychol.* 3 (1939), 37–60 [In C. H. Schiller (trans.), *Instinctive Behavior. The Development of a Modern Concept*. International Universities Press, New York, 1957.]

Turkel, J., and Wallman, J. Oscillatory eye movements with possible visual function in birds. *Soc. Neurosci. Abstr.* 3 (1977), 158.

Van Gisbergen, J. A. M., and Van Opstal, A. J. Models. In R. H. Wurtz and M. E. Goldberg (Eds.), *The Neurobiology of Saccadic Eye Movements* (Vol. 3 of *Reviews of Oculomotor Research*). Elsevier, Amsterdam, 1989, pp. 69–98.

Wallman, J., and Pettigrew, J. D. Conjugate and disjunctive saccades in two avian species with contrasting oculomotor strategies. *J. Neurosci.* 5 (1985), 1418–1428.

Wallman, J., and Velez, J. Directional asymmetries of optokinetic nystagmus: Developmental changes and relation to the accessory optic system and to the vestibular system. *J. Neurosci.* 5 (1985), 317–329.

Westheimer, G. Eye movement responses to a horizontally moving visual stimulus. *Arch. Ophthalmol.* 52 (1954), 932–41.

Wylie, D., and Frost, B. J. Purkinje cells in the vestibulocerebellum of the pigeon respond best to either translational or rotational visual flow. *Exp. Brain Res.* 86 (1991), 229–232.

15 Sensorimotor Mechanisms and Pecking in the Pigeon

H. Philip Zeigler, Ralf Jäger, and
Adrian G. Palacios

The pigeon's pecking response mediates both its ingestive behavior (eating and drinking) and a conditioned behavior (key pecking), which is among the most widely used response measures in psychology. For students of conditioning, key-pecking functions as a convenient *indicator* response in studies of reinforcement schedules, detection, or discrimination. For this reason the focus of most key-pecking studies is on response rate, since it provides an easily quantifiable index of behavioral control (cf. chapter 16). However, in nature, the pigeon's pecking behavior functions primarily to transport a prehensile effector organ (the jaw) toward biologically significant targets like food or water (*peck localization*) and to generate jaw movement patterns (*grasping, manipulation*) whose topography is appropriate to the stimulus properties of the target. Both types of pecking involve the same effector systems—the neck and the jaw—and the same movement patterns—a transport component (head movement) and a gape component (jaw movement). Moreover the coordination of these two response components is an essential feature of the pecking response.

Early studies of pecking response topography were based on the use of high-speed cinematography. Recent advances have come from the development of instrumentation for the "on-line" monitoring of head and jaw movements (figure 15.1), which, in combination with conditioning paradigms, has enabled us to bring both the transport and gape components under experimental control (Deich et al., 1985; Allan and Zeigler, 1989; Bermejo et al., 1993).

The rapidity with which pecking is localized to the key using conditioning paradigms indicates its susceptibility to control by associative mechanisms, and developmental studies suggest a role for such mechanisms in the ontogeny of pecking (Graf et al., 1985; Deich and Balsam, 1993). Moreover, whether acquired under a classical (respondent) or an instrumental (operant) conditioning paradigm, the form of the conditioned response is strikingly similar to that of the ingestive response to the reinforcer (Wolin, 1968; Jenkins and Moore, 1973; Allan and Zeigler, 1993). The presence of such similarities suggests that ingestive and

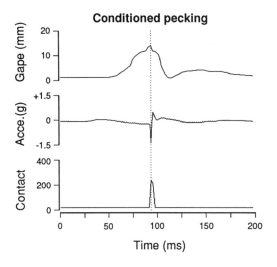

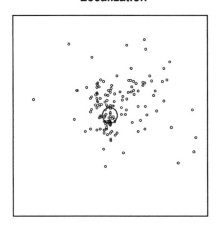

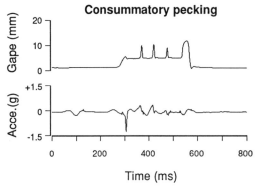

Figure 15.1 "On-line" monitoring of head movements, jaw movements and peck localization during a single conditioned pecking response trial (both CS and US periods). Top (conditioned pecking): Head and jaw movement components of the conditioned key peck. The dotted line indicates the moment of contact with the touch screen. Trace 1 (*Gape*) is the output of a magnetosensitive transducer mounted on the upper beak, which

conditioned pecking share a common neural substrate, are mediated by similar sensorimotor processes, and involve conjoint control by visuo-motor and associative mechanisms. This conclusion implies, first, that the conditioned key-pecking response may serve as a "model system" for the study of the sensorimotor control of ingestive behavior, and, second, that analyses of the topography and sensory control of ingestive pecking may be useful to students of conditioning. These conclusions are explored in this and the following chapter.

INGESTIVE PECKING: TOPOGRAPHY AND KINEMATIC ANALYSIS

Ingestive behavior (eating, drinking), requires the organization of several distinct movement patterns into an adaptive behavioral sequence (figure 15.2). *Eating* begins with the eyes open, the beaks almost closed, and the head poised above the (target) seed. It may be divided into pecking, grasping, and mandibulation components, the latter two of which are prehensile responses. *Pecking* consists of a series of saccade-like head movements, punctuated by several fixation pauses (Goodale, 1983), during the last two of which (F1, F2) the head is kept in position above the target at relatively constant distances (F1: mean = 97 mm; F2: mean = 56 mm). Head descent begins after F2. *Grasping* is integrated into the pecking response, and is divisible into opening and closing phases. Jaw-opening begins 25–30 msec after the start of head descent, followed within 5–10 msec by eye closure, and continues throughout head descent. Peak gape (interbeak distance) immediately prior to contact varies directly with seed size. The closing phase of grasping is initiated at contact and terminates with the seed held firmly between the beak tips and the eyes fully open. The entire pecking/grasping sequence lasts about 60 msec. Manipulation of the seed within the oral cavity requires several additional movement phases. *Stationing*, the first phase of mandibulation, consists of one or more jaw opening and closing movements, which function to reposition the seed prior to its subsequent transport within the oral cavity. *Intraoral transport* of small seeds involves a linqual transport mechanism ("slide-and-glue") in

produces a voltage proportional to the magnetic field induced by a magnet mounted on the lower beak. The output of the system is a continuous record of variations in gape (interbeak distance: Deich et al., 1985). Trace 2 (*Acce.*) shows the output of a head-mounted accelerometer. The duration of the peck is indicated by the width of the *Contact* trace. Middle (localization): Location of pecks made to a computer-generated, stimulus display (large circle) whose size and location may be varied on each trial. Peck locations are recorded on the *x, y* coordinate system of a "touch-sensitive" device. The black dots represent the distribution of terminal peck locations over a series of trials, with respect to the location of the stimulus feature on that trial. Bottom (consummatory pecking): Data from acceleration and gape transducers recorded during the US period are replotted, using a time base that permits high resolution monitoring of the ingestive response to the reinforcer. From Bermejo et al. (1993).

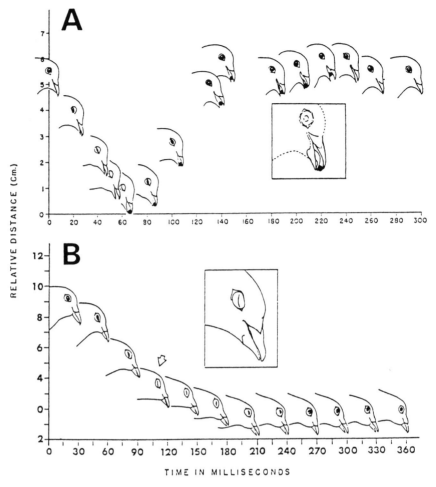

Figure 15.2 Ingestive behavior in the pigeon. (A) Eating behavior. Inset shows the position of the tongue at the start of *intraoral transport*. (B) Drinking behavior. Arrow indicates point of contact with water surface (see inset). Based on cinematographic records taken at 100 frames/sec. From Zeigler et al. (1980).

which mucous secretions from intraoral glands cause the seed to adhere to the dorsal surface of the tongue, which conveys it from the beak tips to the caudal palate and pharynx. With larger seeds, an inertial transport ("catch and-throw") mechanism is used, which combines a head jerk and a complete gape cycle, while the tongue is kept retracted. During stationing and intraoral transport, jaw movements are adjusted to both the size and location of the seed (Zeigler et al., 1980; Zweers, 1982b).

During eating, periods of visual scanning alternate with bouts of pecking (see chapter 18). The accuracy of peck localization (Zeigler et al., 1975; Levine and Zeigler, 1981; Jäger and Zeigler, 1991), its discriminative control by seed targets (Moon and Zeigler, 1979), and the amplitude scaling of gape size to seed size (Zeigler et al., 1980; Deich et al., 1985) suggest that pecking is elicited and guided primarily by visual inputs.

Visuomotor Mechanisms

Grasping must involve both visual and somatosensory inputs, while transport of the seed within the oral cavity is elicited and guided by trigeminal somatosensation. However, we have shown that removal of trigeminal orosensation by deafferentation disrupts all three components of the ingestive pecking sequence: localization, grasping, and mandibulation (Zeigler et al., 1975; Bermejo and Zeigler, 1989).

Drinking also begins with the head elevated and the beaks almost closed, followed by a period of head descent, which is terminated at contact with the water. Water intake involves rhythmic opening and closing movement of the jaws (Klein et al., 1983; Bermejo et al., 1992), and its intraoral transport is mediated by an active suction mechanism, which creates areas of low pressure within the oral and pharyngeal regions, producing a rostral-to-caudal flow of the liguid (Zweers, 1982a).

Once initiated, drinking movements continue without any obvious phasic inputs; indeed, "dry" drinking movements are sometimes made to the water container itself (Bout and Zeigler, 1993). In contrast, eating movements form a sensorimotor chain, whose links are provided by phasic inputs from the food object (Zeigler et al., 1980). With respect to their response forms, however, the essential differentiating features of the eating response are its episodic character and the scaling of jaw opening amplitude (*peak gape*) to the size of the food object. Drinking is characterized by its rhythmicity and by the relative invariance of peak gape. Thus, differences in jaw movement topography may serve as neurobehavioral markers of hunger and thirst.

During pecking/grasping, head descent is generated by an initial acceleration burst that produces an increase in velocity followed by a period of maintained, and then of decreasing velocity (Klein et al., 1985, figure 3). The adaptive function of this strategy is to produce a braking action on the head movement prior to contact with the target or substrate. Indeed, at its termination, the force of the eating peck may be less than 2–3 g (LaMon and Zeigler, 1988), suggesting that such pecking represents a controlled grasp of, rather than a strike at the seed.

VISUAL CONTROL OF INGESTIVE RESPONSES

Kinematic analyses of head and jaw movements during pecking and grasping indicate that both behaviors come under the control of target size. Head position at the start of pecking is higher for large than for small seeds (Klein et al., 1985). Thus, even though the initial head acceleration is similar for seeds of different sizes, the period of initial velocity increase is longer for the large seeds, producing differences in their peak velocity. During grasping, opening movements of the effector organ (jaw) are scaled to the size of the seed (figure 15.3), for both successful and unsuccessful pecks as well as mandibulation (Bermejo et al., 1989). In this, and other respects, the pigeon's grasping resembles the prehensile behavior of humans (Jeannerod, 1981; Klein et al., 1985).

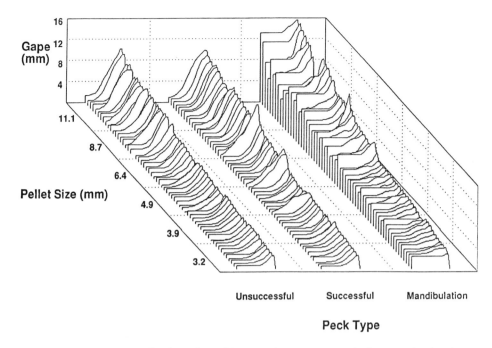

Figure 15.3 Amplitude scaling of jaw opening movements during grasping in pigeon. Jaw movement trajectories as a function of food pellet size for successful and unsuccessful grasping responses, and the stationing component of mandibulation. Note that peak opening amplitude increases with pellet size for all three measures. From Bermejo et al. (1989).

Peck localization and grasping are undoubtedly elicited and guided by visual stimuli from the target. However, given the brevity of the pecking response (< 60 msec), the fact that maximum gape is achieved prior to contact (Deich et al., 1985, figure 1), and that it occurs during a period of gradual eye closure and at head velocities that approximate 165 cm/sec (McFadden, 1991), control of these behaviors is unlikely to involve the processing of visual inputs generated *during* the pecking response. Thus pecking and the opening phase of grasping may involve feedforward control systems (i.e., the response, once intiated, is no longer under the control of visual stimuli from the seed).

VISUAL PROCESSING DURING PECKING/GRASPING

Accurate peck localization and grasping behavior requires the processing of visual information as to the size of the target and its egocentric distance and direction (Collett and Harkness, 1982) When, during the course of the pecking/grasping response, does such processing take place, what type of visual cues are utilized, and which retinal regions are involved?

Goodale (1983) has suggested that the two fixation periods (F1, F2) observed during ingestive pecking could provide intervals for the processing of inputs used to guide pecking. He employed a "feature-positive discrimination" procedure in which the presence on the key of a stimulus feature (a small black dot) was correlated with reinforcement and its absence with a "time-out" (Jenkins and Sainsbury, 1970). Key pecks on both positive and negative trials were found to include fixation pauses similar to those observed during eating. Because of the similarity in the distance of the first fixation pause on positive and negative trials, Goodale suggested that the decision to peck (or not to peck) was made during these initial fixations, while the final (F2) fixation was used to process information about seed size and location. This hypothesis is consistent with the observation that the improvement in pecking accuracy seen with repeated testing parallels changes in the F1 and F2 distance (McFadden, 1991).

VISUAL CUES TO DISTANCE AND THE PIGEON'S PECKING BEHAVIOR

The accuracy of the pigeon's pecking behavior suggests that it makes efficient use of visual cues to distance, but provides no evidence as to their nature or relative contribution. *Accommodation*, a monocular cue, is related to adjustments in the shape of the cornea or lens; *convergence*, a binocular cue, is related to simultaneous adjustments of both eyes. Both adjustments serve to maintain a sharp image of the object on the photoreceptors as the object's distance varies (see chapters 1 and 3).

To assess the relative contribution of the two mechanisms, Martinoya et al. (1984b) used optical manipulations to control the apparent distance of the object from the pigeon. When a pair of negative (concave) lenses or a pair of negative (base-out) prisms is mounted so as to coincide with the normal line of sight, they produce a "virtual" image of the grain whose distance varies with the optical properties of the devices, that is, the grain will appear closer than its actual location. The extent to which the pigeon's pecking behavior is modified by these manipulations provides some evidence of the extent to which either an accommodation or a convergence cue is used to estimate distance. For each peck made to a single grain of corn, the experimenters calculated both the final fixation distance (F2) and the pecking error (amount of undershoot).

Figure 15.4 illustrates, schematically, the organization of pecking responses under both control and experimental conditions. For both prisms or lenses, F2 distances were higher than in the control condition, pecks tended to undershoot the grain, and one or more additional fixations and pecks were necessary for successful localization of the grain. Moreover, for both lenses and prisms, the F2 values increased systematically with increases in the refractive properties of the devices, implying a compensatory adjustment to the apparent distance of the "virtual" image of the grain. These results suggest that *both* accommo-

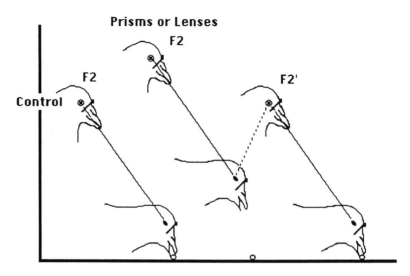

Figure 15.4 Schematic diagram of pecking behavior under the control and optical manipulation (lenses, prisms) condition. F2 corresponds to the last fixation prior to head descent (continuous line. Note that when prisms or lenses are worn, the peck undershoots the seed, and that additional fixations (F2') and descents (dotted line) are required to obtain the seed. From Martinoya et al. (1984b).

dation and convergence mechanisms may provide distance cues for peck localization in pigeons.

RETINAL MORPHOLOGY AND THE VISUAL CONTROL OF PECKING

Identification of the retinal regions mediating the initial stages of processing during pecking has been a persistent problem for students of visuomotor mechanisms (see part I of the present volume). The pigeon's retina contains two morphologically distinct areas that might participate in such processing: a red field and a yellow field. These morphological differences are correlated with differences in the refractive properties and visual representations of the two areas. The projection of the yellow field in the external world corresponds to the *monocular* (lateral) visual field and its optics are characterized by emmetropia; that is, the horizontal and lateral portions of the field receive well-focused images of objects over a wide range of distances. The projection of the red field corresponds to the *monocular* frontoventral visual field and its optics are characterized by emmetropia for the horizon and upper portion of the field and a gradient of increasing myopia (nearsightedness) in the lower portion. This variation in refractive properties may be an adaptation permitting the simultaneous monitoring of the horizon and upper visual field for predators while keeping objects on the ground in focus during foraging, without the necessity of accommodation. Finally the yellow and red retinal fields each contains a specialized region of high ganglion cell density: the *fovea centralis* and the *area dorsalis*, respectively (for details, see chapters 1 and 2).

The frontal and lateral visual fields appear to differ significantly in function. Nye (1973) found that performance on simple discriminations (pattern, color, intensity) falls to chance as the location of the stimuli is gradually shifted from the frontal to the lateral visual fields. Nye hypothesised that "pigeons do not seem to possess the neural capability required to learn to use information contained in laterally located stimuli to *directly* control pecking behavior" (1973, p. 570). Subsequent studies have demonstrated that when frontally directed key pecking is used as an indicator response, pigeons can discriminate between laterally presented stimuli. Using a "behavioral fixation" procedure, in which the stimuli were tachistoscopically presented for brief (250–300 msec) intervals to control for head movements, the lateral and frontal fields were shown to differ with respect to visual acuity and movement discrimination (Bloch et al., 1982; Martinoya et al., 1983).

However, in these experiments visual input is used to control the presence or absence of the peck rather than its terminal location, that is *whether*, rather than *where* to peck. When pigeons are required to peck and grasp seeds with both frontal fields occluded, they seem initially to peck at random then adopt a strategy in which the head is turned sideways to target the seed with the lateral field, and then thrust forward in its general direction. Under these conditions pecking accuracy deteriorates drastically, dropping from 1–2 to 40–50 pecks/seed (Martinoya et al., 1984a). This finding has been confirmed using an operant (response differentiation) procedure in which the terminal location of each peck was monitored electronically and subjects were reinforced only for pecks localized to a 2.5-cm^2 target area at the center of a larger response surface (Jäger and Zeigler, 1991). When viewing with the lateral fields alone, subjects had difficulty locating the food hopper and, even with considerable training, the terminal location of their peeks approximated a random distribution (figure 15.5).

These findings are consistent with Nye's hypothesis, since they indicate that input from the frontal visual field is critical for accurate guidance of peck localization behavior. However, they provide no evidence as to the relative contribution of monocular or binocular cues, or for the existence of a retinal area specialized for the visuomotor control of pecking and grasping. A large body of optical and behavioral observations suggests that the "red field" of the retina, and specifically, its *area dorsalis*, may serve this function. Cinematographic studies of head movement during feeding (Goodale, 1983; Erichsen et al., 1989) have shown that the first (F1) fixation is made with the seed about 10° below the eye-bill axis, while the final (F2) fixation is made with a small (1–2°) segment of the visual field located "just in front of and/or slightly above the bill tip" (Erichsen et al., 1989, p. 276). This "pecking field" (Galifret, 1968) is viewed by the superior temporal portion of the pi-

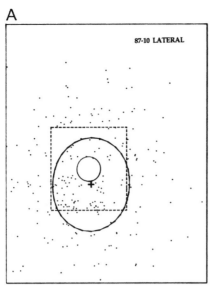

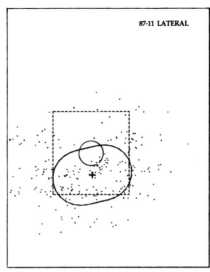

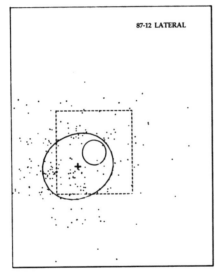

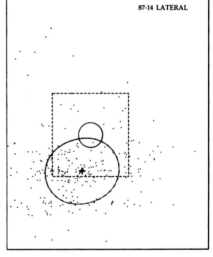

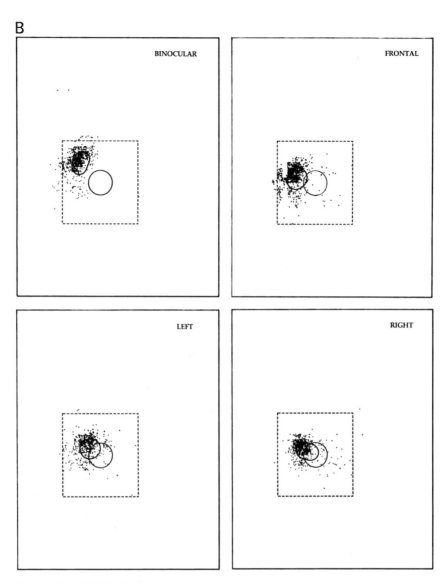

B

BINOCULAR

FRONTAL

LEFT

RIGHT

Figure 15.5 (A) Distributions of pecking responses made to a circular target by four pigeons, using only the lateral visual field (frontal field occluded). (B) Distribution of pecking response made to a circular target under the viewing conditions indicated. Binocular (top left), frontal (top right: lateral fields occluded), and monocular (bottom left and right). In these plots the target stimulus (0.8 cm in diameter) is shown as an open circle centered within a contingency area (dashed line). Pecks falling within this area were reinforced. The terminal location of each peck is indicated by a dot, the mean of the distribution by a cross and its SD is represented in eight axes with their endpoints connected to form an ellipse. From Jäger and Zeigler (1991).

Zeigler et al: Sensorimotor Mechanisms and Pecking

geon's "red field," i.e., the portion whose visual representation is characterized by lower-field myopia.

In contrast to the lateral fields, which are monocular, the frontal visual fields of the pigeon possess an area of bilateral overlap of approximately 30° which is symmetrical about the eye-beak axis, with a peak width at about 10° below that axis (McFadden, 1991). During pecking, frontally presented stimuli elicit coordinated convergence movements, which are evident even when one eye is occluded (Martinoya et al., 1984a). When comparable amounts and direction of eye movement are simulated in anesthetized pigeons, they bring the red field into the binocular region with the *area dorsalis* pointing into the midsagittal plane, 10° below the beak, an outcome highly adaptive for the visual control of pecking (Nalbach and Wolf-Oberhollenzer, 1990: see chapter 2).

While these observations suggest that pecking/grasping normally involves binocular inputs, other behavioral evidence indicates that binocular input is not critical. Monocular occlusion of the frontal field or blocking the overlap of one eye produces a transient reduction in the accuracy of pecking at grain, and a permanent reduction is reported after section of commissural pathways mediating binocular interaction (Martinoya et al., 1984a; McFadden et al., 1986; McFadden, 1991). However, both these deficits, though significant, are slight. Moreover, the studies reporting these deficits used "pick-up" tests of pecking accuracy, which do not distinguish between localization and grasping deficits.

When this distinction is made operationally, there is no significant difference in the localization accuracy of pecks made under binocular or monocular conditions (Jäger et al., 1992, figure 3). Under both conditions, more than 95% of the pecks initiated were well localized (i.e., terminated in contact with the seed). Moreover, pecking accuracy on an operant (response differentiation) test of peck localization (Jäger and Zeigler, 1991) was comparable under binocular and monocular conditions (see figure 15.5) Finally, the scaling of jaw opening amplitude to target size during pecking/grasping (figure 15.6) is as precise under monocular as under binocular viewing conditions (Jäger et al., 1992).

Because grasping errors constitute a high proportion (ca. 44%: McFadden, 1991) of errors on "pick-up tests," such tests may *overestimate* the contribution of binocular inputs to the control of pecking. On the other hand, because the target area in the operant localization task is considerably larger than a seed, it requires less precise localization. Moreover, the "touch-screen" devices used to monitor peck locations in these experiments will not record pecks that fall short of the response surface and so will miss errors due to "undershooting," which are quite common during normal pecking and might be expected to increase under monocular viewing conditions. Results obtained with "touch-sensitive" devices may thus *underestimate* the contribution of binocular inputs. Taken together the conditioned and ingestive pecking studies confirm the critical role of the frontal visual fields. However, they sug-

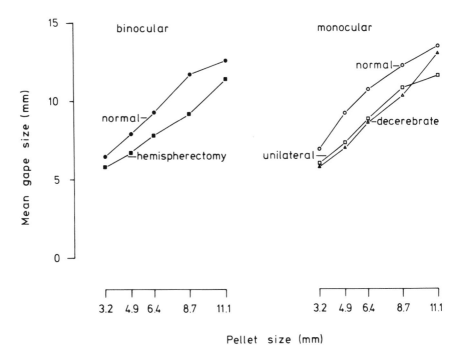

Figure 15.6 Amplitude scaling of *gape* in normal and hemispherectomized pigeons. Functions relating pellet size to gape size for normal and hemispherectomized subjects, tested under different viewing conditions. Note that for the normal subjects, the functions are similar for binocular and monocular viewing. The unilateral and decerebrate testing conditions are explained in the legend of figure 15.7. From Jäger et al. (1992).

gest that input from the monocular frontal field is sufficient for the adaptive control of the pigeon's pecking and grasping behavior. The convergence signal provided during binocular viewing may be more important for depth perception than for egocentric distance perception (Martinoya et al., 1988; McFadden, 1991).

THE VISUAL FOREBRAIN AND PECKING/GRASPING BEHAVIOR

Although central pathways involved in the somatosensorimotor control of the jaw have been identified (Wild and Zeigler, 1980; Berkhoudt et al., 1982; Wild et al., 1985; Arends and Zeigler, 1989), little is known about central visuomotor mechanisms mediating these behaviors. Lesions of thalamic visual relays and telencephalic visual projection areas disrupt visual detection and discrimination behaviors (see chapters 4 and 8), but with rare exceptions (e.g., Jarvis, 1974) such lesions do not disrupt peck localization, and there are no reports of grasping deficits. Classic studies of the decerebrate pigeon have reported "permanent" loss of ingestive pecking after bilateral removal of the telencephalon. However, if care is taken to avoid damaging the diencephalon, ingestive pecking recovers within a few months (Brunelli et al., 1972), and both acquisition and retention of an operant key-pecking task have been demonstrated in the decerebrate pigeon (DeSouza-Celena et al., 1990).

The differential contributions of visual forebrain structures to the control of pecking and grasping may be assessed using a procedure for reversible "visual decerebration" (figure 15.7). The procedure is based upon the observation that each side of the pigeon's visual forebrain (thalamus + telencephalon) receives its visual inputs primarily from the contralateral eye, and that *unilateral* hemispherectomy does not disrupt either ingestive or conditioned pecking behavior. In a unilaterally hemispherectomized subject, the eye contralateral to the intact hemisphere has (unilateral) access to the entire visual system, while for the eye opposite the ablated hemisphere, visual processing is restricted to the structures caudal to the forebrain. Thus, by alternately occluding the eye ipsilateral to the intact, and then to the ablated hemisphere, a subject may be tested first as visually "normal" and then as visually "decerebrate" (Jäger et al., 1992).

When tested under binocular conditions, unilaterally hemispherectomized subjects are as accurate in their peck location as normal sub-

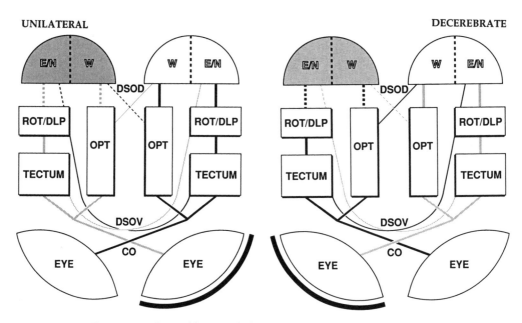

Figure 15.7 Reversible "visual decerebration" in the pigeon. Organization of visual inputs in the unilateral condition (left), with the eye *contralateral* to the ablated (shaded) hemisphere occluded; and in the "decerebrate" condition (right) with the eye *ipsilateral* to the ablated hemisphere occluded. CO, optic chiasm; DSOD, DSOV, dorsal and ventral supraoptic decussations; tectum, optic tectum; OPT, principal optic nucleus of the thalamus; ROT/DLP, nuclei rotundus and dorsolateralis posterioris of the thalamus; E/N, ectostriatum/neostriatum; W, Wulst. Thick solid lines = tectofugal and thalamofugal pathways; thin solid lines = ipsilateral recrossing pathways (tectorotundal): OPT-Wulst. Shaded areas = telencephalic ablations; dashed/shaded lines = nonfunctional connections. From Jäger et al. (1992).

jects. However, their monocular performance depends critically on which eye is occluded. When tested with the eye contralateral to the intact hemisphere, the pigeon's peck localization is normal (misses < 5%); when tested as a "visual decerebrate," not only does its performance deteriorate (misses, 40–80%), but it makes large numbers of "random" pecks at the floor or wall. Comparable results were seen using an operant measure of peck localization (figure 15.8). In contrast, the adjustment of jaw opening size to pellet size is not disrupted in the "visual decerebrate" (see figure 15.6). These results indicate that pecking and grasping are mediated by structures at different brain levels.

CONCLUSIONS

Although it has generally been treated as a unitary response, the pigeon's ingestive behavior may be dissociated into distinct components (pecking, grasping, mandibulation), elicited by different sensory cues, mediated by different effector systems and controlled by different brain structures. This dissociation is a first step in identifying sensorimotor control mechanisms for each component, and may also be useful in clarifying the associative control of pecking (cf. chapter 16).

ACKNOWLEDGMENTS

The research on which this report is based was supported, in part, by research grants from the National Science Foundation and the National Institutes of Health to H.P.Z., by a travel grant from the Deutscher Akademischer Austauschdienst to H.P.Z., and by a Fellowship to R.J. from the Deutsche Forschungsgemeinschaft.

REFERENCES

Allan, R. W., and Zeigler, H. P. Measurement and control of pecking response location in the pigeon. *Physiol. Behav.* 45, (1989), 1215–1221.

Allan, R. W., and Zeigler, H. P. Conditioning of the jaw movement (gape) response during autoshaping of the pigeon's key peck. *J. Exp. Anal. Behav.*, in press.

Arends, J. J. A., and Zeigler, H. P. Cerebellar connections of the trigeminal system in the pigeon. *Brain Res.* 75 (1989), 1215–1221.

Berkhoudt, H. J., Klein, B. G., and Zeigler, H. P. Afferents to the trigeminal and facial motor nuclei of the pigeon (*Columba Livia*): central connections of jaw motoneurons. *J. Comp. Neurol.* 109 (1982), 301–312.

Bermejo, R., and Zeigler. H. P. Trigeminal deafferentation and prehension in the pigeon. *Behav. Brain Res.* 35 (1989), 55–61.

Bermejo, R., Allan, R. W., Deich, J. D., Houben, D., and Zeigler, H. P. Prehension in the pigeon I: Descriptive analysis. *Exp. Brain Res.* 75 (1989), 569–576.

Bermejo, R., Remy, M., and Zeigler, H. P. Beak movement kinematics and jaw muscle (*EMG*) activity during drinking in the pigeon. *J. Comp. Physiol.* 170 (1992), 303–309.

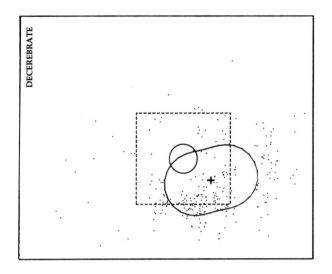

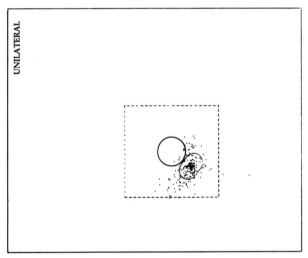

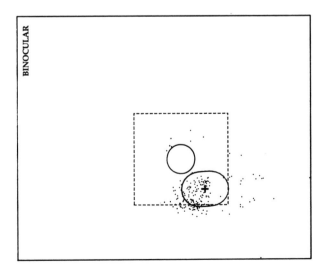

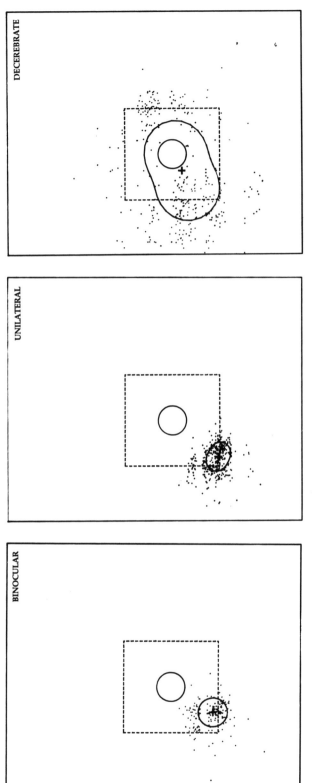

Figure 15.8 The visual forebrain and peck localization. Distribution of terminal pecking response locations in two hemispherectomized subjects. Left (binocular); middle (unilateral: using the eye contralateral to the intact hemisphere); right ("decerebrate": using the eye contralateral to the ablated hemisphere). Conventions as in figure 15.6. From Jäger et al. (1992).

Bermejo, R., Houben, D., and Zeigler, H. P. Dissecting the pigeon's key-pecking response. *J. Exp. Anal. Behav.* (1993), in press.

Bloch, S., Rivaud, S., and Martinoya, C. Comparing frontal and lateral viewing in the pigeon. I. Tachistocopic visual acuity as a function of distance. *Behav. Brain Res.* 5 (1982), 231–234.

Bout, R. G., and Zeigler, H. P. Drinking behavior and jaw muscle (EMG) activity in the pigeon. *J. Comp. Physiology A,* submitted.

Brunelli, M., Magni, F., Moruzzi, G., and Musumeci, D. Brainstem influences on waking and sleep behaviors in the pigeon. *Arch. Ital. Biol.* 110 (1972), 285–321.

Collet, T., and Harkness,L. Depth vision in animals. In D. J. Ingle, M. A. Goodale, and R. J. W. Mansfield (Eds), *The Analysis of Visual Behavior.* MIT Press, Cambridge, MA, 1982, pp. 111–176.

DeSouza-Celena, M. Z., Britto, L. R. G., and Ferrari, E. A. Key-pecking operant conditioning in detelencephalated pigeons (*Columba Livia*). *Behav. Brain Res.* 38 (1990), 223–232.

Deich, J. D., and Balsam, P. D. Development of prehensile feeding in ring dove (*Streptopella risoria*): Learning under organismic and task constraints. In P. Green and M. Davies (Eds.), *Perception and Motor Control in Birds.* Springer-Verlag, Heidelberg, in press.

Deich, J. D., Houben, D., Allan, R. W., and Zeigler, H. P. A microcomputer-based system for the monitoring of jaw movements in the pigeon. *Physiol. Behav.* 35 (1985), 307–311.

Erichsen, J. T., Hodos, W., Evinger, C., Bessette, B. B., and Phillips, S. J. Head orientation in pigeons—postural, locomotor and visual determinants. *Brain Behav. Evol.* 33 (1989), 268–278.

Galifret, Y. Les Diverses aires fonctionelles de la retine du pigeon. *Z. Zellforsch.* 86 (1986), 535–545.

Goodale, M. A. Visually guided pecking in the pigeon (*Columba livia*). *Behav. Brain Evol.* 22 (1983), 22–41.

Graf, J. S., Balsam, P. D., and Silver, R. Associative factors and the development of pecking in ring doves. *Dev. Psychobiol.* 18 (1985), 447–460.

Jäger, R., and Zeigler, H. P. Visual fields and peck localization in the pigeon. *Behav. Brain. Res.* 45 (1991), 65–69.

Jäger, R., Arends, J. J. A., Schall, U., and Zeigler, H. P. The visual forebrain and eating in pigeons (*Columba livia*). *Brain. Behav. Evol.* 39 (1992), 153–168.

Jarvis, C. Visual discrimination and spatial localization deficits after lesions of the tectofugal pathway in pigeons. *Brain Behav. Evol.* 9 (1974), 195–228.

Jeannerod, M. Intersegmental coordination during reaching at natural objects. In J. Long and A. Baddely (Eds.), *Attention and Performance IX.* Erlbaum, Hillsdale, NJ, 1981, pp. 153–168.

Jenkins, H. M., and Moore, B. R. The form of the autoshaped response with food or water reinforcers. *J. Exp. Anal. Behav.* 20 (1973), 163–181.

Jenkins, H. M., and Sainsbury, R. S. Discrimination learning with the distinctive feature on positive or negative trials. In D. I. Mostofsky, (Ed.), *Attention: Contemporary Theory and Analysis.* Appleton-Century-Crofts, New York, 1970.

Klein, B., LaMon, B., and Zeigler, H. P. Drinking in the pigeon: Response topography and spatiotemporal organization. *J. Comp. Psychol.* 97 (1983), 178–181.

Klein, B. G., Deich, J. R., and Zeigler, H. P. Grasping in the pigeon: Final common path mechanisms. *Behav Brain Behav.* 18 (1985), 201–213.

LaMon, B., and Zeigler, H. P. Control of pecking response form in the pigeon: Topography of ingestive behaviors and conditioned responses for food and water reinforcers. *Anim. Learn. Behav.* 16 (1988), 256–267.

Levine, R. R., and Zeigler, H. P. Extratelencephalic pathways and feeding behavior in the pigeon (*Columbia livia*). *Brain Behav. Evol.* 19 (1981), 56–92.

Martinoya, C., Le Houezec, J., and Bloch, S. Depth resolution in the pigeon. *J. Comp. Physiol. A.* 163 (1988), 33–42.

Martinoya, C. Rivaud, S., and Bloch, S. Comparing frontal and lateral viewing in the pigeon. II. Velocity threshold for movement discrimination. *Behav. Brain Res.* 8 (1983), 375–385.

Martinoya, C., Le Houezec, J., and Bloch, S. Pigeon's eyes converge during feeding: Evidence for frontal binocular finxation in a lateral-eyed bird. *Neurosci. Lettr.* 45 (1984a), 335–339.

Martinoya, C., Palacios, and Bloch, S. Participation of eye convergence and frontal accommodation in programming grain pecking in pigeons. *Neurosci. Lett. Suppl.* 18 (1984b), S-233.

McFadden, S. A. Eye design for depth and distance perception in the pigeon: An observer orientated perspective. *Int. J. Comp. Psych.* 3 (1991), 1–22.

McFadden, S. A., Lemeignan, M., Martinoya, C., and Bloch, S. The effect of commissurotomy on pecking and eye convergence in the pigeon. *Neurosci. Lett.* 26 (1986), 572.

Moon, R. D., and Zeigler, H. P. Food preferences in the pigeon (*Columba livia*). *Physiol. Behav.* 22 (1979), 1171–1182.

Nalbach, H-O., Wolf-Oberhollenzer, F., and Kirschfeld, K. The pigeon's eye viewed through an ophthalmoscopic microscope: Orientation of retinal landmarks and significance of eye movements. *Vision Res.* 30 (1990), 529–540

Nye, P. W. On the functional differences between frontal and lateral visual fields of the pigeon. *Vision Res.* 13 (1973), 559–574.

Wild, J. M., and Zeigler, H. P. Central representation and somatotopic organization of the jaw muscles within the facial and trigeminal nuclei of the pigeon (*Columba livia*). *J. Comp. Neurol.* 94 (1980), 783–794.

Wild, J. M., Arends, J. J. A., and Zeigler, H. P. Telencephalic connections of the trigeminal system in the pigeon (*Columba livia*): A trigeminal sensorimotor circuit. *J. Comp. Neurol.* 234 (1985), 441–464.

Wolin, B. R. Difference in manner of pecking a key between pigeons reinforced with food and with water. In C. C. Catania (Ed.), *Contemporary Research in Operant Behavior.* Scott-Foresman, Chicago, 1968.

Zeigler, H. P., Miller, M. G., and Levine, R. R. Trigeminal nerve and eating in the pigeon: neurosensory control of the consummatory response. *J. Comp. Physiol. Psych.* 89 (1975), 845–858.

Zeigler, H. P., Levitt, P., and Levine, R. R. Eating in the pigeon: response topography, stereotypy and stimulus control. *J. Comp. Physiol. Psychol.* 94 (1980), 783–794.

Zweers, G. A. Drinking in the pigeon (*Columba livia*). *Behaviour* 80 (1982a), 274–317.

Zweers, G. A. Pecking of the pigeon (*Columba livia*). *Behaviour* 81 (1982b), 173–230.

16 Control of Pecking Response Topography by Stimulus-Reinforcer and Response-Reinforcer Contingencies

Robert W. Allan

In some classic experiments with pigeons and rats, Skinner observed that smooth, characteristic patterns of behavior could be produced and maintained by brief food deliveries, which were made contingent on closing a microswitch behind a bar or key (Skinner, 1938; Ferster and Skinner, 1957). Because of the clear, consistent control established over these responses Skinner concluded that he had uncovered one of the "natural lines of fracture along which behavior and the environment actually break" (Skinner, 1938, p. 33). Indeed, the pigeon's pecking response has become a focus of behavioral analysis, and rate of responding has proven a useful measure of the respondent and operant control of behavior.

Recent research has suggested that the pecking response itself contains potential "lines of fracture," along which environment and behavior may be separated, and which may have considerable analytic utility for those seeking to correlate response topography with underlying neurological events. Using an autoshaping paradigm (Brown and Jenkins, 1968) Jenkins and Moore (1973) observed that without differentially reinforcing any specific response topography, the form of the pigeon's classically conditioned pecking response resembled the form of their ingestive responses. Food-deprived pigeons pecked episodically, with relatively large gapes, at both food and response keys; the key-pecking of water-deprived pigeons, like their drinking behavior, was characterized by rhythmic jaw movements and small beak openings. Subsequently, LaMon and Zeigler (1984, 1988) identified two topographical components of the pecking response, head transport and beak opening (gape), that varied systematically with deprivation state and reinforcer type. These findings suggest that these characteristic response components might be brought under experimental control using various conditioning paradigms. After precise control is established then neurobehavioral work can begin to delineate the pathways that mediate this well-defined environment-behavior relation.

If we assume that the pecking system is in a constant state of behavioral flux, then determining where the pigeon pecks, with what gape amplitude, and with what frequency requires that we understand and disentangle the contribution of several potentially critical causal factors. These include (1) deprivation state, (2) visual stimuli exerting discriminative control over transport and gape, and (3) the past history of the organism with respect to (a) similar stimuli and (b) differential contingencies specifying particular transport locations or gape values (these contingencies could be real, i.e., programmed by the experimenter, or superstitious, i.e., a function of adventitious contiguity between responses of a particular type and subsequent reinforcement—see Herrnstein, 1966). This chapter will discuss some recent conditioning work designed to isolate environmental factors controlling the head transport and gape response components.

HEAD TRANSPORT

Although key-pecking experiments demand that pigeons peck at a particular location, response keys are essentially dimensionless, i.e., they detect responses only at a single location; off-key responses are not recorded. For studies of response rate, the dimensionless key is an adequate manipulandum; in nature, however, peck localization may be more important than rate. The problem with a dimensionless key is that localization accuracy cannot be calculated unless the positions of all pecks are known. To resolve this difficulty unidimensional response surfaces (typically horizontal arrays of keys) have been used to expand the area of response detection. Herrnstein (1961) and Eckerman and Lanson (1969) examined the distribution of peck locations under various schedules of reinforcement and extinction. They reported that, without any explicit differential reinforcement, pigeons pecked at particular locations in a rather stereotyped fashion, and that in extinction responding became more variable along the response dimension. The location of pecking could be manipulated by differentially reinforcing responses falling within a criterion area. As the criterion position was changed, the location of the pigeons' pecks followed (Eckerman et al., 1980; see also Hori and Watanabe, 1987; Galbicka and Platt, 1989). Taken together, these studies suggest that the location of pigeons' pecks along a single dimension can be affected by several contingent relations (see also Chase et al., 1974; Dunham et al., 1969; Wildemann and Holland, 1972).

The advent of computer-assisted response monitoring has made it feasible to examine the effects of similar contingencies on the accuracy of pecking responses occurring along two, and even three dimensions (Pisacreta and Rilling, 1987; Allan and Zeigler, 1989; Morrison and Brown, 1990; Allan, 1992; see also Pear et al., 1989). Computer touchscreens, the most widely used of these devices, return x,y coordinate values each time the subject pecks at the stimulus display. If the coordinates of the stimulus are known then response locations can be related to individual elements of that stimulus. In addition, contingencies may be programmed on the basis of individual response locations. The growing utilization of touch-screen devices is providing a clearer picture of the lines of fracture between response location and environmental conditions.

Stimulus-Reinforcer Control of Response Localization

Using an autoshaping preparation, Allan (1993) presented, on a computer monitor for 6 sec, a circular stimulus (2.54 cm diameter) in the same position from trial to trial. After as few as 20 trials, pigeons began pecking at the projected stimulus, however, as many as 62% of the responses were located off the stimulus, sometimes by as much as 3–4 cm. By simply decreasing stimulus size to 1.5 cm, the percentage of on-stimulus responding increased dramatically. Thus a simple pairing of stimulus and reinforcer is sufficient to elicit and sustain localized pecking responses.

When the 1.5 cm stimulus appeared in one of seven predetermined positions, on successive trials, the location of pecks tracked the position of the stimulus as it changed from trial to trial, indicating good stimulus-reinforcer control of the location of responding. In a final experiment, the stimulus was animated on the computer monitor, moving from left to right during a 30-sec interreinforcer interval. On reaching the right side of the monitor the stimulus disappeared and a reinforcer was presented (see Hearst and Jenkins, 1974, p. 11). Within 50–100 trials, naive subjects began pecking at the stimulus with increasing rates after it had reached the middle of the monitor. Figure 16.1A plots these results in three dimensions with the x and y axes representing response locations along the horizontal and vertical dimensions respectively while the z-axis plots response probability. The highest probabilities are those associated with the stimulus positions closest to reinforcement. Figure 16.1B plots response position as a function of stimulus position—a measure of accuracy, and indicates that the bulk of the responses actually led (landed in front of) the stimulus by a fraction of a centimeter (see discussion below of Rilling and LaClaire, 1989). The finding common to all these studies is that, in the absence of any contingency specifying changing response position (in fact, in the absence of any response contingency) there is considerable organization of the location of responding relative to stimulus position.

Noncontingent stimulus control of response location had previously been reported using operant schedules involving discriminative control by some small feature of the positive stimulus that signaled reinforcement availability (e.g., Jenkins and Sainsbury, 1970). In this "feature-positive" paradigm, a relatively constant stimulus projected onto a response key was altered periodically by the addition of a "feature" (e.g., a 1/8-inch-

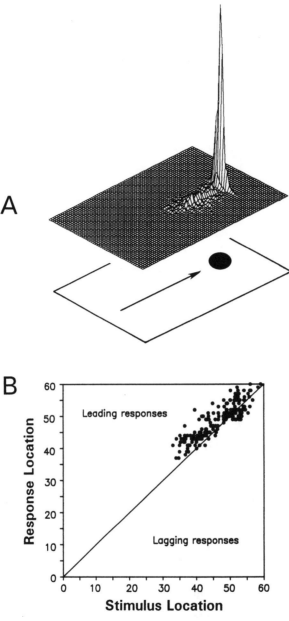

Figure 16.1 (A) Probabilities of responding (z-axis) at each location, as recorded by a touch screen, when a circular stimulus is moved from left to right across a computer monitor. (B) Response location as a function of relative stimulus location with the diagonal representing a match between response and stimulus position.

diameter black dot, superimposed on the stimulus). In the presence of this feature, responding (anywhere on the key) was reinforced. Pigeons not only responded when the feature was present, but they also tracked its location by pecking at the feature.

Allan (1990) used a touch screen to detect peck locations on a multiple variable-interval 20 sec, extinction schedule (MULT VI20 sec EXT), with four filled squares signaling the EXT component and a filled triangle replacing the square in one of the four positions signaling reinforcer availability. In the presence of the triangle, pecking anywhere on the monitor was reinforced during the VI20-sec schedule. Figure 16.2 presents the probabilities of responding at each response location as a function of the five possible types of stimulus arrangement. Again, although reinforcement was not contingent on pecks to a specific location, each subject characteristically tracked the location of the "feature" triangle. During the EXT component, responses at each of the four locations were at very low levels, suggesting good discriminative control of responding.

In a second experiment using a more "natural" set of stimuli (e.g., Herrnstein and Loveland, 1964; see Watanabe et al., this volume), pigeons were trained to peck a rather large (22 × 15 cm) touch sensitive response panel onto which photographic stimuli were back-projected (Allan, 1990). Stimuli were a set of 40 color slides, some with, and some without human figures. Using a MULT VI20 sec EXT schedule, a discrimination was arranged such that the VI components (feature positive) were signaled by slides containing one to three human figures grouped somewhere in the picture; the EXT component was signalled by the absence of humans. Every 30 sec the slides changed, without respect to responding, and again, there was no location response contingency. Birds learned rapidly to respond only when humans were present in the slides. As figure 16.3 indicates, responding was localized by the positive feature, i.e., the presence of human forms, even in the absence of any explicit differential reinforcement for pecks at those locations. When novel slides were presented, pigeons continued to track the humans, minimizing the likelihood that the results reflected superstitious reinforcement (although such an adventitiously reinforced response could generalize to new discriminative instances).

It is clear that stimulus-reinforcer relations (whether or not they are maintained by superstitious contingencies) can have a powerful effect on *where* pigeons peck. The nature of the stimuli signaling reinforcer availability does not seem to matter. When correlated with either response-contingent or noncontingent reinforcer delivery, simple geometric forms or complex "natural" stimuli, presented either under "static" (nonmoving) or "dynamic" (moving) conditions, seem to elicit and direct pecking behavior.

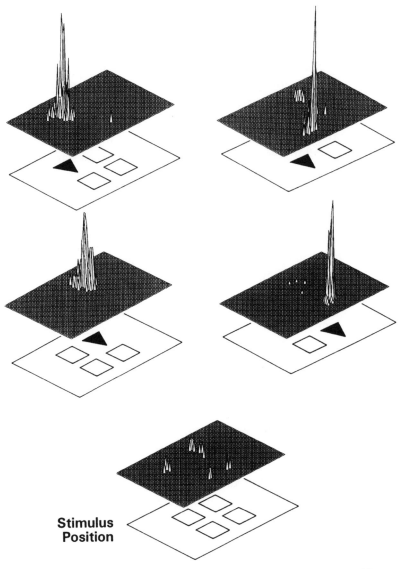

Figure 16.2 Probabilities of responding at each location in the presence of five possible stimulus displays. With a triangle present in one of four positions, responses anywhere on the screen were reinforced on a VI schedule. In each case responding tended to track the triangle's position. When four squares were present responding was ineffective; in this case very few responses were emitted.

Response-Reinforcer-Control of Response Localization

If stimulus-reinforcer relations (or superstitious contingencies) can control response location so well then certainly explicit operant contingencies should control peck localization quite precisely (cf. Eckerman et al., 1980). An experiment by Allan and Zeigler (1987) examined the extent to which the precision of peck localization is increased by the introduc-

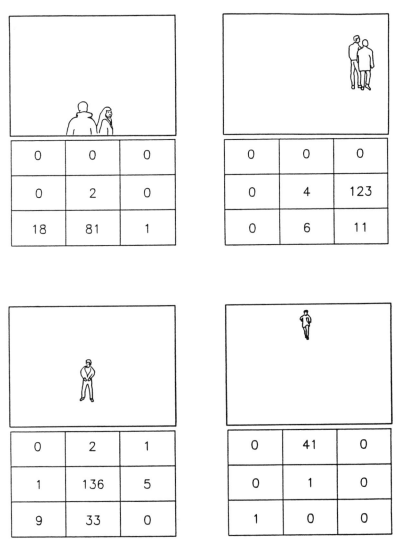

Figure 16.3 For each of four "natural" stimuli presented to a pigeon, the lower panels present response frequencies in nine equal-area segments associated with locations on that slide. The location of the pigeon's responses tracked the position of the humans in these slides.

tion of such a contingency. In the first phase of the study, unconstrained pecking to a circular stimulus was maintained (for separate groups) on either fixed ratio (FR) or variable interval (VI) schedules. In the second phase, a positive feature (a 3-mm dot) was superimposed on the circle and testing continued. Finally, with the feature removed, a location-dependent differential reinforcement contingency was introduced. On discrete trials a peck within the boundaries of the stimulus was followed by stimulus offset and reinforcement. Responses outside of the stimulus boundaries were also followed by stimulus offset but no reinforcement (a timeout condition). The data from subjects under both FR and VI conditions are illustrated in figure 16.4.

Under the VI and FR condition, there was considerable variability in response location, with less than 20% of all responses directed to the circular stimulus. With the addition of the positive feature, on-stimulus pecking was as high as 52%. After three to four sessions (40 reinforcers each) of exposure to the differential-reinforcement-of-response-location (DRLoc) schedule, approximately 70–80% of pecks were directed to the stimulus, with very few responses recorded further than 1 cm from the stimulus boundaries. In some sessions, subjects produced perfect performances, but over 230 sessions of DRLoc, rather high levels of variability continued, and performance accuracy seemed to wax and wane. Pigeons appeared to peck at the stimulus border rather than its center, and even inaccurate, or off-stimulus responses were actually located very near the stimulus. Since pecks are usually made with an open beak, responses to the stimulus edge would increase the likelihood of "misses."

The effect of adding an FR requirement to the DRLoc schedule was examined by exposing birds to FRx[DRLoc] schedules in which x took on values of 1, 2, 4, 6, 8, and 10 responses (Allan et al., 1988). Fixed ratio strings of accurate responses were reinforced, while an off-stimulus response resulted in stimulus offset, a 4-sec timeout and a resetting of the FR counter. Figure 16.5 depicts response frequencies for a single subject, originally trained on a location-independent FR50 schedule. Most of this bird's responses centered on the lower-right edge of the circular stimulus, with 76% of it responses, off-stimulus. With the introduction of the FR1[DRLoc] schedule, the peak of the response distribution shifted and became centered directly over the stimulus (figure 16.5, as labeled). This shift continued with increasing FR requirements, although as the lower panel in figure 16.5 shows, under an FR10[DRLoc] there remained a small population of pecks (to the lower right of the stimulus) that extended the session by terminating many strings of accurate responses before reinforcement.

It is clear from these data that the DRLoc contingency can achieve a high level of control over the spatial distribution of pecking responses, but the continued maintenance of a small population of off-stimulus responses is puzzling. These "errors" may reflect open beak responses to the stimulus boundaries. Alternatively, such residual response variability may serve an important role in maintaining subject contact with changing contingencies under differential reinforcement conditions (Allan, 1987).

Rilling and LaClaire (1989) had pigeons track a dynamic stimulus, reinforcing only responses intercepting a small moving box. Not only was the percentage of "catches" by the two subjects small (22% and 12%), but most responses (70% and 62%) lagged the stimulus, with only a small number of leading responses (8% and 26%). These obser-

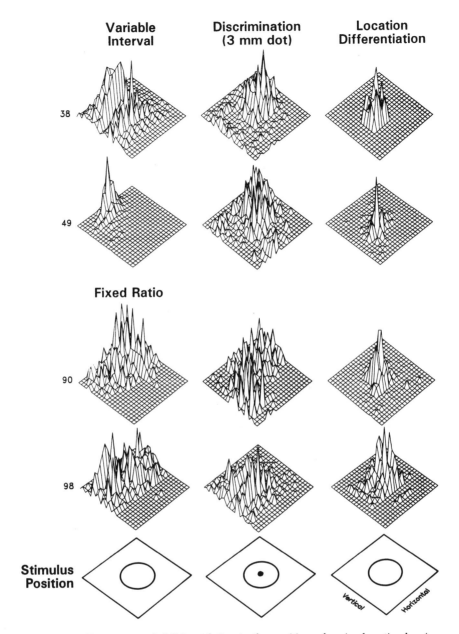

Figure 16.4 Response probabilities relative to the position of a circular stimulus (as indicated) for VI-trained birds (38 and 49) and for FR-trained birds (90 and 98). The first column presents data from their unconstrained VI and FR performances, with center and right columns depicting the shift in response location under discrimination and location differentiation schedules, respectively. During the discrimination schedule a small 3-mm dot was superimposed on the circular stimulus, as depicted in the lower stimulus position panel.

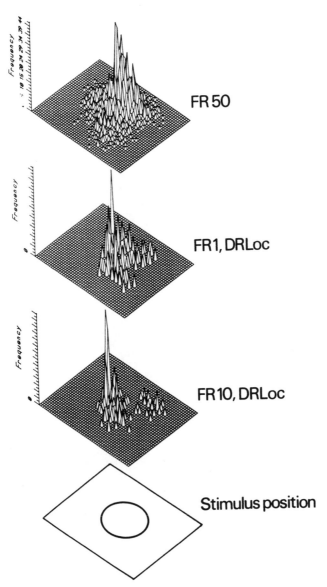

Figure 16.5 Response probabilities relative to the position of a circular stimulus (as indicated) when responding was maintained during a location-independent FR50 schedule and two fixed ratio (FR), differential-reinforcement-of-location (DRLoc) schedules with requirements of either 1 or 10 accurate responses. These differential contingencies clearly centered the location of responding over the stimulus position.

vations are the converse of the stimulus "leading" responses observed by Allan (1993, above) under response independent conditions and with a circular moving stimulus. This difference in control may be due to the addition of a response-reinforcer contingency in the Rilling and LaClaire study.

Recent work has also shown that pecks at touch screen locations that are unsignaled (i.e., there is no projected target) can be differentially reinforced. Rectangular "landmark" stimuli were presented in some spatial relation to the unmarked target area, but pecks at the "landmarks" were never reinforced (Spetch et al., 1992). When the position of the "landmark" was shifted, the location of responses tended to shift in a similar, relative direction although the shift was generally a bit less than the "landmark" shift. In addition, response location changes were largest when the "landmark" was shifted parallel to the closest computer monitor edge (suggesting that the computer monitor edge also served as a "landmark").

Taken together, these experiments suggest that the "natural" levels of variability in peck localization can be brought under relatively precise control by adding localizable discriminative stimuli and by differentially reinforcing response location, with or without an explicit pecking target. Continued analysis utilizing sophisticated monitoring devices should provide useful data on response-independent and response-dependent control of the transport (localization) component of the pigeon's peck.

GAPE RESPONDING

Although Jenkins and Moore (1973) noted that gape is an essential topographic feature distinguishing food-reinforced and water-reinforced key pecking, the behavioral analysis of this response has been neglected, in part because of the limitations of "off-line" measurement techniques (e.g., LaMon and Zeigler, 1984, 1988; Smith, 1974; Zweers, 1982). The development of an "on-line" gape transducing system (see figure 15.1) has made it possible to study this response in real-time, to examine stimulus-reinforcer relations, and to program gape-related response-reinforcer contingencies (Deich et al., 1985, 1988). Recent experiments have examined the contingencies controlling both the rate of beak opening and the distance between the beaks (amplitude).

Stimulus-Reinforcer Control of Gape

Figure 16.6A presents sample gape records taken from food- and water-deprived subjects exposed to an autoshaping procedure in which a keylight was present for 6 sec on the average once every minute, followed by delivery of the appropriate food or water reinforcer (Allan and Zeigler, 1993). These records present quantitative confirmation that

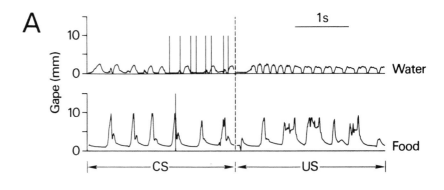

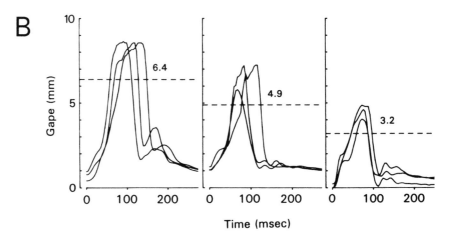

Figure 16.6 (A) Autoshaping trial gape records taken when individual birds were either water or food deprived (as indicated). The conditioned stimulus (CS) and unconditioned stimulus (US, or reinforcer) periods are indicated and a time scale is provided. (B) For three different birds, each receiving a different size pelleet (6.4, 4.9, or 3.2 mm, as indicated), 3 gape records collected during the CS are superimposed. It is clear that the highest beak openings exceed but appear to be scaled as a function of pellet size.

gape topography in food-or-water deprived pigeons is controlled by the type of reinforcer offered.

The extent of stimulus-reinforcer control of gape responding by the reinforcer is evident in figure 16.6B. Three birds were offered different pellet sizes as reinforcers in an autoshaping preparation. During the keylight period over many trials, many pecks and their accompanying gapes were produced. This figure plots, for each bird receiving different pellet sizes, three complete beak opening records. The highest gape values approximated or generally exceeded the size of the indicated food pellet (dashed line). This tracking of pellet size by gapes produced during presentation of the keylight stimulus occurred in the absence of any explicit contingency with respect to gape.

The temporal organization of gaping responses exhibits a pattern very similar to that of the transport component; i.e., generally when pigeons peck they also gape. When the interresponse time (IRT) of peck N is plotted against the IRT of peck $N + 1$, there is a cluster of points at roughly 0.3 sec, suggesting that the rhythm of gaping in these unconstrained conditions parallels previously reported temporal patterns of head transport IRTs (Blough, 1963; Palya, 1992; Weiss, 1970).

It should be noted that control of gape by stimulus-reinforcer contingencies is also seen in operant conditioning situations (figure 16.7A) in which pigeons received either food or water reinforcers on VI schedules (Allan, 1992; see also LaMon and Zeigler, 1984). These data confirm the original observations of Wolin (1968).

Response-Reinforcer Control of Gape

By appropriately arranging reinforcement contingencies, it is possible to directly control either increases or decreases in gape amplitudes produced during key pecking. Deich et al. (1988) used a computer-controlled, discrete-trial procedure in which the peak gape associated with each key peck was measured and compared to a preset criterion value. During *baseline* sessions, gapes were monitored noncontingently, although reinforcers were contingent on key pecking. During an *up* condition, if the peak gape exceeded the established criterion, a rein-

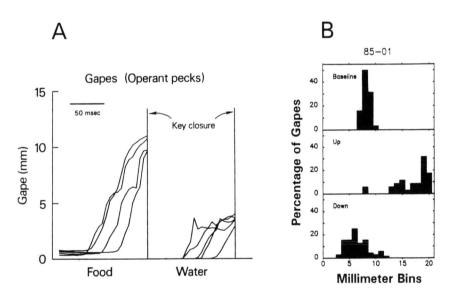

Figure 16.7 (A) Four food and water gape records collected just prior to key closure. A single subject was either food or water deprived and pecked for that reinforcer on a VI schedule. Beak openings during food deprivation are larger than during water deprivation. A time scale is provided. (B) Frequency distributions of peak gapes taken during differential reinforcement of gape size. Emitted gapes had to be greater than an experimenter-selected criterion in the Up condition, and less than a criterion in the Down condition. Baseline data was taken when key contact was the only required response.

Allan: Control of Pecking Response Topography

forcer was delivered; otherwise, a time-out was imposed. During a *down* condition, peak gapes less than the criterion were reinforced. As figure 16.7B indicates, both *up* and *down* conditions produced appropriate shifts, from baseline levels, in the distribution of gapes, suggesting operant control of gape size.

CONCLUSIONS

Skinner (1938, p. 432) noted that "The contribution that a science of behavior makes to neurology is a rigorous and quantitative statement of the program before it." An essential part of that program must be the analysis of mechanisms controlling the temporal and spatial organization of adaptive behavior. The studies reviewed in this chapter suggest that behavior analytic techniques are critical to the process of elucidating the causal control of one such behavior, the pigeon's pecking response.

REFERENCES

Allan, R. W. The control of behavior: The differentiation of response location. *Assoc. Behav. Anal. Abstr.* Nashville, TN (1987).

Allan, R. W. Concept learning and peck location in the pigeon. *Assoc. Behav. Anal. Abstr.* Nashville, TN (1990).

Allan, R. W. Technologies to reliably transduce the topographical details of pigeons' pecks. *Behav. Res. Meth. Instru. Comput.* 24 (1992), 150–156.

Allan, R. W. Stimulus-reinforcer control of response location in the pigeon. *J. Exp. Anal. Behav.* (1993), submitted.

Allan, R. W., and Zeigler, H. P. The control of peck location. *East. Psychol. Assoc. Abstr.* 58 (1987), 41.

Allan, R. W., and Zeigler, H. P. Measurement and control of pecking response location in the pigeon. *Physiol. Behav.* 45 (1989), 1215–1221.

Allan, R. W., and Zeigler, H. P. Autoshaping the pigeon's gape response: Acquisition and topography as a function of reinforcer type and magnitude. *J. Exp. Anal. Behav.* 1993, accepted for publication.

Allan, R. W., Valentine, S., and Zeigler, H. P. Some effects of schedules of partial reinforcement on peck location. *East. Psychol. Assoc. Abstr.* 59 (1988), 44.

Blough, D. S. Interresponse time as a function of continuous variables: A new method and some data. *J. Exp. Anal. Behav.* 6 (1963), 237–246.

Brown, P. L., and Jenkins, H. M. Autoshaping of the pigeon's key peck. *J. Exp. Anal. Behav.* 11 (1968), 1–8.

Chase, S., Geller, E. A., and Hendry, J. S. On the establishment of a continuous repertoire. *Bull. Psychonom. Soc.* 4 (1974), 14–16.

Deich, J. D., Houben, D., Allan, R. W., and Zeigler, H. P. "On-line" monitoring of jaw movements in the pigeon. *Physiol. Behav.* 35 (1985), 307–311.

Deich, J. D., Allan, R. W., and Zeigler, H. P. Conjunctive differentiation of gape during food-reinforced key-pecking in the pigeon. *Aniimal. Learn. Behav.* 16 (1988), 268–276.

Dunham, P. J., Mariner, A., and Adams, H. Enhancement of off-key pecking by on-key punishment. *J. Exp. Anal. Behav.* 12 (1969), 789–797.

Eckerman, D. A., and Lanson, R. N. Variability of response location for pigeons responding under continuous reinforcement, intermittent reinforcement, and extinction. *J. Exp. Anal. Behav.* 12 (1969), 73–80.

Eckerman, D. A., Heinz, R. D., Stern, S., and Kowlowitz, V. Shaping the location of a pigeon's peck: Effect of rate and size of shaping steps. *J. Exp. Analy. Behav.* 33 (1980), 299–310.

Ferster, C. B., and Skinner, B. F. *Schedules of Reinforcement*. Appleton-Century Crofts, New York, 1957.

Galbicka, G., and Platt, J. R. Response-reinforcer contingency and spatially defined operants: Testing an invariant property of phi. *J. Exp. Anal. Behav.* 51 (1989), 145–162

Hearst, E., and Jenkins, H. M. Sign tracking: The stimulus-reinforcer relation and directed action. *Monograph Psychonom. Soc.* Austin, Tex. 1974.

Herrnstein, R. J. Stereotypy and interrmittent reinforcement. *Science* 133 (1961), 2067–2069.

Herrnstein, R. J. Superstition: A corollary of the principles of operant conditioning. In W. K. Honig (Ed.), *Operant Behavior: Areas of Research and Application.* Appleton-Century-Crofts, Englewood Cliffs, NJ, 1966, pp. 33–51.

Herrnstein, R. J., and Loveland, D. H. Complex visual concept in the pigeon. *Science* 146 (1964), 549–551.

Hori, K., and Watanabe, S. An application of the image processing system for detecting and controlling pigeon's peck location. *Behav. Brain Res.* 26 (1987), 75–78.

Jenkins, H. M., and Moore, B. R. The form of the autoshaped response with food or water reinforcers. *J. Exp. Anal. Behav.* 20 (1973), 163–181.

Jenkins, H. M., and Sainsbury, R. S. Discrimination learning with the distinctive feature on positive or negative trials. In D. I. Mostovsky (Ed.), *Attention: Contemporary Theory and Analysis.* Appleton-Century-Crofts, New York, 1970.

LaMon, B., and Zeigler, H. P. Grasping in the pigeon: Stimulus control during conditioned and consummatory responses. *Animal Learn. Behav.* 12 (1984), 223–231.

LaMon, B., and Zeigler, H. P. Control of pecking response form in the pigeon: Topography of ingestive behaviors and conditioned key-pecks with food and water reinforcers. *Animal Learn. Behav.* 16 (1988), 256–267.

Morrison, S. K., and Brown, M. F. The touch screen system in the pigeon laboratory: An initial evaluation of its utility. *Behav. Res. Methods . Instrum. Computers* 22 (1990), 123–126.

Palya, W. L. Dynamics in the fine structure of schedule-controlled behavior. *J. Exp. Anal. Behav.* 57 (1992), 267–287.

Pear, J. J., Silva, F. J., and Kincaid, K. M. Three-dimensional spatiotemporal imaging of movement patterns: Another step toward analyzing the continuity of behavior. *Behav. Res. Methods, Instrum. Computers* 21 (1989), 568–573.

Pisacreta, R., and Rilling, M. Infrared touch technology as a response detector in animal research. *Behavior Res. Methods, Instrum. and Computers* 19 (1987), 389–396.

Rilling, M. E., and LaClaire, T. L. Visually guided catching and tracking skills in pigeons: A preliminary analysis. *J. Exp. Anal. Behav.* 52 (1989), 377–385.

Skinner, B. F. *Behavior of Organisms.* Prentice-Hall, Englewood Cliffs, NJ, 1938.

Smith, R. F. Topography of the food-reinforced key peck and the source of 30-millisecond interresponse times. *J. Exp. Anal. Behav.* 21 (1974), 541–551.

Spetch, M. L., Cheng, K., and Mondloch, M. V. Landmark use by pigeons in a touch screen spatial search task. *Animal Lear. Behav.* 20 (1992), 281–292.

Weiss, B. The fine structure of operant behavior during transition states. In W. N. Schoenfeld (Ed.), *The Theory of Reinforcement Schedules.* Appleton-Century-Crofts, New York, 1970, pp. 277–311.

Wildemann, D. G., and Holland, J. G. Control of a continuous response dimension by a continuous stimulus dimension. *J. Exp. Anal. Behav.* 18 (1972), 419–434.

Wolin, B. R. Differences in manner of pecking in pigeons reinforced with food and water. In A. C. Catania (Ed.), *Contemporary Research in Operant Behavior.* Scott Foresman, Glenview, IL, 1968, p. 286.

Zweers, G. A. Pecking of the pigeon (*Columba livia*). *Behaviour* 81 (1982), 173–230.

17 Visual Mechanisms of Prey Capture in Water Birds

Gadi Katzir

Predation on fish ("piscivoury") is common among several orders of birds. In certain orders, such as sphenisciformes (penguins) or pelecaniformes (pelicans, gannets, cormorants) the trait may be common to all the species. In other cases it is confined to certain genera or species within an order, as with certain kingfishers (coraciiformes) or osprey and sea eagles (falconiformes; Welty and Baptista, 1988). Piscivorous birds vary in their fishing techniques (Ashmole, 1971), yet all of them share the need to cope with two different optical media: air and water. On the basis of the visual environment in which they operate two broad groups may be distinguished (Lythgoe, 1979). The first group includes birds that pursue fish underwater and that must therefore shift from aerial to aquatic vision (Walls, 1967). The second includes birds that plunge-dive into the water, or wade in shallow water to strike at submerged prey with their bill. They locate prey and commence their capturing movements, with their eyes above the water and must cope with both the reflection and the refraction of ambient light (see chapter 1).

BIRDS THAT FEED UNDERWATER

Because the refractive index of the cornea is greatly reduced under water, penguins, cormorants, and other "underwater feeders" that pursue their prey with their eyes submerged are confronted by a major optical/visual problem (Walls, 1967; Sivak, 1976; Sivak et al., 1977, 1978, 1979, 1985; Howland and Sivak, 1984; Martin and Young, 1984). Although it was earlier suggested that penguins are adapted to water and are myopic in air, later observations indicated that in air there is little refractive error, with only a trend toward slight myopia (less than 2 diopters, D), while in water there is a moderate hyperopia (8–13 D). Indeed, the most recent studies suggest that penguins may well be emmetropic (i.e., without any refractive error) in both air and water (Sivak et al., 1987) In contrast, plunge-divers such as the brown pelican

(*Pelecanus occidentalis*) are emmetropic in air, and highly hyperopic in water.

The relatively small alteration in the refractive state of the penguin's submerged eye (compared with approximately 40 D change for the human eye) is attributed to the unique shape of the cornea, which, in penguins, is small in diameter and abnormally flat relative to the overall size of the eye. This corneal flattening may be an adaptation that minimizes the loss of accomodative power accompanying submergence (cf. Sivak and Milodot, 1977).

Cormorants (*Phalacrocorax carbo*) were found to be emmetropic when not accommodating, but highly myopic (40–50 D) during accommodation (Hess, 1910, cited in Levy and Sivak, 1980). This may involve primary control of the lens by the sphincter muscle of the iris, rather than the ciliary muscle, a phenomenon also found in other diving species such as the black guillemot (*Cepphus grylle*) and hooded merganser (*Mergus cucullatus*). In diving ducks such as the redhead duck (*Aythya americana*) and in the merganser, a 50 D change was observed within a time span of 30 sec, lasting up to 4 min (Levy and Sivak, 1980). Contraction of the iris sphincter produces a rigid disc with a central pupil, while the contraction of the ciliary muscle pushes the malleable lens against the iris disc and the central lens bulges through the pupil. Using this iris control mechanism, diving ducks can accommodate the 70–80 D needed to focus light on the retina when the eye is submerged (Sivak et al., 1979, 1985).

The requisite intraocular musculature, and the ability to compensate for the refractive loss are also seen in penguins. However, the flattened cornea of penguins considerably reduces the amount of accommodation needed to focus light on the retina, increasing the length of the accommodative periods for the ciliary muscles, thus meeting the requirements of the long dives taken by penguins (Sparks and Soper, 1968).

BIRDS THAT PLUNGE-DIVE OR STRIKE THROUGH THE WATER SURFACE

Birds that plunge-dive or strike at submerged prey must take into account prey position and movement, underwater depth and distance to the substrate, their own height above the water, their dive or strike speed, and the moment of contact with the water surface and with the prey (Lee and Reddish, 1981). All these calculations must be made while the bird's eyes are still above the water, in a complex visual environment. The visual world of these diving birds is dominated by ambient light reflected from the surface, refracted after penetrating the water (Lythgoe, 1979; Jenkins and White, 1976) or visually modulated by movements of the water surface.

Reflection

Surface reflectance comprises light reflected from the sun and sky as well as the inherent radiance of the water volume (Lythgoe, 1979). The spectral composition of surface reflectance (glare) is similar to that of the sky, while light rising from the water has a spectral radiance dominated by the absorption and scatter of the water itself. To see well through the surface glare, which reduces visual contrasts, birds should be more sensitive to wavelengths in which the sky reflections are relatively poor and the reflected light is relatively rich. Water absorbs light strongly at wavelengths (λ) greater than $\lambda 575$ nm, making reflections from the sky at these wavelengths often brighter than the reflected radiance. Through-surface visibility would be best at $\lambda 425$–525 nm for blue water, at $\lambda 500$–550 nm for blue-green water, and at $\lambda 520$–570 nm for green water. A receptor mechanisms most sensitive to wavelengths greater than $\lambda 575$ nm will allow clear viewing of very shallow, but not deep, objects (Lythgoe, 1979).

Refraction

As figure 17.1 indicates, light rays at the air–water interface are "bent" toward the normal, relative to the incident ray (Snell's law). Thus, to an aerial observer, an underwater prey will appear displaced to some point along the line of refraction, i.e., somewhat higher than it actually is (Jenkins and White 1976; Dill, 1977; Horvath and Varju, 1990). Moreover, refraction distorts the image and has a magnifying effect that reduces the apparent brightness of a submerged object, and affects the

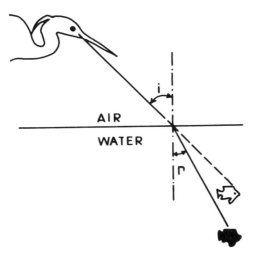

Figure 17.1 Light refraction at the air/water interface in accordance with Snell's law (sin i/sin $r = 1.33$, $i > r$) causes the apparent image (white fish) to be seen somewhere along the line of refraction, i.e., above the real fish (black). From Katzir and Intrator (1987).

directional distribution of underwater light through water surface movement (see below; Lythgoe, 1979).

Surface Movement

Surface movement from ripples and wavelets fragments reflected light into a multitude of glitter points. Wavelets act as cylindrical lenses of constantly changing curvature, projecting a network of bright lights into the water (Schenck, 1957). In clear, shallow water, periodic bright bands of light produced by the refraction of sunlight at the wavy surface sweep across the bottom at surface wave velocity (McFarland and Loew, 1983; Loew and McFarland, 1990). In addition, the constantly changing "surface lenses" cause the image of a stationary subsurface object to be continuously distorted and displaced (in both the vertical and horizontal planes).

COPING WITH LIGHT REFLECTION AND WITH SURFACE MOVEMENT

The oil droplets of avian retinal cones (see chapter 2) provide a mechanism that may minimize the effects of reflected light by serving as chromatic filters (cf. Martin, 1985). On the basis of cone distribution, Muntz (1972) distinguished two groups of sea birds. The first group includes species with relatively few (ca. 20%) red and orange oil droplets, e.g., razorbills, shearwaters, and cormorants. The second group includes species with relatively large proportions (ca. 50–80%) of red and orange oil droplets, e.g., gulls and terns. The first group pursue fish underwater while birds of the second group plunge-dive, leading Muntz to suggest that the higher sensitivity to shorter wavelengths aid in seeing objects well beneath the surface, while the richness in long-wave sensitive cones aids in seeing better through the water. Another possible explanation is that a higher concentration of carotenoid-containing oil droplets is correlated with the birds' feeding habits. Birds that need to detect black and white-plumaged conspecifics over long distances, through a hazy atmosphere, may benefit from this chromatic filter (Lythgoe, 1979). Unfortunately, empirical support for this hypothesis is lacking.

Reflected skylight is brighter near the horizon than when looking directly downward, while in general the brightest feature on a calm surface is the reflection of the sun (Lythgoe, 1979). It might thus be expected that birds will adopt behavioral strategies designed to reduce the effects of reflected light. However, there is little evidence that birds point away from the sun, or prefer to strike at prey that is directly beneath them. Great blue herons (*Ardea herodias*), for example, tilt their head toward the sun in order to minimize glare (Krebs and Partridge, 1973). In contrast, azimuthal directions of the body axis of a hovering pied kingfishers, *Ceryle rudis,* are determined more by wind direction than by sun direction (Katzir, unpublished) and little egrets, *Egretta garzetta garzetta,* do not seem to prefer vertical to acute sighting angles (see below).

Surface movement also affects prey capture success. An increase in surface ripples results in an initial increase and then a decrease in prey captures in terns, *Sterna* spp. (Dunn, 1973), and in a continuous decrease in osprey, *Pandion haliaetus* (Grubb, 1976, 1977). However, under these conditions it is difficult to distinguish the effect of surface movement on the birds' ability to detect and aim at the prey, from its effects on the response of the prey itself.

COPING WITH REFRACTION: EVIDENCE FROM HERONS

The ability to correct for refraction was first demonstrated not in birds but in archerfishes (*Toxotes* spp.), which are capable of hitting aerial insects with a jet of water droplets, after aiming at them with their eyes submerged (Dill, 1977). However, the need to cope with light refraction at the air–water interface is probably more widespread and more vital in birds than in any other group of terrestrial vertebrates. It has been demonstrated in reef herons, *Egretta garzetta schistacea,* little egrets, squacco herons *Ardeola ralloides* (Katzir and Intrator, 1987; Katzir et al., 1989; Lotem et al., 1991; Katzir et al., 1993) and pied kingfishers (Labinger et al., 1991; Katzir et al., 1993).

Egrets and herons (ardeidae) stalk submerged prey while wading in shallow water. Capture is by a rapid strike, which commences with their head held above the water (Hancock and Kushlan, 1984). If the egret's eyes are not directly above the prey, there will be a disparity between the prey's apparent and real position. The magnitude of the disparity, which is determined by the egret's eye position relative to the prey at the moment of strike, may exceed 10 cm, even for a medium sized bird such as little egret. How do egrets cope with this problem?

PREY CAPTURE BY LITTLE EGRETS AND BY REEF HERONS

In the field, little egrets succeed in capturing fish in 40 to 90% of their attempts (Hafner et al., 1982; Lotem et al., 1991). If refraction is not corrected for, a lower success would be expected at larger disparities, i.e., at more acute angles, and at deeper strikes. However, of the successful strikes observed in a recent study (Lotem et al., 1991), only 25% were vertical, while 75% were acute (figure 17.2). Furthermore, capture success increased with increased acuteness of strike angles, while variations in strike depth had no apparent effect on success. Little egrets are thus capable of correcting for light refraction. The increase in capture success at more acute strike angles may stem from the fact that to a fish, an aerial predator close to the horizon will appear dimmer and

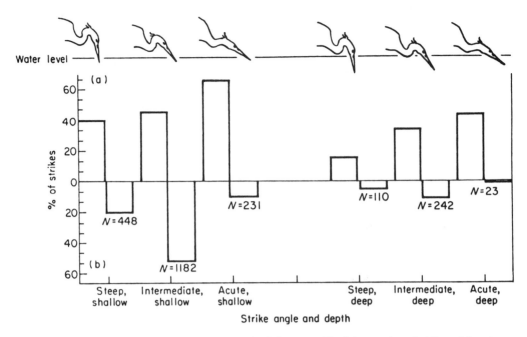

Figure 17.2 (a) Capture success by little egrets (% of the number of strikes of the given combination of angle and depth); (b) frequency of use of the different strikes (% of the total observed). n = the number of strikes observed. From Lotem et al. (1991).

smaller relative to a similar object overhead, being at the edge of its "Snell's window" (Walls, 1967).

Under natural conditions, the magnitude of the refraction problem cannot be computed, as the relative spatial positions of the bird and the prey are unknown. Moreover, environmental factors (e.g., water turbidity) and prey factors (e.g., size, color, and movement), which are most important in determining prey capture success, are not controlled for. The net effect of disparity is thus obscured. To determine the magnitude of the disparity problem and the strategy used during prey capture, we developed techniques for the study of these behaviors under more controlled conditions, which allowed us to present small, stationary underwater "prey" (fish) at different depths and distances from the bird, in clear water with minimal surface movement (Katzir and Intrator, 1987). Our subjects were reef herons *Egretta garzetta schistacea* (Hancock and Kushlan, 1984; but see Cramp and Simmons, 1977, and Voisin, 1991, for a different classification).

In the testing situation, success rate was maintained at high levels over a very wide range of prey positions. During the approach and strike two phases could be distinguished: a "prestrike" and a "strike" (figure 17.3). During prestrike, the head moved forward, on a straight path, with the bill kept horizontal or pointing slightly downward. At a certain point, the point of strike (STR), a rapid straightening of the neck began and the head was thrust directly forward and downward. Bill

A

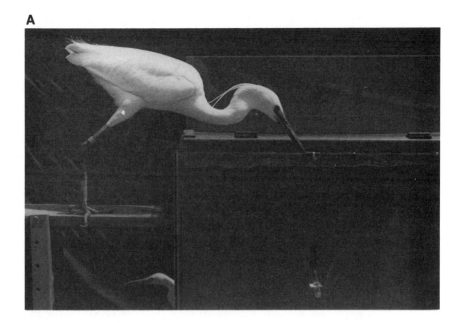

B

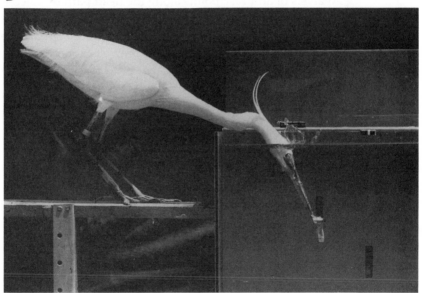

Figure 17.3 Striking of underwater prey by a reef heron. (a) Approach and aiming; (b) prey capture. From Katzir and Intrator (1987).

opening began only 1/60 to 1/30 sec before contact with the prey. Pre-strike and strike differed significantly in terms of path angle (the angle relative to the vertical) and velocity (mean prestrike velocity 49 cm/sec, mean path angle 60°, mean strike velocity 269 cm/sec, mean path angle 33°). From STR, the bill tip path led straight to the real prey position without passing through the point of the apparent prey position.

The point of strike (STR) was considered by Katzir and Intrator (1987) as that in which final corrections for refraction were made. The acceleration of movement beyond this point (70 m/sec^{-2}) and the velocities attained are likely to preclude further motor corrections. Also, under-water vision must have been impaired by the nictitating membranes over the eyes, and by air bubbles drawn in by the penetration of the bill into the water. At STR, angle α, the eye-bill angle, and angle β, the angle between eye and apparent prey (figure 17.4), were correlated with prey depth and with prey distance as well as among themselves. The line of sighting to the prey was ca. 7.5° below the bill. Furthermore, apparent prey depth and real prey depth were linearly correlated. As gape size was not correlated with prey parameters, the herons probably did not compensate for greater disparities by striking with a wider gape. Analysis of arbitrary points along the head path revealed no other point with such clear features, confirming the uniqueness of STR. Interestingly, in the archerfish the relationship between apparent prey elevation relative to the fish's eyes and real prey elevation relative to the nose at the points from which it spits a jet of water is also linear (Dill, 1977).

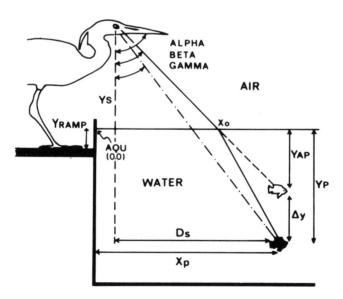

Figure 17.4 Certain parameters measured for herons and egrets. X axis determined by the water surface. Y_p, prey depth; D, horizontal distance between eye and prey (D at the moment of strike is denoted D_s); alpha (α), angle of eye-bill line; beta (β), angle of sighting of apparent prey. Y_{ap}, apparent prey position ($Y_{ap} = X/\tan i$). From Katzir and Intrator (1987).

Given these findings, one may ask whether the visuomotor pattern during strikes is unique to submerged prey, i.e., do reef herons respond differently to unsubmerged prey? In fact, the two types of strike do differ. While a diffuse point of strike (STR) is seen, for unsubmerged prey, the difference between prestrike and strike is smaller (mean prestrike velocity 64 cm/sec, mean path angle 48°; mean strike velocity 163 cm/sec, mean path angle 42°). Also, the path of the bill tip was directed at the prey from relatively far away, eye path during strikes followed the straight line between STR and prey position, and the angle of sighting of the unsubmerged prey at STR was only 2.5° below the eye-bill line compared with an α of 7.5° when the prey was submerged (Katzir et al., 1989).

The existence of a clear "point of change" was observed not only in reef herons but also in squacco herons, *Ardeola ralloides*, which are considerably smaller than little egrets, and feed only on aquatic organisms. Under experimental conditions an apparent STR is observed during submerged prey capture, a linear correlation between apparent prey depth (Y_{ap}) and real prey depth (Y_p) is observed at STR, and the herons keep angle α at about 10° above angle β.

CATTLE EGRETS—A SPECIES NOT COPING WITH REFRACTION

One heron species, the cattle egret *Bubulcus ibis*, is strictly terrestrial (Cramp and Simmons, 1977); it feeds on terrestrial vertebrates and invertebrates and, rarely, on aquatic species. When presented with submerged prey, cattle egrets demonstrate a pattern of prey capture that differs from that of the acquatic species. Their frequency of unsuccessful strikes at submerged prey is significantly higher and they show no clear point of strike.

A MODEL FOR THE HERON'S ABILITY TO CORRECT FOR REFRACTION

The visual information available to the heron for calculating the prey's real position includes, its own eye height above the water, apparent prey depth, and the angle of sighting the apparent prey. Katzir and Intrator (1987) developed a model to account for the ability of acquatic feeding herons to correct for the disparity between real and apparent prey images. The model (figure 17.5) is based on the the relationship between real and apparent prey positions, observed in the herons' strike and on the index of refraction of air–water. For any given apparent prey depth, real prey depth is calculated according to the empirical equation ($Y_{prey} = 1.4 \times y_{apparent} - 1.7$) and the point on the water surface, X_0, which fulfills the requirement of the ratio $\sin i / \sin r = 1.33$ (Snell's law) is determined. The collection of points that fulfills the observed relationships lies on a straight line (which is the extrapolation of the line

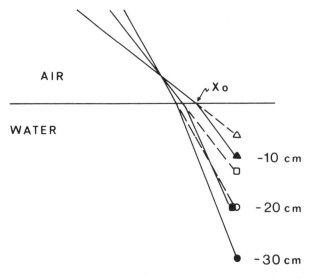

Figure 17.5 A model for the heron's ability to correct for refraction. Lines predicted by a model, for which $Y_p = 1.4 \times y_{ap} - 1.7$ and $\sin i/\sin r = 1.33$ (see text). Broken lines, trajectories of the refracted rays. Black figures, real prey positions; open figures, corresponding apparent positions. From Katzir and Intrator (1987).

X_0–Y_{ap} (figure 17.5). The lines corresponding to different prey depths converge on a given area, which may be the critical point for determining the herons' point of strike. If, for example, a heron determines the rate of change of the visual angle to the apparent prey at the retina, it may then employ its "equation" to strike at the real prey.

When reef herons were experimentally restricted to sighting stationary submerged prey at acute angles only, the proportion of misses increased markedly compared with the unrestricted situation (Katzir et al., 1989). As sighting angles became more acute, the frequency of unsuccessful captures increased. Although real prey depth and apparent prey depth were still correlated under these conditions, the correlations for successful strikes differed from those of unsuccessful strikes. As predicted, for any given prey depth, the larger the difference between the observed and the predicted apparent prey depth, the greater the probability of missing a prey.

VISUALLY GUIDED PLUNGE-DIVES IN THE PIED KINGFISHER

To capture fish, pied kingfishers (*Ceryle rudis;* aves, cerilinae; Cramp and Simmons, 1977) plunge-dive from a hovering flight several (up to 12–15) meters above the water, or from a perch (Douthwaite, 1976; Reyer et al., 1988). While hovering, the pied kingfisher keeps its head stable relative to movements of its body and wings (Lee and Young, 1986). Information related to the prey (movement, size, depth, and distance from the bottom), and to its own body (height above the water, spatial azimuth, dive speed, wing position) must be obtained during the hover or the dive, i.e., prior to entering the water (Lee, 1980; Lee and Reddish, 1981). Other species frequently perform estimation of prey distance, for example, from a perch with the prey on the ground (Moroney and Pettigrew, 1987).

COPING WITH REFRACTION AND ESTIMATING PREY DEPTH

Pied kingfishers determine underwater prey depth during the course of the hover and/or the dive. As the depth of a small, stationary submerged prey was varied, (0 to −60 cm) the form of the dive differed in several respects (Katzir and Schechtman, 1993). With increased prey depth, dive angles became increasingly more vertical. In dives to prey presented 15 cm underwater or deeper, an initial slower and rather curved phase was followed by a relatively straight and more rapid descent. The height of the point of change, like the STR of herons, increased with prey depth, as did the speed of the final descent. When prey was at the surface, diving speed was approximately 2 m/sec, while for prey at 30 and 45 cm underwater, diving speeds showed a twofold increase to over 4.5 m/sec. Obviously, dives at acute angles necessitate corrections for disparity, which the kingfishers are able to make.

Estimating Prey Size

Control of prey selection by use of visual cues to size is an important aspect of foraging (cf. Werner and Hall, 1974). Decision as to size may have to be made while hovering several meters above the water. When presented simultaneously with two stationary prey, differing only in size (size range: 1.0–3.0 cm at increments of 0.2 and 0.5 cm), pied kingfishers predominantly choose the larger prey. Such "selectivity" was found to be positively correlated with the relative size difference between the prey, and to increase with increased prey depth (Labinger et al., 1991).

Effect of Prey Movement on Capture Success

In the wild, pied kingfishers succeed in capturing prey in 10 to 50% of their dives (Douthwaite, 1976; Migongo, 1978; Jackson, 1984; Katzir, unpublished). Like herons, kingfishers tested under experimental conditions with stationary prey very rarely missed (Labinger et al., 1991; Katzir and Camhi, 1993). When tested with a single live fish in an experimental aquarium with clear water and with minimal surface movement, prey was captured in only 50% of the dives (Katzir and Camhi, 1993). Fish depth, fish size, dive angle, and dive speed seemed unrelated to capture success. Fish movement, however, did have a clear effect. In unsuccessful dives, movement occurred significantly earlier

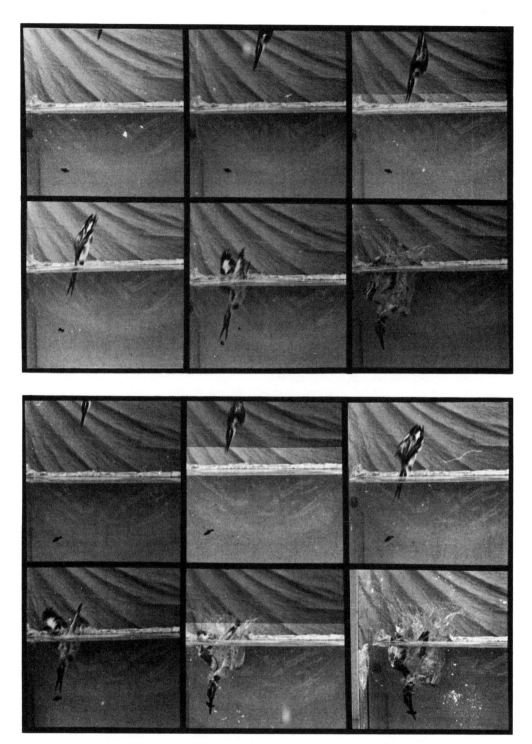

Figure 17.6 (Top) Consecutive fish and pied kingfisher positions at termination of an unsuccessful dive (i.e., fish escaped; from a 16-mm film taken at 64 frames/sec). From top left to top right, the fish was parallel to front glass of aquarium. At bottom left, the fish's body turned at 90°. At bottom right the fish is seen near base of kingfisher's bill. S, water surface. (Bottom) As above, but for a successful dive (i.e., fish captured), with the fish showing no apparent movement. From Katzir and Camhi (1993).

(when the bird was 0.025 sec away) than in captures (with the bird 0.01 sec away). For successful catches, both the distance traveled by the fish between its first observable movement and capture and its initial swimming speed (0.4 cm and 24 cm/sec, respectively) were significantly smaller than for unsuccessful attempts (2.0 cm and 60 cm/sec, respectively; figure 17.6). Prey movement thus plays an important role in determining the kingfishers' ability to hit its prey. As yet there are no indications that the birds are intercepting their prey or are indeed capable of doing so.

REFERENCES

Ashmole, N. P. 1971. Sea bird ecology and the marine environment. In D. S. Farner and J. R. King (Eds.), *Avian Biology*, Vol. I. New York, Academic Press, pp. 224–286.

Cramp, S. T., and Simmons, K. E. L. 1977. (chief eds.). *Handbook of the Birds of Europe, the Middle East and North Africa*, Vol. 1. Oxford University Press, Oxford,

Dill, L. M. 1977. Refraction and the spitting behavior of the archerfish (*Toxotes chatareus*). *Behav. Ecol. Sociobiol.* 2, 169–184.

Douthwaite, R. J. 1976. Fishing techniques and foods of the pied kingfisher on lake victoria. *Ostrich* 47, 153–160.

Dunn, E. 1973. Changes in fishing abilities of terns associated with wind speed and sea surface conditions. *Nature (London)* 244, 520–521

Grubb, T. C. 1976. Why ospreys hover. *Wilson Bull.* 89, 149–150.

Grubb, T. C. 1977. Weather dependent foraging in ospreys. *Auk* 94, 146–149.

Hafner, H., Boy, V., and Gory, G. 1982. Feeding methods, flock size and feeding success in little egrets, *Egretta garzetta* and squacco heron *Ardeola ralloides* in Camargue, southern France. *Ardea* 70, 45–54.

Hancock, J., and Kushlan, J. 1984. *The Herons Handbook*. Croom Helm, London.

Horvath, G., and Varju, D. 1990. Geometric optical investigation of the underwater visual field of aerial animals. *Math. Biosci.* 102, 1–19.

Howland, H. C. 1974. Optimal strategies for predator avoidance. *J. Theoret. Biol.* 47, 333–350.

Howland, H. C., and Sivak, J. G. 1984. Penguin vision in air and water. *Vision Res.* 24, 1905–1909.

Jackson, S. 1984. Predation by pied kingfishers and white breased cormorants on fishes in the kosi estuary system. *Ostrich* 55, 113–132.

Jenkins, F. A., and White, H. E. 1976. *Fundamentals of Optics*, 2nd ed. McGraw-Hill, New York.

Katzir, G., and Camhi, J. 1993. Escape response of black mollies (*Poecilia sphenops*) from predatory dives of a pied kingfisher (*Ceryle rudis*). *Copeia*, in press.

Katzir, G., and Intrator, N. 1987. Striking of underwater prey by reef herons, *Egretta gularis schistacea*, *J. Comp. Physiol. A* 160, 517–523.

Katzir, G., and Schechtman, E. 1993. Dive patterns of pied kingfishers, *Ceryle rudis*, to prey at different depths. In preparation.

Katzir, G., Lotem, A., and Intrator, N. 1989. Stationary underwater prey missed by reef herons, *Egretta gularis:* head position and light refraction at the moment of strike. *J. Comp. Physiol. A* 165, 573–576.

Katzir, G., Strod, T., Arad, Z., and Benjamini, Y. 1993. Striking at submerged prey by herons: Cattle egrets, *Bubulcus ibis,* cannot correct for light refraction. In preparation.

Krebs, J. R., and Partridge, B. 1973. The significance of head tilting in the great blue heron. *Nature (London)* 245, 533–535.

Labinger, Z., Katzir, G., and Benjamini, Y. 1991. Prey size choice by captive pied kingfishers, *Ceryle rudis L. Animal Behaviour* 42, 969–975.

Lee, D. N. 1980. The optic flow field: The foundation of vision. *Phil Trans R. Soc. London B* 290, 169–179.

Lee, D. N., and Reddish, P. E. 1981. Plummeting gannets: A paradigm of ecological optics. *Nature (London)* 293, 293–294.

Lee, D. N., and Young, D. S. 1986. Gearing action to the environment. *Exp. Brain Res. Ser.* 15, 217–230.

Levy, B., and Sivak, J. G. 1980. Mechanisms of accommodation in the bird eye. *J. Comp. Physiol. A* 137, 267–272.

Loew, E. R., and McFarland, W. N. 1990. The underwater visual environment. In R. H. Douglas and M. B. A. Djamgoz (Eds.), *The Visual System of Fish.* Chapman and Hall, London.

Lotem, A., Katzir, G., and Schechtman, E. 1991. Capture of submerged prey by little egrets, *Egretta garzetta garzetta:* Strike depth, strike angle and the problem of light refraction. *Animal Behav.* 42, 341–346.

Lythgoe, J. N. 1979. *The Ecology of Vision.* Clarendon Press, Oxford.

Martin, G. R. 1985. Eye. In A. S. King and J. McLelland (Eds). *Form and Function in Birds,* Vol. 3. Academic Press, London.

Martin, G. R., and Young, S. R. 1984. The eye of the Humboldt penguin, *Spheniscus humboldti:* visual fields and schematic optics. *Proc. R. Soc. London B* 223, 197–222.

McFarland, W. N., and Loew, E. R. 1983. Wave produced changes in underwater light and their relation to vision. *Env. Biol. Fish* 8, 3/4, 173–184.

Migongo, E. 1978. Environmental factors affecting the distribution of malachite and pied kingfishers in lake Makuru national park. Unpublished MSc Thesis. University of Nairobi.

Moroney, M. K., and Pettigrew, J. D. 1987. Some observations on the visual optics of kingfishers (Aves, Coraciformes, Alcedinidae). *J. Comp. Physiol A* 160, 137–149.

Muntz, W. R. A. 1972. Inert absorbing and reflecting pigments. In H. J. A. Dartnall (Ed.), *Handbook of Sensory Physiology,* Vol. VII/1. Springer-Verlag, Berlin, pp. 529–565.

Reyer, H-U., Migongo-Bake, W., and Schmidt, L. 1988. Field studies and experiments on the distribution and foraging of pied and malachite kingfishers at lake Nakuru (Kenya). *J. Animal Ecol.* 57, 595–610.

Schenck, H. 1957. On the focusing of sunlight by ocean waves. *J. Opt. Soc. Am.* 47, 653–657.

Sivak, J. G. 1976. The role of the flat cornea in the amphibious behaviour of the blackfoot penguin (*Spheniscus demersus*). *Can. J. Zool.* 54, 1341–1346.

Sivak, J. G., and Milodot, M. 1977. Optical performance of the penguin eye in air and water. *J. Comp. Physiol. A* 119, 241–247

Sivak, J. G., and Vrablic, O. E. 1979. The anatomy of the eye of the adelie penguin with special reference to optical structure and intraocular musculature. *Can. J. Zool.* 57, 346–352.

Sivak, J. G., Bobier, W. R., and Levy, B. 1978. The refractive significance of the nictitating membrane of the bird eye. *J. Comp. Physiol. A* 125, 335–339.

Sivak, J. G., Hildebrand, T., and Lebert, C. 1985. Magnitude and rate of accommodation in diving and nondiving birds. *Vision Res.* 25, 925–933.

Sivak, J. G., Howland, H. C., and McGill-Harelstad, P. 1987. Vision in the Humboldt penguin (*Spheniscus humboldti*) in air and water. *Proc. R. Soc. London B* 229, 467–472.

Sparks, J., and Soper, T. 1968. *Penguins.* Angus & Robertson, Sydney.

Voisin, C. 1991. *The Herons of Europe.* T. and A. D. Poyser, London.

Walls, G. L. 1967. *The Vertebrate Eye and Its Adaptive Radiation.* Hafner, New York.

Weihs, D., and Webb, P. W. 1984. Optimal avoidance tactics in predator prey interactions. *J. Theoret Biol.* 106, 189–206.

Welty, C. J., and Baptista, L. 1988. *The Life of Birds,* 4th ed. Saunders College Publishing, New York.

Werner, E. E., and Hall, D. J. 1974. Optimal foraging and the size of prey by the bluegill sunfish (*Lepomis macrochirus*). *Ecology* 55, 1042–1052.

V Vision and Cognition

Introduction

Jacky Emmerton

This section examines various aspects of visual cognition. In recent years there has been increasing interest in cognitive approaches to studying animals' behavior. Essentially, the cognitive approach looks at the ways in which animals actively process the wealth of information available in their environments. In laboratory experiments at least, animal cognition owes much of its methodology and theorizing to the development of objective ways of testing human cognition—how we experience and think about our world. In turn, the modern approach to studying human cognition can be traced back to the development of information theory in the field of technical communications.

Animal cognition in general considers how different species acquire information about their environment, how they learn and remember that information, and how present and past information is utilized in adaptive behavior. The first stage, the acquisition of information, refers to the uptake and encoding of stimuli. As applied to vision, the term "cognition" overlaps with many aspects of perception. Whereas perception includes studying how the visual system responds to very simple dimensions—the sensations of brightness or color, for instance—cognition concentrates more on the encoding of abstract properties or features of rather complex stimuli. The stored codes for external stimuli (events, objects, places, conspecifics, etc.) are referred to as internal representations and it is postulated that these internal codes can undergo further transformations and become associated with other internal codes, representing different aspects of the environment. This set of stored information can then guide an animal's subsequent behavior, even if the original encoded stimulus is no longer present.

Thus animal cognition covers studies of animals' abilities to recognize objects, their memory capacities, the strategies they use in solving problems, and their formation of concepts. This list is not exhaustive, however, and the following chapters deal with some specific aspects of how birds process complex visual information and discuss, in part, how they might utilize this information in ecological settings.

Andrew and Dharmaretnam (chapter 18) look at the uptake of visual information by domestic chicks. More specifically, they discuss the viewing strategies used by chicks when their task is to recognize various objects in their environment. Of particular interest in birds is the pronounced lateralization of the visual system, which is also reflected in their visually guided behavior. Birds have visual fields that are functionally differentiated. Nevertheless, at some point they must be able to integrate what they have seen in one part of their environment with either the same or different information seen in another part of their visual surroundings. This problem is addressed in chapter 19 by Remy and Watanabe, who discuss the extent to which birds have access to information they obtain from different parts of their visual field, and consider the mechanisms that underlie the internal transfer of this information.

The next two chapters deal more with the nature of the internal codes by which features of the environment and objects are represented. Watanabe, Lea, and Dittrich (chapter 20) argue that birds, along with other higher animals, have evolved to recognize objects in their environment, rather than the simpler sensory dimensions of which these objects are comprised. Although objects are highly variable, birds nevertheless often respond to them in similar ways, as if objects fall into common classes or categories. Their chapter considers the cognitive and perceptual mechanisms that underlie birds' abilities to discriminate concepts or categories. They also look at the extent to which two-dimensional pictures, often used to test birds' cognitive abilities in laboratory experiments, actually represent real, three-dimensional objects to them. Chapter 21, by Emmerton and Delius, explores in more detail the concept of an internal representation as it is applied in a number of cognitive tasks. They discuss the ways that birds encode abstract properties of complex and variable perceptual stimuli, as well as the different ways in which this information may be stored in memory.

The final chapter in this section, by Bingman, examines the role of brain mechanisms, in particular the hippocampus, in birds' ability to integrate visual features of the environment to form a "cognitive map" of their surroundings. He shows how this spatial map may be essential for pigeons' ability to orient themselves and home accurately in their natural environment, and how this type of spatial learning can be studied under laboratory conditions.

18 Lateralization and Strategies of Viewing in the Domestic Chick

R. J. Andrew and M. Dharmaretnam

Birds make conspicuous head movements as they look around or examine objects. Little is known of the way in which head and eye movements work together in visual search and examination: there has been no study in which both types of movement have been simultaneously measured while a bird looks at stimuli of known position and character. Nevertheless, a good deal can be learned from head position alone, under conditions when eye movements appear to be unimportant. In the chick there is indirect evidence (below) that the eyes often remain diverged in the primary position of gaze (Wallman and Pettigrew, 1985), while the head is moved to bring particular retinal fixation points to bear.

Head movements and head positions are discussed here for two visual strategies: sustained viewing of stimuli of especial interest to a chick and visual search. Sustained viewing in mammals such as ourselves almost invariably involves the single fovea of each eye used binocularly in a characteristic stare. Birds, in contrast, have a choice between lateral and binocular fixation (Rochon-Duvigneaud, 1943). Lateral fixation is assumed to make use of the high acuity of the lateral fovea. The domestic chick has a relatively unspecialized retina: the area centralis (used in lateral fixation) lacks a foveal pit. However, it does have a somewhat enhanced density of receptors (Ehrlich, 1981), which are arranged in regular columns, which radiate out from the center, forming an "aster" (Morris, 1982). Both enhanced density and regularity of arrangement are likely to increase visual acuity, and so cause the area centralis to be used for fixation.

The findings discussed here suggest that a second lateral fixation point also exists in the chick. As a result, when the fixation point used during binocular viewing is taken into account, there are likely to be at least three preferred points of fixation within each eye. When the eyes are in the primary position of gaze, and so diverged, or when they are moving independently (below), all three points are potentially available in each eye for use in fixation. When a chick is interested in a small nearby object, it converges its eyes for binocular fixation: an almost owl-like stare results.

It will be argued here that the choice of fixation point for sustained viewing is affected not only by properties of the fixation points themselves (such as enhanced acuity) but also by the pattern of involvement of the (differently specialized) right and left cerebral hemispheres in visual analysis. (The term "hemisphere" is used throughout for the sake of brevity. Visual structures elsewhere in the brain may well be involved in the differing specializations of right and left visual systems.) Use of left lateral fixation points, for example, provides direct visual input to the right hemisphere, but largely excludes the left hemisphere. Direct but restricted input to the ipsilateral hemisphere does occur by return crossover between thalamus and forebrain (Boxer and Stanford, 1985); however, its most likely function is to provide binocular input to neurons fed from the frontal visual fields, when convergence of the eyes allows binocular vision. There is apparently very poor cerebral access (if any) to information from the ipsilateral lateral visual field (below).

Visual search is also likely to have features in birds like the chick that differ sharply from human experience. Independent but synchronous eye movements are usual in the chick (Wallman and Pettigrew, 1985). Their most obvious use is the independent and simultaneous examination of objects, which are situated to the right and the left of the head. The small to moderate amplitude of such eye movements (15° maximum, Turkel and Wallman, 1977) means that they will usually need to be supplemented by head movements. Unless a target has been identified within one or other visual field, such head movements are presumably designed to displace the search areas of both eyes in some standard and appropriate manner. When a very large area has to be scanned, chicks turn the head in long series of regular movements, first to one side and then to the other. The pauses between them are so brief that eye movements are probably unimportant.

In this extreme condition, as in sustained viewing, the primary position of gaze may well be used throughout. Clearly it is necessary for each view of the visual world to be related to that which results from the next head turn. One possibility is that the regular amplitude of head turns helps analysis by causing sections of the panoramic view, which is being built up, to transfer in a predictable and standard way from one zone of the retina to another.

HEAD POSITIONS WHEN VIEWING

Viewing patterns were studied in chicks that were presented with a highly valent stimulus (e.g., a live hen, a live rat, a small flashing light) that had not been seen before. Each chick was constrained only in that in order to view the stimulus, it had to put its head out of the test cage through a hole; dorsal and frontal views of the head were recorded by video. Chicks tended to assume one of two lateral head positions during sustained viewing (figure 8.1). When all data for all three stimuli and all ages of test were considered together, most viewing fell into one of two peaks, 34–39° and 61–66°; there was in addition a slight tendency for binocular viewing. Both lateral head positions involve monocular fixation; the limits of binocular vision are reached at about 27° (estimated from the point at which the cornea ceased to be visible in recordings taken from directly in front of the chick). The chick is not unique amongst ground feeding birds in using a 60° head position: Bischof (1988) notes that zebra finches commonly fixate food grains with the head at about 60°.

The constancy of the two preferred head positions strongly suggests that the eyes are in a standard position throughout (presumably the primary position of gaze), and that two different specialized retinal fixation points are therefore being used. (Present evidence does not exclude the use of small eye movements to transfer the retinal fixation point between features of the fixated stimulus.) The 61–66° head position probably involves a fixation point ("main lateral," ML, figure 18.2) within the area centralis. The pupillary axis in the chick (which virtually

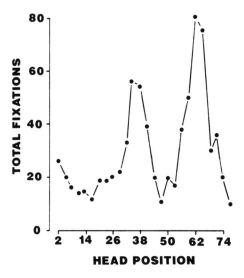

Figure 18.1 A fixation was measured only when the head was held still for more than 3 sec. Fixations are assigned in the figure to bins of 3° (1–3°, 4–6°, and so on). The graduations shown for "head position" are labeled with the middle degree of the first, fifth and ninth bins, continuing in the same series. The two peaks thus each involve two bins. The first peak extends from 34 to 39° and the second from 61 to 66°; the center points of the peaks are therefore 36.5° and 63.5°. For statistical analysis, fixations were considered in blocks of 10° (0–9°, 10–19°, and so on): the two peaks in consequence fell in the 30–39° and 60–69° blocks sectors. The distribution of fixations across sectors was not random ($G = 273.3$, df 7, $p < 0.001$). This remained true when the 30° or the 60° sector was excluded ($G = 244.8, 74.8$ respectively; both $p < 0.001$). However, distribution was random when both 30° and 60° sectors were excluded ($G = 60$).

Andrew & Dharmaretnam: Lateralization in the Chick

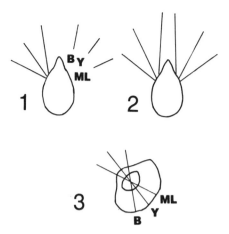

Figure 18.2 Potential lines of sight associated with the three fixation points B, Y, and ML (text) are shown for the primary position of gaze (1) and for convergence of the eyes to allow binocular fixation (2). The arrangement of fixation points on the retina is shown diagrammatically in 3. It is assumed that the three fixation points are separated by two equal steps of 27°.

coincides with the optical axis) lies at about 64° (Wallman and Velez, 1985); it more or less coincides with the position taken up by the eyes under anesthesia. Miles (1972) gives about 60° for the optic axis of anesthetized chicks. It is thus likely that when the head is in the 60° sector during viewing, the eyes are in the "primary position of gaze" to which birds tend to return their eyes after saccadic excursions (Wallman and Pettigrew, 1985). Comparison with foveate birds suggests that the main lateral fixation point of the chick should lie on the pupillary axis, and so be used when the head is at 61–66° to the stimulus. The only discrepancy is with Ehrlich's (1981) report of the main high-density region of ganglion cells (presumably the area centralis) at 80–90° in freshly killed chicks. A belt of enhanced density extended into the temporal retina from this zone of highest density for about 60–70°; it almost certainly stopped short of the binocular field, which is unexpected, in that comparison with bifoveate birds suggests that the binocular fixation point should lie at the end of such a belt (Walls, 1942, p. 187). Both discrepancies would be explained if the eyes were diverged beyond the primary position of gaze, for some reason, in this study.

At first sight, the simplest explanation of the 34–39° head position is that the binocular fixation point (i.e., the point, B, figure 18.2, used in binocular fixation when the eyes are converged) is being used with eyes diverged. However, to allow binocular fixation, this would require the eyes to converge by 34–39° as the head moves through the same angle. In the chick, Turkel and Wallman (1977) record 15° as the maximum excursion during a single eye movement. Direct measurements of the angle through which the eye is moved during convergence from the primary position of gaze to binocular fixation of an object close to the bill tip are available for two other species. In the pigeon this angle is 17° (Bloch et al., 1987) and in the zebra finch 10–15° (Bischof, 1988). It is unlikely that the chick differs greatly; note that a lesser angle would be required for binocular fixation of a more distant object. It thus seems likely that there is a preferred point of fixation on the retina between ML and B; it will be referred to here as Y.

HEAD MOVEMENTS DURING SEARCH

Some clues as to the way in which different retinal fixation points may be used can be obtained from the head movements used in visual search. However, before considering how a stimulus may be captured by one fixation point and then transferred to another, it is necessary first to consider how far information about the stimulus obtained at the first fixation may be available after transfer to another fixation point. Evidence, discussed elsewhere (see chapter 19), shows that in pigeons information does not always transfer freely. "Intraocular transfer" is asymmetric: information first acquired laterally is subsequently available frontally, but not vice versa. "Interocular transfer" is successful with frontal but not with lateral stimulus presentation. Interocular transfer is good in the chick also, for frontal presentation (for review, see Andrew, 1991).

These striking asymmetries were revealed by tests involving retrieval from memory; however, it seems likely that they were caused by corresponding asymmetries during the early elaboration of a visual record. On this interpretation, information is readily available from the previous fixation when a stimulus is transferred from lateral fixation to frontal. This would be appropriate when a stimulus is detected in the lateral visual field, and then moved to frontal fixation, followed by convergence of the eyes, so as to bring the frontal fixation points into register for binocular fixation. Clearly, when a stimulus is captured in this way for binocular fixation by rapid large head movements, it is important that the stimulus should be identified after each move, so that it can be positioned accurately by the next move.

Stimulus capture of this sort can be seen during food search. Rogers and Andrew (1989) trained chicks to feed on black foodgrains made cryptic by their placement on the black squares of a floor with a chessboard pattern. At test only three single grains were present, widely spaced. The point of detection of a grain was easily recognized. The chick paused, and fixated monocularly, often first turning the head further to the side so as to bring the grain to a position that was quite far lateral. After detection, the head was turned to point directly at the grain and the chick ran straight toward it. Here binocular fixation was clearly employed; it seems likely that ocular convergence occurred with the head turn to point the bill at the target. The target stimulus is thus sometimes shifted nasally within the lateral retina before transfer to binocular fixation, presumably in order to place it on a specialized fixation point such as ML. This may help identification; it also means that standard head movements are then needed to bring the stimulus on to B.

During food search, head movements vary in amplitude, presumably because a potential target may be detected almost anywhere in the visual field; at least the initial head movement is therefore likely to vary in amplitude. When a chick is placed in a novel environment, scanning movements of the head are much more regular (Andrew, 1975). There is little locomotion; the animal may turn on the spot, apparently in order to continue the head turns to the right or left. The median of the mean number of head turns in a series for a large population of individuals was 3.15. Such a series carries the head from a position well over to one side to beyond the midline. Longer series take the head so far over as to require turning of the body as well. No accurate measurements of the size of the head turns have been made, but they are probably roughly 30° (and certainly less than 50°). Fixation periods between head turns are so brief that it is unlikely that they are further divided and abbreviated by eye saccades.

It is interesting to compare this estimate of angle of head turn with estimates of angular separation of the fixation points which are used in sustained viewing. If the eyes are in the same standard position during use of the 30° and the 60° sectors, then ML and Y are separated by about 27°. The separation of Y and B is likely to be close to the same value, since the head turn of 36–37°, which will bring the bill to point directly at the stimulus from viewing using Y, is probably accompanied by an opposing movement of the eye, as a result of binocular convergence. If Y and B were separated by 27°, this opposing eye movement would be about 10° (which agrees quite well with estimates for the zebra finch, above). Standard head movements through this angle (i.e., 27°) during stimulus capture or regular scanning would mean that a feature that initially fell on ML would be transferred first to Y and then to B; equally, the segment of the visual world surrounding the feature that was transferred in this way would retain the same spatial relations to each fixation point in turn.

Such a standard pattern of transfer might be important not only in efficient visual capture of a stimulus, but also in the analysis of the panorama that is seen during wide scanning. There is of course no evidence as to the relative importance of (say) the area centralis and the rest of the belt of high receptor density in such analysis, but it would clearly be more effective, given an eye like that of the chick, to build up a central record of a novel visual world using information from the relatively large fields of view within which acuity is adequate, rather than concentrating on a small area, like that covered by the human fovea. During scanning, each head turn changes the position of the scene on the retina by a substantial amount (and deletes a strip at one end of the panorama, while adding another strip at the other end). Efficient analysis would require rapid recognition of features seen in the previous fixation, following each head turn, so that the series of overlapping snapshots could be correctly aligned. This in turn would require that information from the view seen before the head turn should be available when the same view is transferred to a new retinal position. If the flow of information is indeed predominantly from lateral to frontal fixations, then each hemisphere would build up a record of the visual world while the environment moved over the contralateral retina in this direction. The two hemispheres would therefore work alternately.

As has already been noted, binocular fixation is assumed in food search, once a target has been detected. It may sometimes be sustained during search itself: in the study by Rogers and Andrew (1989) the strategy of search was strikingly changed when attention was stabilized by testosterone (see also Andrew, 1983a). Such chicks chose target areas before detecting a grain and would often circle back to squares on which they had previously found a food grain. More commonly they chose an adjacent black square. As a result, grains were usually detected on a square that the chick was already approaching. Often a target was incorrectly identified and the run ended with a peck at an inconspicuous speck on the square. As a result many detections (48% as against 5–6% for control chicks) were made within the binocular field (conservatively defined as 15° or less on either side of the bill). It is probable that such chicks began binocular fixation as soon as they had chosen a target area, spending most of their time during test in this phase of searching.

One reason for binocular fixation of a distant target before approach is almost certainly that the head is in line with the body during rapid direction locomotion. This presumably makes easier the analysis of visual flow fields. However, the assumption of binocular fixation during search can also be viewed as marking the shift from independent analysis by each hemisphere to the assumption of a single joint strategy (i.e., approach to a particular target).

Finally, if the angle between Y and B were about 27°, then an interesting consequence of eye convergence to allow binocular fixation would be that Y would lie on the edge of the binocular visual field (also estimated as about 27°: above). It is possible therefore that Y lies just inside the edge of the area within which (after convergence) binocular disparity can be calculated. This would be compatible with the possibility that fixation at Y during sustained viewing may allow some direct access of information about the fixated stimulus to the ipsilateral hemisphere in a way that is not possible during fixation at ML. This is considered further in the next section.

AGE-SPECIFIC SHIFTS IN HEMISPHERIC DOMINANCE AND STRATEGIES OF VIEWING

Shifts in hemispheric dominance during the development of the chick are considered here, since they reveal strategies of eye use which would otherwise have been difficult to demonstrate. Age-dependent changes in hemispheric properties in the domestic chick were first demonstrated by Rogers (Rogers and Ehrlich, 1983; Rogers, 1991) using direct hemispheric insult. In male chicks unilateral injection of cycloheximide produces long-term deficits in visual learning, but only at certain ages: on day 8 only left hemisphere injection is effective, whereas on days 10 and 11 only right hemisphere injection has an effect. Immediately before and after this period and on day 9, injection is without effect, so that it is clear that first the left, and then the right hemisphere go through circumscribed periods of special sensitivity. These periods are accompanied by an unusual and marked degree of control of behavior by the sensitive hemisphere. Thus in a test in which two dead *Tenebrio* beetles were simultaneously advanced from behind into the right and left visual fields, the beetle on the right was pecked first on day 8 but that on the left was taken on days 10 and 11 (Andrew, 1988; Dharmaretnam, 1989). In younger chicks direction of first choice was close to random. Similar age-dependent changes in bias are revealed by tests in which the chick is allowed to view an object (a white ball) on which it is imprinted. The right eye is used in viewing on day 8, and the left eye on day 11; on day 9 there is no bias (Dharmaretnam, 1989; Dharmaretnam and Andrew, 1993). The pattern of bias toward control of response by one or other hemisphere revealed by these and other tests may be conveniently summarized as follows: days without bias are shown in parentheses and days of peak bias are in italics:

(day 7); *day 8:* left hemisphere control; (day 9); day 10 and *day 11*, right hemisphere control

Detailed measurements of head position during viewing are available, as already noted, for the first sight of a hen, a rat or a small flashing light; each point in figures 18.3 and 18.4 is for a separate group of chicks. The patterns of viewing the hen appear to be the outcome of the interaction of a strong overall tendency to use the right eye for viewing a stimulus of this sort, with the age-dependent shifts that have just been described. This can be clearly seen in female chicks (figure 18.3A), which used the right eye predominantly except for day 11, when the left eye was used instead. Almost exactly the same pattern of change over age was shown by males (figure 18.3B), although here the degree of departure from equal use of right and left eye was less throughout. Days 8 and 11 thus show the expected age-dependent biases.

However, day 10 is anomalous: left eye use, not right eye use, is predicted. It is thus striking to find that a unique pattern of viewing

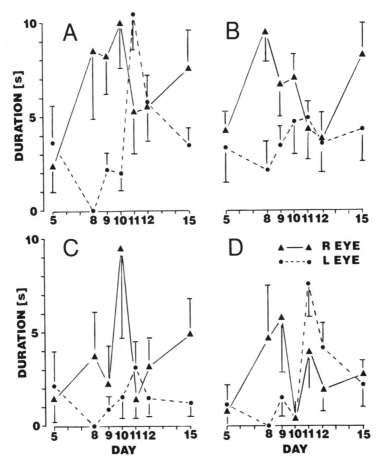

Figure 18.3 (A, B) The mean time spent fixating the hen with the right or the left eye, which is shown here, was defined as the sum of time spent in the 30 and 60 sectors (text). (A) Fixation by males. (B) Fixation by females. The pattern of fixation varied significantly over time (AGE, $F_{6,197} = 3.89$, $p = 0.001$); there were no significant differences between the sexes (SEX, $F_{1,197} = 0.004$; AGE × SEX, $F_{6,197} = 1.39$). (C, D) The mean time spent by female chicks fixating the hen in the 30° sector (C) and in the 60° sector (D).

occurs on day 10 in females. When 30° and 60° sectors were considered separately (figure 18.3C,D), right eye fixation proved predominantly to involve the 30° sector ("R30") on day 10 and only on that day. The R30 sector is thus commonly only on the day that marks the passage from right eye to left eye viewing. A comparable peak of 30° sector use occurred on day 10 in male chicks as well. In view of the apparent overall bias toward viewing the hen with the right eye, it seems likely that R30 use occurs when this overall bias is balanced by increasing age-dependent bias toward right hemisphere control.

Strikingly different patterns of viewing were evoked by the flashing light. The female chicks that were presented with this stimulus showed age-dependent changes in fixation that were almost the mirror image of those obtained with the hen. There was an overall tendency to view

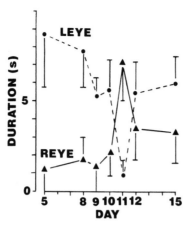

Figure 18.4 The mean time spent fixating the pilot light with right or left eye (defined as in figure 18.3) is shown there for female chicks. The patterns of fixation evoked by the three stimuli (hen, rat, pilot light) differ markedly with age and between stimuli (AGE, $F_{6,208} = 3.43$, $p = 0.003$; STIMULUS, $F_{2,208} = 9.76$, $p < 0.001$; AGE × STIMULUS, $F_{12,208} = 5.56$, $p < 0.001$); the latter effects were caused by the great differences between viewing the pilotlight and viewing the other two stimuli.

with the left eye, which was particularly clear on day 8 (and day 5); only on day 11 was the right eye used instead (figure 18.4). Leaving aside the reversal of eye use, the timings of change were exactly as in the timecourse for the hen: day 11 is again the only day on which viewing is the reverse of that which reaches its peak on day 8. Once again, viewing is clearly affected by the shift from left hemisphere control to right hemisphere control.

On day 11 both age-dependent effects and the nature of the stimulus would be expected to cause use of the left eye. Instead the right hemisphere, which must be presumed to be dominant on both these scores, appears to use its subordinate partner to view for it, using the right eye. Such "reversed viewing" occurs also in males on day 11.

Explanations of reversed viewing of an object like the light must begin by considering its properties. It is a novel feature in a familiar visual environment, which may herald further change. Its own properties are simple and could be recorded by the controlling hemisphere by even brief examination. It is unlikely to evoke the sort of social and attachment responses that are produced by an imprinting object; equally it did not appear to be frightening. Under these circumstances reversed viewing might allow the controlling hemisphere to use its partner (literally) to keep an eye on the light, while freeing itself for other tasks. These might include further processing of the information already gained (perhaps taking into account processing conducted relatively independently by the partner) or search for change elsewhere in the environment.

There are thus at least three strategies of monocular viewing. Two (normal and reversed viewing), since they use the 60° sector, are likely to confine direct input mainly to contralateral visual structures, and so presumably determine that these contralateral structures are predominantly responsible for the immediate processing of information about the stimulus. The third strategy involves use of the 30° sector, and is associated with balance between conflicting tendencies to control behavior by the right, and the left hemispheres. There are two possible complementary explanations of the use of 30R under such conditions. It may represent sustained preparation for a shift to binocular or left eye viewing (which, however, very rarely occurs). Although the head position prevents the left eye from seeing the stimulus it does allow sight of features close to the stimulus. This might make it easier for left eye fixation to be achieved rapidly and accurately. A second possibility is that sustained fixation with Y (that is, with the head in the 30R sector) allows information about the stimulus to reach binocular viewing systems, and so to reach the right hemisphere at least to some extent.

HEMISPHERIC SPECIALIZATION AND VIEWING

The first evidence that chicks may shift between the use of the right and left eyes according to stimulus properties was provided by Workman and Andrew (1986). Chicks presented the right side of the head to a simple model that they courted and mounted for copulation, but the left side of the head to another chick around which they were circling.

It is not at first obvious that hemispheric specialization should impose any differential use of the two eyes. Since important stimuli (e.g., predators, food) could appear equally often on either side of the head, there must be strong selection pressure keeping right and left eyes, and their corresponding visual systems, equally capable of performing difficult detection and recognition tasks. However, since sustained viewing of objects (at least at a distance) is commonly monocular, the choice of right or left eye for such viewing (once detection and initial recognition is over) might be affected by the lateralization of function.

Experiments with left-eyed chicks (LE) suggest special involvement of the right hemisphere (and perhaps visual systems elsewhere on the right side of the brain) in the analysis of novelty and the spatial configuration of the environment. LE chicks have a marked advantage over right-eyed (RE) chicks in the use of both near and distant features to locate food buried at a particular point in a sawdust covered tray (Rashid and Andrew, 1989). They also show dishabituation of pecking when, in a series of presentation of a colored bead, the position in space from which the bead approaches is changed between trials; RE chicks are quite unaffected (Andrew, 1983b, 1991). Similar dishabituation experiments in which the color of the bead is varied also show clear dishabituation in LE birds (Andrew, 1991). Again RE birds ignore this obvious change, even though in discrimination following training with an unpleasant taste they discriminate color more completely than do LE birds (Andrew and Brennan, 1985).

Interest in novelty in LE chicks was also shown in choices between an imprinting object of the sort with which the chick had been living (a red table tennis ball) and a transformation of it (Vallortigaro and Andrew, 1991). The two balls were hung at opposite ends of a runway, in the middle of which the chick was placed. Both RE and LE chicks spent nearly all their time close to one or other ball; there was thus no evidence that there was any difference in attachment. However, LE chicks were much more affected by small or moderate transformations. In one series of experiments the transformation involved rotation of a white bar on the side of the red ball. LE males chose the familiar stimulus as against a ball with 90° rotation of the bar; however, they chose the transformed ball when rotation was only 45°. In both cases RE birds chose at random. Only with large transformations (e.g., removal of bar) did RE choose, and then they always chose the familiar. Similar interest of LE birds in small or moderate change is thus shown when using stimuli that are large and distant, or small and very close; the responses that are evoked may be pecking or social behavior. It is therefore unlikely that the differences between LE and RE birds are predominantly due to motivational or simple perceptual factors. The left eye is thus preferentially used when viewing a stimulus whose most important property is novelty.

The best attested example of a stimulus that tends to be viewed with the right eye is a hen (at least when seen for the first time). There is other evidence that the left hemisphere has a special interest in adult conspecifics: the assumption in chicks reared under natural conditions (Workman and Andrew, 1989) of full left hemisphere control on day 8 is associated with the sudden appearance on that day of periods when chicks stare at (but do not approach) adult conspecifics other than their mother.

In most of the strategies that have so far been discussed, the fixation positions are such as are likely to allow one hemisphere to do most or all of the analysis. Hemispheric collaboration is much more difficult to establish from viewing position alone. Such collaboration seems likely, on the face of it, during binocular fixation. However, indirect evidence from experiments, in which chicks using right, left, or both eyes are compared, suggests that either hemisphere may dominate or both may be involved during binocular fixation, according to the conditions of the task (Andrew, 1991).

One viewing strategy in which it is likely that both hemispheres are involved in analyzing the same stimulus is rapid alternation of lateral fixation between the two eyes. This is obvious when passerine birds are foraging over the ground for invertebrate prey. Presumably such alternation allows the different specializations of both hemispheres to be used in the identification of a potential prey. One of the most interesting topics for future research is the way in which strategies such as this, or the use of the 30° sector, may allow perceptual inputs to the two sides of the brain to be appropriately adjusted to the needs of collaboration between the hemispheres.

ACKNOWLEDGMENTS

We are very grateful to Michael Land and Philip Zeigler for their comments on an earlier draft of this chapter.

REFERENCES

Andrew, R. J. Effects of testosterone on the calling of the domestic chick in a strange environment. *Animal Behav.* 23 (1975), 169–178.

Andrew, R. J. Specific short-latency effects of oestradiol and testosterone on distractibility and memory formation in the young domestic chick. In J. Balthazart, E. Prove, and R. Gilles (Eds), *Hormones and Behaviour in Higher Vertebrates.* Springer-Verlag, Berlin, 1983a, pp. 463–473.

Andrew, R. J. Lateralisation of emotional and cognitive function in higher vertebrates, with special reference to the domestic chick. In J. P. Ewart and D. J. Ingle (Eds), *Advances in Vertebrate Neuroethology.* Plenum, New York, 1983b, pp. 477–509.

Andrew, R. J. The development of visual lateralisation in the domestic check. *Behav. Brain Res.* 29 (1988), 201–209.

Andrew, R. J. The nature of behavioural lateralisation in the chick. In R. J. Andrew (Ed), *Neural and Behavioural Plasticity: the Use of the Domestic Chick as a Model.* Oxford University Press, Oxford, 1991, pp. 536–556.

Andrew, R. J., and Brennan, A. Sharply timed and lateralized events at time of establishment of long term memory. *Physiology. Behav. A* 34 (1985), 347–556.

Bischof, H. J. The visual field and visualy guided behaviour in the Zebra Finch (*Taeniopygia guttata*). *J. Comp. Physiol. A* 163 (1988), 329–337.

Bloch, S., Lemignan, M., and Martinoya, C. Coordinated vergence for frontal viewing, but independent eye movements for lateral viewing in the pigeon. In J. K. O'Regan and A. Levy-Schoen (Eds.), *Eye Movements.* Elsevier, Amsterdam, 1987, pp. 47–56.

Boxer, M., and Stanford, D. Projections to the posterior visual hyperstriatal region of the chick: An HRP study. *Exp. Brain Res.* 57 (1985), 494–498.

Dharmaretnam, M. Lateralization of viewing and other functions in the domestic chick. D. Phil. Thesis (1989). University of Sussex, Brighton, U.K.

Dharmaretnam, M., and Andrew, R. J. (1993). In preparation.

Ehrlich, D. Regional specialisation of the chick retina as revealed by the size and density of neurons in the ganglion cell layer. *J. Comp. Neurol.* 195 (1981), 643–657.

Mench, J. A., and Andrew, R. J. Lateralization of a food search task in the domestic chick. *Behav. Neural Biol.* 46 (1986), 107–114.

Miles, F. A. Centrifugal control of the avian retina. I. Receptive field properties of retinal ganglion cells. *Brain Res.* 48 (1972), 65–91.

Morris, V. B. An afoveate area centralis in the chick retina. *J. Comp. Neurol.* 210 (1982), 198–203.

Rashid, N. Y. Lateralization of topographical learning and other abilities in the chick. D. Phil. Thesis (1988). University of Sussex, Brighton, U.K.

Rashid, N. Y., and Andrew, R. J. Right hemisphere advantage for topographical orientation in the domestic chick. *Neuropsychologia* 7 (1989), 937–948.

Rochon-Duvigneaud, A. *Les Yeux et la Vision des Vertébrés.* Masson, Paris, 1943

Rogers, L. J. Development of Lateralisation. In R. J. Andrew (Ed.), *Neural and Behavioural Plasticity: the Use of the Domestic Chick as a Model.* Oxford University Press, Oxford, 1991, pp. 507–535.

Rogers, L. J., and Andrew, R. J. Frontal and lateral visual field use by chicks after treatment with testosterone. *Anim. Behav.* 38 (1989), 394–405.

Rogers, L. J., and Ehrlich, D. Asymmetry in the chicken forebrain during development: A possible involvement of the supraoptic decussation. *Neurosci. Lett.* 37 (1983), 123–127.

Turkel, J., and Wallman, J. Oscillatory eye movement with possible visual function in birds. *Neurosci. Abstr.* 3 (1977), 158.

Vallortigaro, G., and Andrew, R. J. Lateralisation of response to change in social partner in chick. *Anim. Behav.* 41 (1991) 187–194.

Wallman, J., and Pettigrew, J. D. Conjugate and disjunctive saccades in two avian species with contrasting oculomotor strategies. *J. Neurosci.* 5 (1985), 1418–1428.

Wallman, J., and Velez, J. Directional asymmetries of optokinetic nystagmus: developmental changes and relation to the accessory optic system and to the vestibular system. *J. Neurosci.* 5 (1985), 317–329.

Walls, G. L. *The Vertebrate Eye and Its Adaptive Radiation.* Cranbrook Press. Bloomfield Hills, MI, 1942.

Workman, L., and Andrew, R. J. Asymmetries of eye use in birds. *Anim. Behav.* 34 (1986), 1582–1584.

Workman, L., and Andrew, R. J. Simultaneous changes in behaviour and in lateralisation during the development of male and female domestic chicks. *Anim. Behav.* 38 (1989), 596–605.

19 Two Eyes and One World: Studies of Interocular and Intraocular Transfer in Birds

Monika Remy and Shigeru Watanabe

Pigeons are both skilled flyers and effective ground foragers. Their eyes, though laterally placed, are specialized to provide acute near vision at short distances during pecking and nearly panoramic vision at long distances during flight. These different visual functions are mediated by morphologically distinct visual fields; a small region of binocular overlap comprising the frontal visual field and a large area of monocular vision in each lateral visual field. The visual fields, in turn, are related to different retinal areas. The pigeon retina is divided into the dorso-temporal "red field" and the remaining "yellow field." The red fields are stimulated by objects in the lower frontal visual field; the yellow fields are stimulated by objects located above the head or lateral to it. Variations in the refractive state of the eye permit the focused vision of distant objects in the lateral visual field and of near stimuli in the binocular frontal portion of the visual field (see chapter 2).

In most natural situations, there will be a constant flow of stimulation to both eyes impinging on both frontal and lateral visual fields and on different locations within each eye. Somehow, the information from various sources must be centrally accessible if the bird is to be provided with a continually updated and coherent impression of its visual world. Moreover, such integration is a prerequisite for the control of visually elicited and guided movements. Consider, for example, a bird encountering, simultaneously, seeds in both the right and left monocular fields, or, alternatively, a seed in one field and a predator in the other. In both cases the responses evoked are conflicting (peck right, peck left: peck, fly away) and in both cases resolution of the conflict must involve some mechanism for the central integration of the two visual inputs. Indeed, it has been reported that when presented with conflicting information to the two eyes, pigeons respond to the more relevant information (Palmer and Zeier, 1974). Research bearing on this problem has generally involved studies of the interocular (I_rOT) and intraocular (I_aOT) transfer of learned information.

EXPERIMENTAL STUDIES OF INTEROCULAR TRANSFER

The existence of perfect interocular transfer is demonstrated if a response acquired during training with a stimulus presented to one eye is elicited when that same stimulus is presented to the other (previously occluded) eye. The usual experimental paradigm in I$_r$OT studies involve monocular training in a visually guided behavioral task until performance stabilizes and then testing with the previously occluded (untrained) eye. Transfer may be complete or incomplete and performance under the original and transfer conditions may differ qualitatively or quantitatively. Thus pigeons trained monocularly to respond to one color exhibited similar spectral generalization gradients with the trained and untrained eyes, but response rate was lower with the untrained eye (Ogawa, 1966). In both successive and simultaneous discriminations, pigeons made more errors with the untrained eye, even though transfer of the discrimination was clearly present (Watanabe, 1986). Such results may be interpreted in terms of either stimulus or response mechanisms. That is, stimuli viewed by one eye may not appear identical to the same stimuli viewed with the other or, while the stimulus input is identical, different performance may reflect an incomplete transfer at the motor level.

An ubiquitous and particularly striking result in many I$_r$OT experiments is the "mirror image reversal" effect (MIR). Thus, when pigeons were trained monocularly on a mirror-image discrimination (e.g., 45° vs. 135° oblique lines) and then exposed to the stimuli with the untrained eye, they preferred the previously negative (S−) stimulus (Mello, 1965). Watanabe and Ogawa (1973) found that after training with a single oblique line, pigeons showed a bimodal generalization gradient with peaks at both the original oblique angle and its mirror image, and this was true for both the trained and the untrained eye. Such a bimodal gradient was also obtained after binocular training (Beale et al., 1972; Thomas et al., 1966; Vetter and Hearst, 1968). Introduction of S− along the same dimension as S+ changed the bimodal gradient to one having a single peak at S+ with the trained eye and one with a peak at the mirror image of S+ with the untrained eye. These data suggest that pigeons, like many other animals as well as children, have mirror-image confusion (Zeigler and Schmerler, 1965).

To account for MIR, Beale and Corballis (1967, 1968) observed that on a monocular discrimination the pigeon's pecks are directed to the side of the key corresponding to the viewing eye, and that the extent of interocular reversal of an L–R discrimination depends on how much of the stimulus is masked by the head and the beak. They proposed that the masking produced by this "beak shift" changed the part of the monocular stimulus that controlled pecking. Because the left half of an asymmetrical stimulus resembles the right half of its mirror image, MIR would be expected.

Subsequent research has generally supported the "beak shift" hypothesis. Watanabe (1975) employed a line stimulus equivalent to the radius of a pecking key and, by rotating the line stimulus around the center of the pecking key, separated a lateral mirror image, a vertical mirror image and a lateral-vertical mirror image. As would be expected from the "beak shift" hypothesis, MIR was found to occur only at the lateral mirror image. Using a tilted line as a stimulus, Watanabe (1974) divided a tilted line into left and right halves and, after monocular discrimination training, carried out interocular transfer tests with these stimuli. After training with the right eye, pigeons often responded to the right half of S+ with the trained (right) eye and to the left half of S− when tested with the untrained (left) eye. After training with the left eye, similar relationships between the side of the viewing eye and the parts of the stimuli that controlled responding were seen. If the bird discriminates the orientation of the stimulus with reference to their visual field, a line tilted to "the right" means a line tilted to "the lateral" for the right eye, while a line tilted to "the lateral" is a line tilted to the left for the left eye. Tiemen et al.(1974) gave pigeons an artificial reference cue by fitting a partial cover on goggles worn by the birds. They were able to produce both lateral MIR and up-down MIR by shifting the partial cover from left to right or dorsal to ventral, respectively. The latter finding is not easily interpretable by other than a "masking" hypothesis.

One of the most intriguing findings in the IOT literature is the phenomenon of interocular conflicting discrimination. In this paradigm, one of a pair of discriminative stimuli is S+ when viewed with one eye and S− when viewed with the other (Catania, 1965; Levine, 1945a; Konermann, 1966). Successful performance on this task could reflect either the formation of separate memories in the two hemispheres, or a conditional discrimination, in which use of the viewing eye itself serves as a conditional cue.

To distinguish between these alternate accounts, Watanabe (1980) trained pigeons on four different conflicting tasks (figure 19.1). In the first, monocularly trained, task the S+ (vertical line) for one eye with the S− (horizontal line) for the other. In the second task, one discrimination was learned monocularly and via only one eye, whereas the reverse discrimination was acquired binocularly. In the third task, one discrimination was acquired monocularly, but with each eye alternately, while the reverse discrimination was acquired binocularly. In task 4, three different discriminations were acquired; one binocular and two monocular. In the binocular condition, S+ and S− were vertical and horizontal lines, respectively. In one monocular condition, S+ was the horizontal line and S− a blank key; in the other monocular condition, S+ was the blank key and the S− the horizontal line. Thus all three viewing conditions were conflicting. Successful learning of task 1 can be accounted for by either the "separate memories" or "conditional

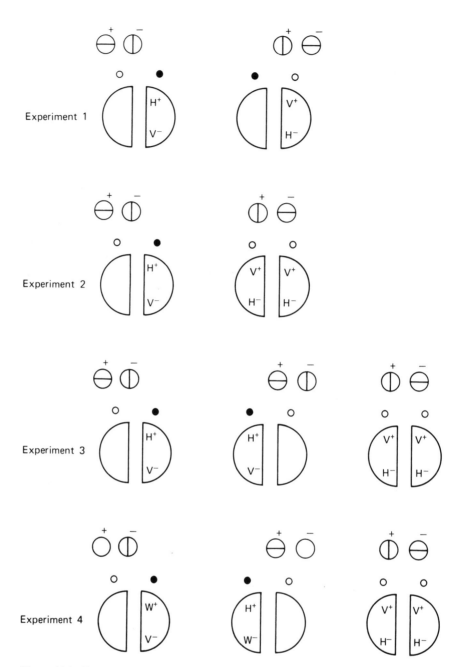

Figure 19.1 Experiments on interocular conflicting discrimination. Experiment 1: Monocular training on horizontal–vertical discrimination with one eye and the reversed discrimination with the other. Experiment 2: Monocular training on one discrimination with one eye; binocular training on the reversed discrimination. Experiment 3: Monocular training with each eye, alternately plus binocular training on the reversed discrimination. Experiment 4: Three conflicting discriminations, two acquired monocularly and one binocularly. + and − indicate reinforcement and nonreinforcement, respectively. H, V, and W indicate horizontal, vertical and white key, respectively. Small black dot indicates the location of the visual occluder. Details in text. Modified from Watanabe (1980).

Vision and Cognition

discrimination" hypotheses. Although the separate memories hypothesis might account for successful acquisition of task 2, it predicts failure of acquisition for tasks 3 and 4, whereas the conditional discrimination hypothesis predicts success for these last two tasks.

Performance on task 1 alternated between good and poor as the occluder was switched from the trained to the untrained eye, but the task was eventually learned. The binocular discrimination in task 2 was learned more rapidly than the monocular discrimination. Task 3 was also learned, but without evidence of binocular superiority. Task 4 required extended periods of training but was finally learned. The results support the conditional discrimination hypothesis and imply that the bird's viewing condition (one vs. two eyes; left vs. right eye) can be the cue for its choice of stimuli.

CONDITIONS FACILITATING THE OCCURRENCE OF INTEROCULAR TRANSFER

The behavioral conditions for successful transfer have been extensively explored. Using a jumping stand, Levine (1945a,b) found successful transfer of shape and brightness discriminations when stimuli were presented in a horizontal position (on the jumping stand platform) but not when they were vertically presented (on a wall behind the platform). These observations were later confirmed for pigeons (Graves and Goodale, 1977, 1979; Goodale and Graves, 1980), ring doves (Siegel, 1953a,b), and geese (Konermann, 1966).

In the jumping stand, stimuli presented in the horizontal position both elicit the response and control its direction, but this is not true for the stimulus in the vertical position. One interpretation of these findings suggests that the spatial arrangement of the stimulus and response locations is an important variable in the occurrence of successful transfer. This interpretation is supported by a variety of operant conditioning studies of I,OT. In a conventional operant discrimination paradigm, the discriminative stimulus on the key not only elicits the pecking response but directs it. That is, the "discriminandum" and the "manipulandum" share the same spatial location. Under such conditions, successful transfer is reported (Catania, 1965; Ogawa, 1966; Ogawa and Ohinata, 1966). However, no transfer was seen in a conditional spatial discrimination in which pigeons had to peck left when both keys were green and peck right when both keys were red (Green et al., 1978). To test the spatial location hypothesis, Watanabe (1986) arranged three conditional spatial tasks, employing two keys arranged either vertically or horizontally (figure 19.2). In the first two tasks, the keys were arranged vertically. In task 1, the discriminative stimulus was presented on the upper key and the response key was the lower one; in task 2 this situation was reversed. In task 3 the keys were arranged horizontally. For birds trained with the left eye, the stimulus key was the left one and vice

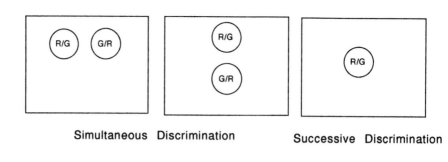

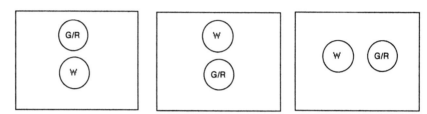

Separation of discriminandum and Operandum

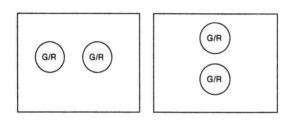

Conditional Spatial Discrimination

Figure 19.2 Experiments on the conditions facilitating interocular transfer. Spatial arrangements of the discriminative stimuli. The upper panels are conventional simultaneous (left, middle) and successive (right) discriminations. In the middle panels, the pecking key (white) is spatially separated from the discriminative stimuli, presented successively. In the bottom panels, pecking at a key is conditional upon its color. Details in text. From Watanabe (1986) and Watanabe and Weiss (1984).

versa. In all three situations, pecks at the response key (manipulandum) were conditional on the color of the stimulus key (discriminandum). Under these conditions, the pigeons failed to show I_rOT. However, excellent transfer was seen both for successive discriminations using a single key or simultaneous discriminations, with the two keys arranged either vertically or horizontally.

Watanabe (1986) has interpreted the absence of transfer under such conditions as resulting from a failure of sensorimotor integration related to the spatial separation of discriminandum and manipulandum and has extended this interpretation to the results of the jumping stand experiments. An alternative interpretation of the jumping stand findings was suggested by Goodale and Graves (1980, 1982). Taking into account the organization of the pigeon's retinal areas and their relation to its visual fields, they noted that stimuli presented horizontally on a jumping stand impinge on the dorsoposterior part of the retina (the red field), but this is not the case for vertically presented stimuli. They proposed that the location of the stimulus within the bird's visual field is a powerful determinant of the success or failure of interocular transfer.

Unfortunately, it is not possible to specify the retinal location of discriminative stimuli in freely moving birds. However, it is hard to attribute the absence of IOT in the Watanabe (1986) study to differences in retinal areas because the identical spatial arrangement of stimuli was employed in these experiments. The pigeons might see discriminative stimuli in their monocular field in the horizontally arranged keys, but were unlikely to have seen them on their lateral visual field with vertically arranged keys.

An experimental test of the retinal area hypothesis was carried out in the head-fixed pigeon (Mallin and Delius, 1983), using jaw movements (mandibulation) as an operant (indicator) response and manipulating the retinal locus of the colored stimuli. Despite the spatial separation of stimulus and response in this preparation, subjects showed transfer of a monocularly learned discrimination task when the stimuli were presented frontally in the binocular visual field, but not when they were presented laterally in the monocular visual field (figure 19.3). Although these findings appear to support the "retinal locus," it should be noted that the pigeons did not need to spatially direct their response (mandibulation). Furthermore, the pigeon's beak was oriented to the position of the discriminative stimuli in the frontal position, whereas in the lateral presentation they were distant from the beak orientation.

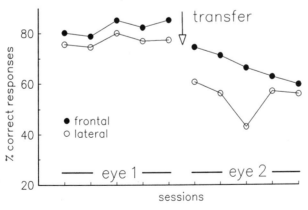

Figure 19.3 Interocular transfer of a color discrimination in the head-fixed pigeon. Performance during the last five training and first five transfer sessions. Transfer was significantly better when the stimuli were presented in the frontal than in the lateral visual fields. After Mallin and Delius (1983).

The relation between the two interpretations, "retinal locus" and "sensorimotor integration," is currently unclear. Moreover, there are a number of I$_r$OT findings that do not fit easily under either rubric. Thus, tasks in which transfer was absent include a pattern discrimination using heat reinforcement (Gaston, 1979) and avoidance of the visual cliff (Zeier, 1970), both in chicks, as well as search for the location of stored food in marsh tits (Sherry et al., 1981). Successful transfer was demonstrated in cardiac conditioning (Mihara and Watanabe, 1982), in the conditioned withdrawal response of pigeons, chickens, and gulls (Stevens and Klopfer, 1977), and in taste aversion studies with chicks (Bell and Gibbs, 1979; Cherkin, 1970; Gaston, 1978, 1980). Moreover, most of the pigeon discrimination experiments have involved training of the motor response (pecking) under binocular conditions prior to monocular training on the experimental task. For example, in one study reporting successful I$_r$OT of autoshaping, subjects had received binocular magazine training prior to monocular autoshaping. It is therefore interesting that when the eye is occluded during initial acquisition of the pecking response, pigeons did not show transfer of the motor response to the untrained eye (Stevens and Kirsch, 1980). Similarly, subjects trained with one eye on a fixed interval (FI) schedule did not show transfer of the typical FI scallop response pattern when tested with the untrained eye (Watanabe, 1985b). Additional studies of I$_r$OT of the motor response would be useful.

Watanabe has suggested that the "retinal locus" and "sensorimotor integration" hypotheses may not be contradictory. Following McLeary (1960), Watanabe proposed that I$_r$OT is not a unitary process and distinguished between "sensory" and "visuomotor" transfer. Retinal locus may be crucial when a task does not require sensorimotor integration (as in the Mallin and Delius study, above) However, if a task requires sensorimotor integration, I$_r$OT will not occur even when the discriminative stimuli impinge on the binocular field. While this account is plausible, it should be kept in mind that retinal location remains a potentially important variable and must be thoroughly controlled before higher order mechanisms are invoked to explain the results of interocular transfer experiments.

BRAIN STRUCTURES MEDIATING INTEROCULAR TRANSFER

The anatomical substrate for transfer involves both the retina and the central visual pathways. The two visual pathways receive inputs from different retinal areas, have distinctly different relays, and terminate on different telencephalic projection fields. Almost all the retinal ganglion cell axons comprising the thalamofugal pathway originate in the yellow field; those of the tectofugal pathway originate in the red field. Because there is virtually complete crossing of the retinal ganglion cell axons in the optic chiasm (Cowan et al., 1961), visual information derived from one eye is (primarily) conveyed to the contralateral hemisphere of the telencephalon. However, the presence of a crossed optic chiasm, commisural connections (tectal and posterior), and recrossing projections in the dorsal and ventral supraoptic decussations (DSOD, thalamofugal; DSOV, tectofugal) make it possible for ipsilateral visual inputs to have access to each hemisphere (Benowitz and Karten, 1976; Cuenod, 1974; Engelage and Bischof, 1988; Meier et al., 1974; Perisic et al., 1971). Figure 19.4 presents a schematic summary of the organization of the pigeon's visual system.

Interocular transfer may be conceptualized as involving at least two distinct processs: the formation of a some sort of "memory engram" and its "read out" into behavior. For successful transfer, the engram must either be laid down bilaterally, so that it may be "read out" from either eye, or laid down unilaterally and read out bilaterally. A variety of disruptive manipulations have been carried out at almost every level of the visual pathway to identify central structures mediating interocular transfer and clarify their contribution to the "engram formation" and "read out" processes.

Although birds lack a corpus callosum, alternate substrates for interocular transfer are provided by the tectal, posterior, and anterior commissures and by the supraoptic decussations. The logic of the "split

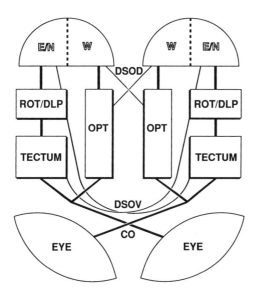

Figure 19.4 The anatomical substrate for interocular transfer. Organization of visual inputs in the pigeon. CO, optic chiasm; DSOD, DSOV, dorsal and ventral supraoptic decussations; tectum, optic tectum; OPT, principal optic nuclei of the thalamus; ROT/DLP, nuclei rotundus and dorsolateralis posterioris of the thalamus; E/N, ectostriatum/neostriatum; W, Wulst. Thick solid lines indicate tectofugal and thalamofugal pathways; thin solid lines indicate ipsilateral recrossing pathways (tectorotundal, OPT-Wulst). From Jäger et al. (1992).

brain" experiments used to investigate the contribution of these structures is shown in figure 19.5. Sections of the tectal and posterior commissures in pigeon disrupted I$_r$OT of autoshaping and habituation of a head-orienting response, but had no effect on I$_r$OT of color and form discrimination (Cuenod and Zeier, 1967; Meier, 1971; Essock-Vitale, 1979; Hamassaki and Britto, 1987). The results suggested that these commissures are important in the transfer of sensorimotor, but not of sensory processes.

Studies of DSO section take their rationale from the fact that its two divisions, the dorsal (DSOd) and ventral (DSOv) supraoptic decussations, are components, respectively, of the thalamofugal and tectofugal visual systems (Hunt and Kunzle, 1976; Karten et al., 1973). Because it is not feasible to restrict DSO sections to one or the other component, Watanabe (1985a) compared the effect of total DSO section with that of damage restricted to the dorsal portion. While section of the dorsal component had no effect, lesions damaging both parts disrupted I$_r$OT of a horizontal-vertical line discrimination (see also Maier, 1976; but see Goodale, 1985). The disruption of I$_r$OT seen after complete DSO section implies that monocular training lays down an "engram" only on the single (contralateral) side that cannot be accessed directly from the untrained eye. The finding thus supports the unilateral memory hypothesis.

The results of the DSO experiments also suggest tectofugal rather than thalamofugal involvement. They are consistent with the observation that unilateral lesions of thalamofugal structures such as the thalamic OPT complex or Wulst are without effect while unilateral damage

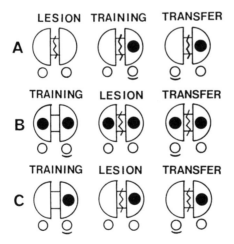

Figure 19.5 Schematic representation of the split-brain experiment. Half circles represent the hemisphere, small circles the eyes, and black circles the lateralized "engram." (A) Commissure section prior to monocular training. (B) Commissure section after monocular training. If the "engram" is formed bilaterally (B) the untrained eye can access it; if the "engram" is lateralized (C), the untrained eye cannot access it. From Watanabe (1985a).

to the tectofugal relay (nucleus rotundus) severely impair I$_r$OT (Francesconi et al., 1982; Watanabe, 1986, 1988, 1991; Watanabe et al., 1986). An interesting aspect of the Watanabe studies is the light they shed on the contributions of the tectofugal pathway to the "memory" and "read out" processes involved in I$_r$OT (figure 19.6).

In these studies, unilateral lesions were made in either OPT or rotundus, varying both with respect to the laterality of the lesion (trained vs. untrained side) and the stage of training (before or after acquisition) of the monocular discrimination. OPT lesions had no effect under any of these conditions. Nucleus rotundus lesions of the trained (contralateral) side disrupted I$_r$OT if they were made after acquisition of the discrimination; lesions made before acquisition, while they increased the time required to learn the discrimination, did not prevent transfer. In these subjects, the discrimination must have been learned with the remaining (ipsilateral) visual system but its readout must have involved the intact visual system contralateral to the viewing eye.

The disruption of I$_r$OT seen with lesions made after acquisition suggests that during acquisition of the original monocular discrimination, the information is processed in tectofugal visual structures contralateral to the viewing eye. The disruption of I$_r$OT seen in this situation must be due to lesion effects on "memory" processes located in these structures. Rotundal lesions in the untrained hemisphere caused transfer deficits regardless of the temporal relation between surgery and original training. The I$_r$OT deficits seen in these subjects reflect the fact that the visual structures used for "read out" by the untrained eye was damaged,

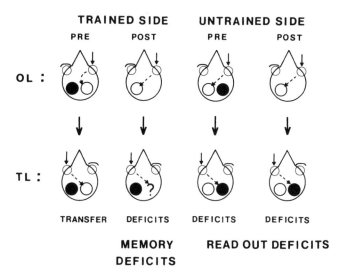

Figure 19.6 Unilateral rotundal lesions and interocular transfer. Top (OL, original learning) Lesions are placed in either the trained (left) or untrained (right) side, either prior to (pre) or after (post) monocular learning. Bottom (TL, transfer learning) Presence (transfer) or absence (deficits) of interocular transfer. Filled circle indicates rotundus lesion. From Watanabe (1991).

and may thus be interpreted as "sensory" deficits. Taken together with the DSO studies, these data suggest that information from one eye appears to be basically processed in the contralateral hemisphere, but it may be "read out" from either hemisphere if conditions are appropriate. The data are consistent with the hypothesis that interocular transfer is mediated by mechanisms involving lateralized memory and its bilateral readout. It is this mechanism that generates one world from the input to two separate eyes, and it appears to involve the tectofugal, rather than the thalamofugal visual pathway.

At first glance, this conclusion seems paradoxical. I_rOT is generally assumed to involve binocular convergence mechanisms, and the thalamofugal, rather than the tectofugal system has often been viewed as the substrate for binocular integration in birds. However, the studies on which this view is based were performed in frontal-eyed birds like the owl (Bravo and Pettigrew, 1981; Pettigrew and Konishi, 1976), and the situation may be quite different in lateral-eyed birds like pigeons. In these species, inputs from the central retina arise from the monocular, not the binocular portions of the visual field and are conveyed to the Wulst via the thalamofugal pathway (Remy and Güntürkün, 1991). However, this does not preclude binocular integration mechanisms as the substrate of I_rOT. There is a substantial projection from the red retinal fields to the optic tectum in pigeons (Clarke and Whitteridge, 1976), and a recrossing pathway from tectum to nucleus rotundus. Moreover, electrophysiological experiments in zebra finch show that the telencephalic target of the tectofugal pathway (the ectostriatum) can be activated by ipsilateral stimulation (Engelage and Bischof, 1988 and chapter 8). Thus, in lateral-eyed birds, the tectofugal mediation of binocular convergence remains a possibility to be explored.

Finally, it should be noted that I_rOT occurs between the binocularly stimulated red fields of the retina but not between the monocularly stimulated yellow fields (Goodale and Graves, 1980, 1982). The asymmetry of interocular transfer demonstrated in many I_rOT studies may be of functional significance. Objects that may appear in the binocular visual field include seeds or a landing perch. Pigeons can use depth cues such as binocular disparity to improve the accuracy of pecking grain or of a landing maneuver (McFadden and Wild, 1986). Thus I_rOT between the red fields is adaptive. By contrast, the monocular lateral fields may present two quite different and sometimes conflicting stimulus situations (e.g., seeds and a predator). Mechanisms precluding I_rOT between these two fields may reduce such potential conflicts and allow rapid decision making.

EXPERIMENTAL STUDIES OF INTRAOCULAR TRANSFER

Experiments on intraocular transfer in birds are rare and often difficult to interpret, because of the problem of specifying the precise retinal location of stimuli viewed by freely moving subjects. In an early experiment employing a frontally located response key, Nye (1973) reported that color and brightness discriminations acquired to frontally presented stimuli could not be maintained when the stimuli were presented in the lateral field, even though the transition to the lateral field was made gradually over a period of weeks.

Color and pattern discriminations acquired monocularly with training on a jumping stand were lost when the position of the stimuli was changed from subrostral (horizontally below the beak) to anterorostral (vertically in front of the beak), i.e., from the lower frontal to the upper frontal visual field. Levine (1952) interpreted these results as indicating a lack of transfer between functionally independent areas of acute vision within the same eye. Subsequently, Goodale and Graves (1982) reported that pigeons on a jumping stand scanned anterorostral stimuli monocularly in their lateral visual field. In the light of this observation, Levine's results, like Nye's (1973) suggest a lack of transfer from the frontal to the lateral visual field.

Using head-fixed pigeons and an operant indicator response (mandibulation), Mallin and Delius (1983) showed that a color discrimination task acquired to stimuli presented in the frontal field would not transfer to the lateral field. Lateral-to-frontal transfer, though also poor, was about 10% better. However, the transfer tests were carried out under extinction, which may have obscured directional differences in transfer.

An unequivocal demonstration of asymmetry in the direction of intraocular transfer was provided in an experiment by Remy and Emmerton (1991). Two groups of head-fixed pigeons learned to discriminate the presence of a bright light from its absence, in an instrumental conditioning situation using a mandibulation indicator response. For one group, the stimulus was presented in the frontal visual field (red retinal field) for acquisition and shifted to the lateral visual field (yellow retinal field) during transfer testing; for the other group, these conditions were reversed. Intraocular transfer was directionally selective. It occurred when stimulus presentation was changed from lateral to frontal (figure 19.7b) but not when the change was from frontal to lateral (figure 19.7a).

Earlier, Goodale and Graves (1982) had shown that reliable interocular transfer occurs only when the red field has been stimulated. Even when both eyes are unoccluded, no transfer was shown with stimulation of the yellow field (Goodale and Graves, 1980). Thus the "one way" intraocular transfer demonstrated in the Remy and Emmerton (1991) study cannot be based on previously learned information which had been transferred between the two eyes.

The asymmetry demonstrated in these experiments may reflect the natural organization of some visually guided behaviors. In doves and pigeons, the detection of seeds is reported to involve fixation by the

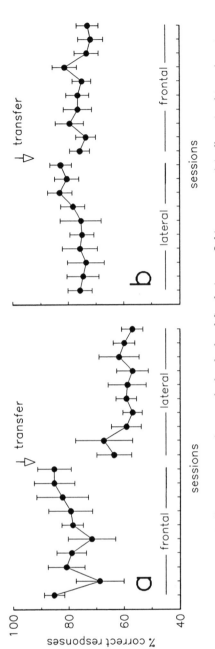

Figure 19.7 Directional effects in intraocular transfer by the head-fixed pigeon. Subjects were originally trained in a detection task with stimuli either in the frontal (a) or lateral (b) field and tested for transfer to the converse visual field. Details in text. From Remy and Emmerton (1991).

lateral visual field and then a refixation with the frontal field to guide pecking (Fridman, 1975). Recall that the refractive state of the pigeon's eye permits focused vision of distant objects in the lateral portion of the visual field and of near stimuli in its binocular frontal portion. This ability, combined with the one-way transfer of information, would facilitate a rapid switch from lateral to frontal vision during foraging or on landing from flight.

REFERENCES

Beale, I. L., and Corballis, M. C. Laterally displaced pecking in monocularly viewing pigeons: A possible factor in interocular mirror-image reversal. *Psychon. Sci.* 9 (1967), 603–604.

Beale, I. L., and Corballis, M. C. Beak shift: An explanation for interocular mirror-image reversal in pigeons. *Nature* 220 (1968), 82–83.

Beale, I. L., Williams, R. J., Webster, D. M., and Corballis, M. C. Confusion of mirror images by pigeons and interhemispheric commissures. *Nature (London)* 238 (1972), 348–349.

Bell, G. A., and Gibbs, M. E. Interhemispheric engram transfer in chick. *Neurosci. Lett.* 13 (1979), 163–168.

Benowitz, L. J., and Karten, H. J. Organization of the tectofugal visual pathway in the pigeon. A retrograde transport study. *J. Comp. Neurol.* 167 (1976), 503–520.

Bravo, H., and Pettigrew, J. D. The distribution of neurons projecting from the retina and visual cortex to the thalamus and tectum opticum of the barn owl, *Tyto alba* and the burrowing owl, *Speotyto cuicularia. J. Comp. Neurol.* 199 (1981), 419–441.

Catania, A. C. Interocular transfer of discriminations in the pigeon. *J. Exp. Anal. Behav.* 8 (1965), 147–155.

Cherkin, A. Eye to eye transfer of an early response modification in chicks. *Nature (London)* 227 (1970), 1153.

Clarke, P. H. G., and Whitteridge, D. The projection of the retina, including the "read area" onto the optic tectum of the pigeon. *Quart. J. Exp. Physiol.* 61 (1976), 351–358.

Cowan, W. M., Adamson, L., and Powell, T. P. S. An experimental study of the avian visual system. *J. Anat.* 95 (1961), 545–563.

Cuenod, M. Commissural pathways in interhemispheric transfer of visual information in the pigeon. In F. O. Schmitt and F. F. Worden (Eds), *Neuroscience*. MIT Press, Cambridge, MA, 1974, pp. 21–29.

Cuenod, P. M., and Zeier, H. Transfert visuel interhemispherique et commissurotomie chez le pigeon. *Schweiz. Arch. Neurol. Neurochir.* 100 (1967), 365–380.

Engelage, J., and Bischof, H-J. Enucleation enhances ipsilateral flash-evoked responses in the ectostriatum of the Zebra finch (*Taeniopyia guttata castanotis*, Gould). *Exp. Brain Res.* 70 (1988), 79–89.

Essock-Vitale, S. M. Pigeon's interhemispheric transfer of autoshaping and other visual discriminations. *Physiol. Behav.* 22 (1979), 1211–1215.

Francesconi, W., Fogassi, L., and Musumeci, D. Interocular transfer of visual discrimination in Wulst-ablated pigeons. *Behav. Brain Res.* 5 (1982), 399–406.

Fridman, M. B. How birds use their eyes. In P. Wright, P. Caryl, and D. M. Vowels (Eds.), *Neural and Endocrine Aspects of Behavior in Birds*. Elsevier, Amsterdam, 1975, pp. 188–204.

Gaston, K. E. Interocular transfer of a visually mediated conditioned food aversion in chicks. *Behav. Biol.* 24 (1978), 272–278.

Gaston, K. E. Lack of interocular transfer of pattern discrimination learning in chicks. *Brain Res.* 171 (1979), 339–343.

Gaston, K. E. Evidence for separate and concurrent avoidance learning in the two hemispheres of the normal chick brain. *Behav. Neural Biol.* 28 (1980), 129–137.

Goodale, M. A. Interocular transfer in the pigeon after lesions of the dorsal supraoptic decussation. *Behav. Brain Res.* 16 (1985), 1–7.

Goodale, M. A., and Graves, J. A. Failure of interocular transfer of learning in pigeons (*Columba livia*) trained on a jumping stand. *Bird Behav.* 2 (1980), 13–22.

Goodale, M. A., and Graves, J. A. Interocular transfer in the pigeon: Retinal focus as a factor. In D. Ingle, M. A. Goodale, and R. Mansfield (Eds.), *Analysis of Visual Behavior*. MIT Press, London, 1982, pp. 211–240.

Graves, J. A., and Goodale, M. A. Failure of interocular transfer in the pigeon (*Columba livia*). *Physiol. Behav.* 19 (1977), 425–428.

Graves, J. A., and Goodale, M. S. Do training conditions affect interocular transfer in the pigeon? In I. S. Russell, M. W. Van Hof, and G. Berlucchi (Eds.), *Structure and Function of Cerebral Commissures*. Macmillan Press, London, 1979, pp. 73–86.

Green, L., Brecha, N., and Gazzaniga, M. S. Interocular transfer of simultaneous but not successive discriminations in the pigeon. *Animal Learn. Behav.* 6 (1978), 261–264.

Hamassaki, D. E., and Britto, L. R. G. Interocular transfer of habituation in pigeons: Mediation by tectal and/or posterior commissure. *Behav. Brain Res.* 23 (1987), 175–179.

Hunt S. P., and Kunzle, H. O. Observations on the projections and intrinsic organization of the pigeon optic tectum: An autoradiographic study based on anterograde and retrograde axonal and dendric flow. *J. Comp. Neurol.* 170 (1976), 153–172.

Jäger, R., Arends, J. J. A., Schall, U., and Zeigler, H. P. The visual forebrain and eating in pigeons. *Brain Behav. Evol.* 39 (1992), 153–168.

Karten, H. J., Hodos, W., Nauta, W. J. H., and Revzin, A. M. Neural connections of the 'visual Wulst' of the avian telencephalon: Experimental studies in the pigeon (*Columba livia*) and owl (*Speotyto cunicularia*). *J. Comp. Neurol.* 150 (1973), 253–278.

Konermann, V. G. Monokulare Dressur von Haugänsen, z.T. mit entgegengesetzter Merkmalsbedeutung für beide Augen. *Z. Tierpsychol.* 23 (1966), 555–580.

Levine, J. Studies in interrelations of central nervous structures in binocular vision. I. The lack of binocular transfer of visual discriminative habits acquired monocularly by the pigeon. *J. Gen. Psychol.* 67 (1945a), 105–129.

Levine, J. Studies in interrelations of central nervous structures in binocular vision. II The conditions under which interocular transfer of discriminative habits takes place in the pigeon. *J. Gen. Psychol.* 67 (1945b), 131–142.

Levine, J. Studies in interrelations of central nervous structures in binocular vision. III localization of the memory trace trade as evidenced by the lack of inter and intraocular habit transfer in the pigeon. *J. Gen. Psychol.* 81 (1952), 19–27.

Maier, V. Effekte unilateraler telencephaler und thalamischer Läsionen auf die monokulare Musterdiskriminationfähigkeit kommissurotomierter Tauben. *Rev. suis. Zool.* 83 (1976), 59–82.

Mallin, H. D., and Delius, J. D. Inter- and intraocular transfer of colour discriminations with mandibulation as an operant in the head-fixed pigeon. *Behav. Anal. Let.* 3 (1983), 297–309.

McClearly, R. A. Type of responses as a factor in interocular transfer in the fish. *J. Comp. Physiol. Psychol.* 53 (1960), 311–321.

McFadden, S. A., and Wild, J. M. Binocular depth perception in the pigeon. *J. Exp. Anal. Behav.* 45 (1986), 149–160.

Meier, R. E. Interhemisphärischer Transfer visueller Zweifachwahlen bei kommissurotomierten Tauben. *Psychol. Forsch.* 34 (1971), 220–245.

Meier, R. E., Mihailovic, J., and Cuenod, M. Thalamic organization of the retino-thalamo-hyperstriatal pathway in the pigeon (*Columba livia*). *Exp. Brain Res.* 19 (1974), 351–364.

Mello, N. K. Interhemispheric reversal of mirror image oblique line after monocular training in pigeons. *Science* 148 (1965), 252–254.

Mihara, M., and Watanabe, S. Interocular transfer of cardiac conditioning in the pigeon. *Behav. Brain Res.* 4 (1982), 411–416.

Nye, P. W. On the functional differences between frontal and lateral visual fields of the pigeon. *Vis. Res.* (1973), 559–574.

Ogawa, T. Interocular generalization on color stimuli in pigeon. *An. Anim. Psychol.* 16 (1966), 87–102.

Ogawa, T., and Ohinata, S. Interocular transfer of color discrimination in a pigeon. *An. Anim. Psychol.* 16 (1966), 1–9.

Palmer, C., and Zeier, H. Hemispheric dominance and transfer in the pigeon. *Brain Res.* 76 (1974), 537–541.

Persic, M., Mihailovic, J., and Cuenod, M. Electrophysiology of contralateral and ispilateral visual projections to the Wulst in the pigeon (*Columba livia*). *Int. J. Neurosci.* 2 (1971), 7–14.

Pettigrew, J. D., and Konishi, M. Binocular neurons selective for orientation and disparity in the visual Wulst of the barn owl (*Tyto alba*). *Science* 193 (1976), 675–678.

Remy, M., and Emmerton, J. Direction dependence of inraocular transfer of stimulus detection in pigeons (*Columba livia*). *Behav. Neurosci.* 105 (1991), 647–652.

Remy, M., and Güntürkün, O. Retinal afferents to the tectum opticum and the nucleus opticus principalis thalami in the pigeon. *J. Comp. Neurol* 304 (1991), 1–14.

Sherry, D. F., Krebs, J. R., and Cowie, R. J. Memory for the location of stored food in Marsh tits. *Animal Behav.* 29 (1981), 1260–1266.

Siegel, A. I. Deprivation of visual form definition in the ring dove. I. Discriminatory learning. *J. Comp. Physiol. Psychol.* 45 (1953a), 115–119.

Siegel, A. I. Deprivation of visual form definition in the ring dove. II. Perceptual-motor transfer. *J. Comp. Physiol. Psychol.* 49 (1953b), 249–252.

Stevens, V. J., and Kirsch, W. R. Interocular transfer in pigeons of color discrimination but not motor response training. *Animal Learn. Behav.* 8 (1980), 17–21.

Stevens, V. J., and Klopfer, F. D. Interocular transfer of conditioning and extinction in birds. *J. Comp. Physiol. Psychol.* 91 (1977), 1074–1081.

Thomas, D. R., Klipec, W., and Lyons, J. Investigations of a mirror image transfer effect in pigeons. *J. Exp. Anal. Behav.* 9 (1966), 567–571.

Tieman, S. B., Tieman, D. G., Brody, B. A., and Hamilton, C. R. Interocular reversal of up-down mirror image in pigeons. *Physiol. Behav.* 12 (1974), 615–620.

Vetter, G. H., and Hearst, E. Generalization and discrimination of shape orientation in the pigeon. *J. Exp. Anal. Behav.* 11 (1968), 753–765.

Watanabe, S. Interocular transfer of stimulus control in pigeons. *An. Anim. Psychol.* 24 (1974), 1–14.

Watanabe, S. Interocular transfer of generalization along line-tile dimension in pigeons: A separation of three types of symmetric stimuli. *Jpn. Psychol. Res.* 7 (1975), 133–140.

Watanabe, S. Visual discrimination studies in pigeons. In Y. Tsukada and B. W. Agranoff (Eds.), *Neurobiological Basis of Learning and Memory.* John Wiley, New York, 1980, pp. 233–247.

Watanabe, S. Interhemispheric transfer of visual discrimination in pigeons with supraoptic decussation (DSO) lesions before and after monocular learning. *Behav. Brain Res.* 17 (1985a), 163–170.

Watanabe, S. Interocular transfer of schedule-controlled behavior in pigeon: Does the change of viewing condition mean a change of the external world for the pigeon? *Hiyoshi Rep. (Keio University)* 12 (1985b), 105–115.

Watanabe, S. Interocular transfer of learning in the pigeon: Visuo-motor integration and separation of discriminanda and manipulanda. *Behav. Brain Res.* 19 (1986), 227–232.

Watanabe, S. Effects of unilateral thalamic lesion upon interocular transfer of visual discrimination in pigeons. I. Lesion in the trained hemisphere (memory access deficits). *Behav. Brain Res.* 29 (1988), 259–265.

Watanabe, S. Effects of unilateral thalamic lesion upon interocular transfer of visual discrimination in pigeons. II. Lesion in the untrained hemisphere (sensory deficits). *Behav. Brain Res.* 43 (1991), 103–108.

Watanabe, S., and Ogawa, T. An experimental analysis of mirror image reversal effects in pigeons. *An. Anim. Psychol.* 23 (1973), 1–13.

Watanabe, S., and Weiss, S. A lack of interocular transfer of spatial conditioned discrimination in pigeons. *Behav. Brain Res.* 12 (1984), 65–68.

Watanabe, S., Hodos, W., Bessette, B. B., and Shimizu, T. Interocular transfer in parallel visual pathways in pigeons. *Brain Behav. Evol.* 29 (1986), 184–195.

Zeier, H. Lack of eye to eye transfer of an early response modification in birds. *Nature (London)* 225 (1970), 708–709.

Zeigler, H. P., and Schmerler, S., Visual discrimination of orientation by pigeons. *Animal Behav.* 13 (1965), 475–477.

20 What Can We Learn from Experiments on Pigeon Concept Discrimination?

Shigeru Watanabe, Stephen E. G. Lea, and
Winand H. Dittrich

THE DISCRIMINATION OF OBJECTS

Most of this book is concerned with the mechanisms by which birds
make rather simple visual discriminations. Mechanism, both physiological and behavioral, is vitally important if we are to understand vision.
But we also need to ask questions about function. What do birds make
visual discriminations *for*? This is not just a question about the use to
which the mechanisms we have unraveled can be put. Behind function
stands selective pressure. It is the uses of discrimination that have
driven its evolution, and hence provide the ultimate explanations for
whatever mechanisms we can discover.

There are several different levels at which we can explore the functions of vision. Most broadly, we can look at the ecology of each species
of bird, and ask what visual challenges it poses. What light do individuals have available, and what objects (prey, predators, shelter, conspecifics) is it adaptive for them to discriminate from the background?
Somewhat more specifically, we can look at the innate response tendencies of the species and the releasers that elicit them; a female bird
whose potential mates have brightly colored feathers that release sexual
receptivity in her when erected must have visual mechanisms that will
detect and discriminate the appropriate colors and forms.

At its narrowest, however, function raises questions that do not call
for answers in terms of particular species' characteristics. Birds' visual
worlds do not consist of the kinds of stimuli typically used in perceptual
and physiological experiments—spots of light, lines, and gratings—and
nor do birds in their natural environment respond to such stimuli. They
respond to objects. Some of those objects may be "coded" as significant
by the presence of strong, simple stimuli; we know from the early
experiments of comparative ethologists that almost any patch of red
will elicit the same response from a territory-holding European robin
as the biologically appropriate object (Tinbergen, 1951). But most significant objects in the bird's world are not coded in any such easy way.
Recognition of many of them, like individual related or neighboring

conspecifics, or individual places of home, food supply, or danger, must necessarily be learned rather than innate. And most of these stimuli have two important properties. First, they are inherently variable, and second, they have many visual features in common with similar objects of quite different significance. The young chicken who approaches the wrong hen will find neither safety nor food (Ramsay, 1951); the female swallow who accepts courtship from a male must behave very differently according to whether he is, or is not, her mate (Møller, 1985).

None of this is to say that the discrimination of elementary stimuli, as both physiological and behavioral psychologists tend to study it in the laboratory, is biologically irrelevant. On the contrary, the discrimination of spots, lines, and even gratings is no doubt what makes the discrimination of objects possible. Object discrimination is what such simpler discrimination is for. However, the problems of object discrimination are not solved when we have established what simple discriminations a particular species can achieve. This is true for two basic reasons. The first is that the aggressive robin with its distinctively colored breast is the exception rather than the rule; most visible objects cannot be recognized by any single necessary or sufficient feature, so we have the problem of how several kinds of information can be integrated to allow recognition. The second is that the feature content of objects is not just complex but variable. The same individual conspecific does not present the same visual features when seen from in front or behind; a cache site seen in winter may look very different from the same site seen when food was stored there in autumn.

Object perception, then, is a problem with three facets. First there is the problem of identifying the simpler discriminations that make it possible. Second, we have to understand how those cues or features are integrated. Finally, we have to ask how variable cue combinations can be correctly categorized. Object perception has more to do with the discrimination of categories of stimuli than of individual, elementary stimuli.

When we consider human vision, object, or pattern perception is normally regarded as part of cognitive rather than perceptual psychology, though the boundary between the two is fuzzy and not very important. But it should be no surprise that studies of object perception in birds locate themselves within the rapidly developing field of "animal cognition." Characteristically, this approach involves taking ideas and methods that have been developed for the study of human and machine cognition, and applying them to other animal species. It assumes that it is appropriate to treat animals as having cognitive processes, and proceeds to investigate what those are. This is in contrast to the "bottom-up" program of the behaviorists, in which the existence of cognitive process was to be proved, if ever, after the analysis of behavior into ever more elementary units and a remorseless application to it of Lloyd Morgan's canon. Over the past 15 years, the study of animal cognition has begun to yield a detailed understanding of a variety of cognitive processes in many species, including bird species. For practical reasons many of the results have been obtained with pigeons. So, in this chapter we shall take it for granted that pigeons can discriminate objects, and ask what cognitive and perceptual mechanisms make it possible.

Taking the cognitive perspective makes apparent one surprising conclusion. What we regard as a simple discrimination may not trigger a simple discrimination process in a bird. If birds naturally discriminate objects, when we present them with simple lines or patches of color, they may initially treat them as complex objects and have to learn about their simplicity. It may even be very difficult for them to abstract a simple line or spot from the object on which it is placed, which in the experimenter's eye is mere background. To the experimenter, perhaps, it is obvious that a pigeon's pecking key is the background to the stimulus projected onto it; but to the pigeon, the key might be foreground and the rest of the experimental chamber the background. Thus discriminations we regard as complex may be learned faster than apparently simpler ones—and, certainly, some discriminations of quite complex natural objects are learned very fast indeed (Vaughan and Greene, 1984). Nor is such a result incompatible with the theory that recognition of complex objects involves, initially, response to simple features. It may not be possible for a bird to bypass, as it were, the cognitive stage in which features are synthesized into objects. So investigating the mechanisms by which birds discriminate complex objects may be the best way to discover how they make much simpler discriminations.

EVIDENCE FOR CATEGORY DISCRIMINATION IN BIRDS

The majority of studies of animal discrimination learning have looked at elementary stimuli, and thus tell us only about one small part of object perception. There is, however, a lively area of research into more complex discriminations, and most of it has used birds as subjects. The tasks investigated can either be called *category discriminations*, emphasizing the fact that many different stimuli are used and the subjects bird's task is to categorize them (normally into positive and negative categories), or *concept discriminations* (Lea, 1984), emphasizing the fact that the categories are usually defined in terms of a human language concept.

The first experiments about category discrimination in birds showed not only that it was possible, but, more surprisingly, that it could be demonstrated with severely impoverished stimuli, that it was learned easily, and that it generalized widely. The core results are long established and well known and we do not need to do much more than list them here. Herrnstein and Loveland (1964) demonstrated that pigeons could learn to peck a key in the presence of color slides that contained pictures of people, and to withhold pecks in the presence of slides that did not contain people. This first experiment on category discrimination remains typical in several ways as regards its procedure:

1. The stimulus sets were defined in terms of natural language concepts held by the experimenter.

2. Many different instances of the positive and negative concepts were used, and there were great differences within the positive and negative sets as well as similarities between them.

3. The instances used were not collected according to any very exact criteria.

4. The stimuli were color photographs of natural scenes, back-projected onto a screen on the wall of an operant test chamber.

5. The subjects were laboratory pigeons.

6. The discrimination task was implemented using a single-key multiple schedule of reinforcement, i.e., at different times different stimuli were presented, and food reward was available for pecking in the presence of some stimuli but not others (cf. Ferster and Skinner, 1957, chapter 10).

Herrnstein and Loveland's major results have also been found to be typical:

1. The birds learned the discrimination quite quickly (in about 10 sessions).

2. After acquisition, the birds showed immediate transfer to new exemplars of the concepts.

Many subsequent experiments, using a great variety of categories, have demonstrated that Herrnstein and Loveland's results were quite general. Features (1) to (6) above have been varied in many ways, but the results (1) and (2) have been replicated in almost every experiment that retains reasonable similarity to the original. This literature has been reviewed several times (e.g., Herrnstein, 1985; Lea, 1984) and there is no need to survey it here. However, it is worth listing briefly some of the categories that have been learned and mentioning some of the exceptions to the typical features listed above. The lists given here do not attempt to be exhaustive in any category.

Among the categories that have been learned are human artifacts vs. natural objects (Lubow, 1974), trees and bodies of water (Herrnstein et al., 1976), pigeons (Poole and Lander, 1971; Watanabe, 1992), cats, flowers, cars, and chairs (Bhatt et al., 1988), kingfishers (vs. other birds) and animals vs. nonanimals (Roberts and Mazmanian, 1988), fish (Herrnstein and de Villiers, 1980), species of moths (Pietrewicz and Kamil, 1977), oak leaves as against other leaves (Cerella, 1979), the patterns of leaf damage due to different species of caterpillars (Real et al., 1984), individual conspecifics (Ryan, 1982a; Watanabe and Ito,

1991), cartoon characters (Cerella, 1980), auditory rhythms (Hulse, et al., 1984), letters of the alphabet (Morgan et al., 1976; Lea and Ryan, 1983,1990), triangles generated by computer graphics (Watanabe, 1991), aerial photographs of different locales (unpublished data of E. M. Gray reported by Herrnstein, 1990), and scenes taken from one camera position rather than another (Honig and Stewart, 1988).

Among the exceptions to the general rules outlined above are the following:

1. Artificially constructed categories have been used, usually to control feature content (Lea and Harrison, 1978; Cerella, 1982; Lea and Ryan, 1990; Lea et al., 1993; Huber and Lenz, 1993; von Fersen and Lea, 1990; Pearce, 1989).

2. Training has been given on a small number of instances of the concept (Cerella, 1979; Huber and Lenz, 1993, Experiment 3; Bhatt et al., 1988; Real et al., 1984).

3. In the case of artificial stimulus sets, exactly controlled feature content was used in most of the cases cited above.

4. Line drawings have been used (e.g., of cartoon characters, Cerella, 1980; of squiggles, Vaughan and Greene, 1984; of letters, Morgan et al., 1976; Lea and Ryan, 1983, 1990; of schematic faces, Huber and Lenz, 1993). Most experiments have projected images onto the pigeon's pecking key itself, instead of the separate screen used by Herrnstein and Loveland. But a few have used larger images, viewed through a transparent pecking key (Ryan 1982b; Ryan and Lea, 1990; von Fersen and Lea, 1990). Video images have also been used, both still (e.g., Pearce, 1989; Watanabe and Tailin, 1993; Wright et al., 1988) and moving (Dittrich and Lea, 1993; Watanabe et al., 1993). There have been several experiments using three-dimensional objects (e.g., Delius, 1992; Watanabe, 1991). Hulse et al. (1984) used auditory rather than visual stimuli in an experiment that otherwise was a fairly typical category discrimination task.

5. Species other than pigeons have been used as subjects, including chickens (Ryan, 1982a,b; Ryan and Lea, 1990), Bengalese finches (Watanabe, et al., 1993), and blue jays (Pietrewicz and Kamil, 1977; Real et al., 1984). There have also been experiments with mammals, mostly primates (e.g., D'Amato and Van Sant, 1988; Dittrich, 1988; Schrier et al., 1984; Yoshikubo, 1985) but these are outside the scope of this chapter.

6. A variety of alternative discrimination situations have been used, including simultaneous discrimination (in which birds have to choose between positive and negative stimuli presented simultaneously, e.g., Lea and Harrison, Experiment 2), conditional discrimination (in which birds have to make one of two responses depending on whether a positive or negative stimulus is currently displayed, e.g., Bhatt et al.,

1988), and discriminative autoshaping (in which food arrives independent of the bird's behavior, but only following positive stimuli, e.g., Pearce, 1989; Dittrich and Lea, 1993).

There have, of course, also been exceptions to the general rule that category discrimination tasks are easy for birds to learn and lead to spontaneous generalization across to new instances of categories. Some of these are discussed in the rest of this chapter, since they are critical for the theoretical questions we raise. But in summarizing this section, we can conclude that the evidence is very strong that birds readily learn to discriminate between pictures of categories of objects defined by natural language concepts, and that this reflects a robust perceptual/cognitive ability.

WHAT DOES CATEGORY DISCRIMINATION IMPLY?

It is also important to realize that there are several things that the body of experimental results so far discussed do not imply. Some of them were considered by Herrnstein (1985, 1990) and Lea (1984):

1. As the experiments have frequently been careful to note, there is no implication that their subjects in any sense recognize the pictures as representations of objects. One or two experiments have tested for transfer from pictures to real objects (Cabe, 1976; Trillmich, 1976), but the evidence about when if ever this occurs is not yet strong enough for us to say whether it is likely to occur in a typical concept discrimination task (see Watanabe, 1993).

2. Herrnstein and Loveland's original paper was entitled, "Higher Order Concept Formation in the Pigeon," and several other early papers have similar titles (e.g., Lubow, 1974; Poole and Lander, 1971). However, this title contains two implications which have since been seen to be premature. First, we do not know whether pigeons have concepts and use them to solve category discriminations. Except for some extreme behaviorist philosophers (e.g., Stemmer, 1980), few would deny that it is useful to talk about a concept "person"; but all we know about it is that it exists in the mind of the experimenter, who uses it to select the members of the stimulus sets.

3. Even if pigeons do have a concept of "person" or "pigeon," we do not know that it is formed in the experiment: it could be innate or exist as a result of preexperimental experience. From the mere fact of concept discrimination, we do not know whether discrimination experiments can establish new concepts. Some of the concepts that have been used make it improbable: Herrnstein and de Villiers (1980) argue that it is unlikely that pigeons would have a preexperimental concept of a fish, for example. But even in this case a preexisting concept could be involved. We cannot prove that the pigeon does not solve the fish concept discrimination by identifying what we see as pictures of fish as instances

of some quite different preexisting concept, to do, say, with the classification of plant parts. If this seems strange, reflect how humans classify unfamiliar classes of objects by reference to more familiar ones—consider, for example, the description of the two stereoisomers of cyclohexane as "chair" and "boat" forms. A pigeon might, similarly, see slides of fish as "seed-like" and slides of nonfish as "leaf-like."

4. The same example demonstrates a further problem. Even if pigeons do recognize colored slides as pictures of objects, and do use concepts to make category discriminations between them, we do not know that their concepts are identical to those of the experimenter (Chater and Heyes, in preparation), and sometimes there is evidence that they are not (Herrnstein et al., 1976; Roberts and Mazmanian, 1988). Postacquisition transfer tests are designed to examine the content of the bird's concept, if it has one; but since they are inevitably limited in scope, our knowledge is correspondingly limited.

5. Finally, the mere fact of concept discrimination tells us little or nothing about the perceptual and cognitive mechanisms underlying it. And, as we explained at the beginning of this chapter, the nature of natural language concepts means that those mechanisms must often be quite complex.

Although none of the above questions are answered just by showing that pigeons can discriminate categories based on natural concepts, this does not mean that they are unanswerable in principle. Most recent work on concept discrimination has been directed at answering the more tractable among them. The three that have been most investigated have been the issue of the role of feature analysis relative to memory for individual instances of the concept, the question of whether birds can be said to possess concepts, and the relation between discrimination of pictures and recognition of the objects they represent. The remainder of this chapter treats these three questions in turn, though of course they overlap substantially and our discussion reflects this.

FEATURE ANALYSIS VS. ABSOLUTE DISCRIMINATION

From the beginning of research on concept discrimination in nonhumans, attempts have been made to discover constant features that might underlie the discrimination of the inherently variable stimulus materials. Lubow's (1974) report on discrimination of artefacts in aerial photographs is typical: he investigated which exemplars were well or poorly discriminated, and deduced that overall luminous flux, straight lines, and angles of approximately 90° must be important cues (though neither necessary nor sufficient) for the pigeon to respond to a photograph as containing an artefact. Cerella (1980, 1982) argued that concepts are represented as large unstructured sets of features, with each exemplar being characterized by a subset of features.

However, feature analysis is not necessarily a part of concept discrimination. The alternative possibility is that the correct response to each individual exemplar is learned; within pattern recognition theory, this corresponds to the template matching theory, and within traditional animal discrimination learning theory, to the continuity theories of Hull as formalized by Spence (1936). Its chief proponents within the field of concept discrimination have been Vaughan and Greene (1983, 1984) who have dubbed it "absolute discrimination"; Herrnstein (1990) calls it "categorization by rote."

At first sight, absolute discrimination seems an impossible mechanism for concept discrimination. Experiments sometimes use hundreds of different stimuli during training (Herrnstein and Loveland's original experiments used over 1200), and in one or two cases have never used any stimulus more than once (e.g., Bhatt et al., 1988). Admittedly, typical experiments use far fewer stimuli (often 40 positive and 40 negative, reflecting the capacity of the slide projectors most commonly used). But as we have already noted, it is routinely observed that after concept discrimination training subjects generalize correctly to new instances of the concepts. Although generalization is better following training with many instances (Bhatt et al., 1988), it still occurs even with very few exemplars used in training, at the limit, only one (Cerella, 1979; Real et al., 1984). This seems inexplicable on the basis of absolute discrimination. Herrnstein (1990) argues that categorization by rote can be extended to deal with open-ended categories through the perceptual similarity between known and novel exemplars; but then one is bound to ask, how is similarity to be measured? Must it not depend on common features? Must not stimulus generalization be along some stimulus dimensions, which are themselves just another name for features?

Despite this logical difficulty with the absolute discrimination hypotheses, Vaughan and Greene (1984, Experiment 4) produced some powerful evidence in its favor. They trained two groups of pigeons in category discriminations. For one group, the positive stimulus set consisted of 40 pictures of trees, and the negative category of 40 pictures not containing trees. These sets can obviously be discriminated by using the concept of a tree, or features common to trees. For the other group, the two stimulus sets each contained 20 pictures of trees and 20 of nontrees. This is what Lea and Ryan (1990) call a "pseudoconcept" discrimination, and the intention is that there should be no underlying concept or common features to facilitate discrimination: the birds have no alternative but to learn the reinforcement contingency associated with each individual stimulus. The surprising result was that the two groups both acquired the discrimination equally fast. The implication is that whatever pictures of trees may have in common, the pigeons in the real concept group made no use of it, and those in the pseudoconcept group were not distracted by it. Feature analysis seems to have played no part in their learning at all. That does not, of course, prove that feature analysis is never important: indeed, in subsequent experiments, pseudoconcept groups have been shown to learn more slowly than real concept groups (e.g., Wasserman et al., 1988; Dittrich and Lea, 1993; Watanabe, 1993). But absolute discrimination is presumably always important when pseudoconcepts are successfully discriminated. The very impressive experiments on long-term memory of Vaughan and Greene (1984), in which pigeons discriminated up to 320 distinct slides and retained the discrimination for up to 2 years, were of this type.

Moreover, other experiments have suggested that absolute discrimination plays at least some part in the discrimination of concepts even where feature analysis would solve the problem very easily. For example, the experiments by Lea and Harrison (1978) and Pearce (1989) used artificial concepts whose feature content was known exactly. No single feature was either necessary or sufficient for discrimination, but a simple linear rule for feature combination would have made perfect discrimination possible. In both cases, the "perfect" exemplars of the concepts, in which all features took their positive values, were withheld during training, and used later in transfer tests. In Lea and Harrison's experiment, the pigeons responded correctly to these perfect exemplars, but with long latencies that implied they recognized them as abnormal; in Pearce's experiment, they did not even respond correctly to them. Similarly, Watanabe (1988) found that pigeons could not abstract a "prototype" from its distorted exemplars, whereas humans easily can. Like the equivalence of pseudo and real concept training, this result is not always obtained: Mackintosh (1991) did obtain what a feature model predicts, namely more accurate responding to the "supernormal" transfer stimuli, probably because they used more different stimuli during training than either Lea and Harrison or Pearce. But there is no doubt that absolute discrimination is sometimes used when feature analysis, apparently the simpler process, would be perfectly sufficient.

Further evidence for this position comes from experiments using another kind of artificial concept, groups of letters (Lea and Ryan, 1983, 1990). Here the feature structure of the stimuli was not prescribed in advance, but Lea and Ryan attempted to deduce it by using multiple regression analysis to predict the response rates to individual letters from the features they contained. This is a more formal version of the approach taken by Lubow (1974), discussed above. Consistent results were obtained across birds (reflecting consistent differences in response rates within the positive and negative stimulus sets as well as between them), and regression models accounted for a high proportion of the variance in the response rates. But even after fitting the best regression models, additional variance could be accounted for by taking into account the group (positive or negative) to which each letter belonged. The feature analysis, in other words, did not fully account for the birds' discriminative performance, and presumably the residual discrimination was due to absolute recognition of the letters. That conclusion was supported in another experiment, when an attempt was made to construct "superletters" based on the features of positive stimuli; as in the experiment of Pearce (1989), such stimuli were rejected by the birds (R. A. Joss, unpublished data). Furthermore, when natural stimuli are used, the features correlated with response rate have often proved impossible to identify. In some cases they must be different from those used by humans, because high response rates or accurate discrimination are recorded to what, to the human observer, are atypical instances (Herrnstein et al., 1976; Roberts and Mazmanian, 1988).

There are further difficulties for the feature analysis account. A number of experiments have used artificial stimuli constructed according to well-specified feature content. The studies of Lea and Harrison (1978) and Pearce (1989), already mentioned, used three two-valued features; Lea and Ryan (1990) briefly describe an experiment using stylized drawings of pigeons that were composed using five two-valued features; Lea et al. (1993) used a similar set of stylized drawings of seeds, illustrated in figure 20.1; and Huber and Lenz (1993) used the Brunswik faces, which involved four three-valued features. Von Fersen and Lea (1990) used a similar design, with five two-valued features, but though their

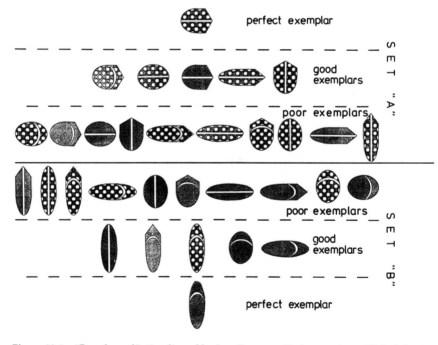

Figure 20.1 "Pseudoseed" stimuli used by Lea, Ryan, and Lohmann (unpublished data). Membership of set A rather than set B depends on possession of three of the following five features: horizontal orientation, low eccentricity, dotted texture, pointed end, and longitudinal split. The perfect exemplars of the two sets have all five relevant features, the good exemplars four of them, and the poor exemplars three.

concepts were artificial their stimuli were not, since they consisted of photographs of natural scenes. Several of these experiments have found difficulty in getting pigeons' keypecking to come under the control of all the available features. One bird in Lea and Harrison's Experiment 2 was much slower to learn one feature than the other two; Lea and Ryan report that all four of their birds learned about only one of the five features in their stylized pigeons, while Lea et al. (1993) found that their pigeons came under control of only two to four of the features of their pseudoseeds. Von Fersen and Lea did get seven out of eight birds under the control of all five features, but only after giving special training to several of them.

Of course it is easy to argue that the problems in these experiments lie with the experimenters' choice of stimuli, differences in salience of the features, and so forth. But this argument misses the point, which is that the artificial concepts with their carefully balanced feature content are meant to be a simplified and idealized model of real, natural concepts (which pigeons discriminate easily). If pigeons cannot get hold of all the features needed to make a good discrimination in these artificial concepts, either we have misunderstood the structure of natural concepts, or feature analysis has no chance of working efficiently under natural conditions, where features are very unlikely to occur in carefully balanced combinations.

It is indeed possible that the experiments of Lea and Harrison (1978), Lea et al. (1993), and von Fersen and Lea (1990) do misrepresent the structure of natural concepts in one important respect. As von Fersen and Lea comment, the similarity space in these experiments is perfectly flat: all feature combinations occur equally often. It is rather likely that natural concepts are not like that; that we have concepts precisely because they identify "lumps" in the similarity space, combinations of features that are particularly likely to occur together (Wasserman et al., 1988). It is significant that Huber and Lenz (1993), using three-valued features, were able to omit a group of intermediate, highly ambiguous stimuli, that had as many positive as negative features, and in consequence the features in their experiment did show some correlation. Unlike all other experiments using artificial stimuli, they were able to show equal use of all the features in their stimuli, even though (as they showed in a control experiment) the features were of quite unequal salience.

There is one other pervading difficulty with the feature analysis theory. What, precisely, should be allowed to constitute a "feature"? We still know too little about early visual processing in birds to insist that features must be properties coded at a particular anatomical or physiological stage. The experiments discussed above have used a great variety of features. Some of them, such as total luminous flux, can plausibly be supposed to be extracted early in visual processing. Others are more complex properties of patterns, such as the length of curved line or the extent of closed space (Lea and Ryan, 1983, 1990). Still others involve some interaction between two or more "primitive" features: the "brow height" feature in the Brunswik faces used by Huber and Lenz (1993) has to be computed from the relative positions of the two eyes and the face outline. Von Fersen and Lea (1990) took this to the extreme, and deliberately used features that they expected to be themselves polymorphous, such as the weather (sunny or cloudy) under which a photograph was taken. Dittrich and Lea (1993), rather similarly, used movement as a feature, and argued that it is itself a complex concept that has to be abstracted from the features of many different kinds of movement.

The peculiar result is that it does not make any obvious difference to the difficulty of the discrimination what kind of feature is used. In the present state of our knowledge, it seems that feature analysis theory is seriously underspecified at the perceptual level, and that feature integration is primarily a cognitive process that is relatively independent of the visual system as such. One of the problems with absolute discrimination as a mechanism for concept discrimination is that it simply pushes the problem back—how do pigeons make absolute discriminations? It hardly seems that feature analysis is in any better case. Both feature analysis and absolute discrimination seem more like aspects of object recognition than theories of its mechanism.

EVIDENCE THAT PIGEONS POSSESS CONCEPTS

As theories of concept discrimination, absolute discrimination, and feature analysis have one thing in common. They offer no place for the possession or formation of concepts. If either of them works completely, they give a complete account of concept discrimination and (subject to the doubts expressed above about absolute discrimination theory) generalization to new exemplars after training.

What, in any case, would it mean for a pigeon to possess a concept? The word has too long a history in the philosophical and psychological study of cognition for any answer to command unanimous assent. Lea (1984) reviewed the possibilities and suggested a definition. He argued that we can say that an animal has a concept if there is some structure in its brain or mind that is active when, and only when, an instance of that concept is present in the external, physical environment. What behavioral criteria would enable us to recognize concept formation in this sense? At least two are possible. The first criterion can be called the "clumping" test. It was used in experiments on imprinting to multiple stimuli by Bateson and Chantrey (1972); Bhatt and Wasserman (1989) point out that it is equivalent to the "secondary generalization" of Hull (1943). It states that once a concept has been formed, it should be more difficult to learn a new task in which different responses are required to different instances of the concept (and the same response to instances of different concepts), than one in which the same response is required to all instances of one concept, and different responses to instances of different concepts. The second criterion was introduced by Lea (1984). It states that if something is learned about one instance of a concept, it should transfer without further training to other instances, and this is usually called "instance to category generalization," to distinguish it from the category to instance generalization that is shown in the usual posttraining transfer tests following concept discrimination. Both criteria follow from the argument that if cognitive processing is occurring at the conceptual level, new learning will be about concepts and not about individual instances. They relate closely to ideas about equivalence classes that have been explored in detail in human operant psychology in recent years (e.g., Fields et al., 1991).

As Herrnstein (1990) points out, the "structure" need not be a single neural entity; concepts are behaviorally defined, not neurophysiologically. Furthermore, in some ways Lea's definition is too restrictive. It does not allow for inaccurate perception or categorization, and it does not allow for a representation of the concept to be excited in the bird's brain or mind by a process of association (Chater and Heyes, in preparation). The first of these processes seems certain to occur, and the second can be demonstrated (Holland and Straub, 1979; Holland and Ross, 1981). However, there does not seem to be any logical difficulty in extending the definition to allow for both possibilities, and this would not undermine the criterion Lea proposed for recognizing when a pigeon has a concept in this sense.

Several experiments have tried to use the criteria proposed above. Bhatt and Wasserman (1989, Experiment 1) tested the clumping criterion in an experiment in which pigeons had to make a four-way conditional discrimination, either between natural concepts or between pseudo-concepts, and then subsequently learned a four-way discrimination between different ratio schedules of reinforcement. All pigeons discriminated between natural concepts at the second stage, but their previous experience made no difference to their speed of learning; thus no evidence of clumping was found.

The instance to category generalization criterion, as Lea (1984) explains, can be used at two levels. The most direct cases of instance to category discrimination involve, literally, individual exemplars that have been used in training. There might, for example, be reversal training to a subset of these stimuli, followed by a test for spontaneous reversal to the remaining members of the category. However, with real concept discriminations, simple feature analysis can explain this case; if birds have learned to respond to all green objects and reject all red ones, then we would not be surprised, or impressed, if reversing them on some green and red objects leads to transfer to the remainder. Lea (1984) suggested that a more acute test would involve deliberately reversing on individual features instead of individual exemplars, and then looking for generalization to other features. Alternatively, it is possible to use reversal on a subset of instances after pseudoconcept training, since in such training there are by assumption no common features that could support transfer.

Bhatt and Wasserman (1989, Experiment 2) tested for instance to category generalization following the four-way categorization procedure just described. They found no evidence for generalization. However, in an unpublished study, Lea, Ryan, and Kirby have found a different result when testing for instance to category generalization following the letter-group discriminations described by Lea and Ryan (1983, 1990). Reversal training was given on a subset of letters (one or two of each of the positive and negative sets), followed by testing on the unreversed letters. Response rates to the unreversed letters were negatively correlated with their prereversal values (figure 20.2). Von Fersen and Lea (1990) also gave reversal training on a subset of stimuli following training on concept discrimination, and clear evidence of generalization of reversal to nonreversed instances was found.

But can such generalization, when it occurs (and Bhatt and Wasserman's evidence shows that it cannot be relied on), be explained by reversal of learning to features? Lea, Ryan, and Kirby tried to show that the instance to category generalization shown in figure 20.2 could not be explained by reversal on individual features, but their evidence

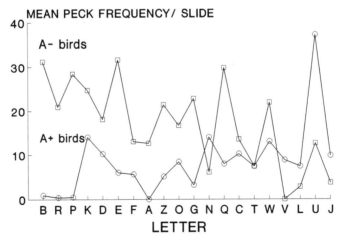

Figure 20.2 Evidence for instance to category generalization following letter-group discrimination (Lea, Ryan, and Kirby, unpublished data). Pigeons were trained to discriminate the two groups of 10 letters shown on the x-axis, and then given reversal training on two from each category. The letters are arranged on the x-axis in the order of their prereversal response rates; the data show immediate postreversal rates for nonreversed letters, which were negatively correlated with prereversal rates. Data are shown separately for two groups, each made up of six birds; in group A+, the originally positive letters were ABDFKNOPR and Z and the originally negative letters were CEGJLQTUV and W; for group A− these contingencies were reversed. The letters chosen for reversal were different for each bird.

was not fully convincing either way because the features in use had to be inferred from a regression analysis of response rates. By using artificial concepts with controlled feature content, von Fersen and Lea (1990) were able to carry out a clearer test. They used for reversal a subset of stimuli that gave information about only a single feature. Reversal generalized only to those other instances in which this feature was relevant. However, an experiment of Vaughan (1988) suggests that instance to category generalization that does not depend on features may be possible. He gave pigeons repeated reversals on a pseudoconcept discrimination, in which all the stimuli were slides of trees. After many reversals, experience of the first few slides was sufficient to produce reversal to all. Unpublished computer simulations by Rick Thompson and Noel Sharkey also suggest that von Fersen and Lea's data may not be conclusive evidence against conceptualization. Thompson and Sharkey attempted to simulate von Fersen and Lea's data using several kinds of learning network. A simple linear model would plainly be sufficient to simulate purely feature-based learning. However, backward propagation networks with a layer of "hidden elements" produced output that was much more similar to von Fersen and Lea's data. While a network model does not have any nodes that quite correspond to a concept as Lea (1984) described it, hidden elements are a distributed version of them: they are elements between the stimulus and the response level that are called into being or into use by the concept discrimination training.

Do pigeons, then, possess or form concepts in the sense described by Lea (1984)? The evidence is not conclusive. Clearly they can manage very impressive discriminations without using concepts to any extent that we can detect (as in the absolute discrimination studies, and perhaps also in the experiments of von Fersen and Lea, 1990). Furthermore, in situations where humans would surely use concepts spontaneously, pigeons do not (e.g., Wasserman et al., 1988). On the other hand, Vaughan's (1988) result seems to establish that concepts can be formed. Vaughan's experiment also suggests that concept formation is slow, almost a cognitive last resort, but it must be recognized that his experiment used pseudoconcept discrimination, about the least favorable condition for concept use. Thompson and Sharkey's simulation results suggest that with subtler analytic techniques we might be able to detect concept formation in simpler situations. The criteria suggested by Lea (1984) were somewhat conservative; both involved putting concepts into situations where they would be expected to be broken down. Perhaps the likeliest conclusion at present is that pigeons can form concepts, but they do not rely on them as much as humans, and their concepts are not as stable as ours. But that conclusion might well change if we can find stimuli of higher ecological relevance to pigeons. Many of the stimuli that have been used have been intended to have such relevance, at least vaguely; but almost all have consisted of photographs. Relevance therefore depends on the pigeons recognizing these representations of the real objects, and we cannot assume that they do so. To this question we now turn.

DO PIGEONS PERCEIVE PICTURES AS REPRESENTATIONS OF OBJECTS?

What Pictures Represent

Cerella (1980) successfully trained pigeons to discriminate figures of Charlie Brown. The birds responded to pictures that were only partial presentations of him after the discriminative training. But they emitted many responses to random mixtures of parts of his body also. These results suggest that what the birds learned was a set of features, associated with reinforcement, of a stimulus that was meaningless to them, rather than an integrated figure of a boy named Charlie Brown. Although we know Charlie Brown is a cartoon figure, we interpret this figure as a representation of a boy. The many possible figures of Charlie Brown constitute a meaningful set for us. But for pigeons the "meaning" of the figures is just that they are stimuli associated with food. In other words Charlie Brown does not differ from any other geometric pattern that is displayed on the birds' pecking key.

When pigeons were trained to discriminate stimuli such as figures of a conspecific that might have more meaning for them, they showed quite different discriminative behavior. Figure 20.3 presents the results of a test comparable to that with a scrambled Charlie Brown, described above. Pigeons were tested with scrambled parts of a pigeon's head after they had received discrimination training between heads of two different individual pigeons (Watanabe and Ito, 1991). The subjects were trained with many colored slides of two real birds displayed on a screen attached to the operant chamber. After training, three types of stimulus, namely, new slides of the S+ head, scrambled parts of the S+ head, and randomly connected parts of the S+ head, appeared in the test. Clearly, the birds did not respond to the scrambled parts of the head, either when the component parts were close to each other or separated. These figures differed from the intact head for the pigeons. What is the essential difference between Charlie Brown and a pigeon's head? Previous experiments have found that pigeons show poor transfer between real objects and line drawings (Cabe, 1976), when the objects are just geometric forms. But the functional meaning of a conspecific is different from that of a cartoon character or a geometric object. Pigeons need to identify another pigeon's head as part of their social activity; they do not need to identify Charlie Brown. In other words, a picture of a pigeon represents a real pigeon for these birds, whereas that of Charlie Brown does not represent a live boy to them. Wittgenstein (1953) described a concept as a tool for communication among members of a

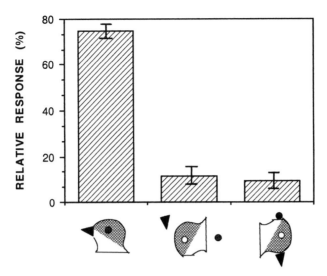

Figure 20.3 Response to colored photographic slides of scrambled parts of a pigeon's head. Six birds were trained to discriminate color slides of two different conspecific individuals, then tested with the full face (left), separated parts (middle), and randomly connected parts (right) of the S+ bird. The stimuli shown in the figure indicate the type rather than the actual stimuli that were used. The birds emitted few responses to abnormal, scrambled figures. Bars indicate standard deviations (Watanabe and Ito, 1991).

society. Without language, it is not obvious how pigeons can use their concepts for communication, but it still seems likely that the concept of a conspecific would have a distinct functional value.

Interaction between the Discrimination of Real Objects and That of Their Pictures

Researchers studying the ability of birds to form natural concepts have typically used photographic slides as stimuli. As we have seen, we cannot assume that birds really see these photographic pictures as representations of real objects. How can we find out? One method is to analyze the interaction between stimulus control by real objects and that by the pictures. The following experiment examines an interaction between the discrimination of photographs and the experience of consummatory behavior.

Experimentally naive pigeons were trained to discriminate colored slides of corn grains and those of nonedible junk objects (stone, paper clip, nut, dice, and maple leaf). The slides were projected on a screen attached to the front panel of an operant chamber. Pecking responses to a transparent rectangular key in front of the screen were reinforced on VI 30 sec when corn appeared but not when nonedible objects appeared. One training session consisted of 30 slides of corn and 30 slides of nonedible objects randomly selected from a stimulus pool of 150 different slides.

After the subjects acquired the discrimination (to a criterion of two successive sessions of more than 90% correct responses) they were tested with slides of artificially colored corn. Natural corn, corn strained red and green with food dye, and corn painted silver appeared on the screen during the test. This test was administered three times. The first test followed the discriminative training directly, the second after 5 days of eating red corn, and the last after 5 days of experience of red corn that had been given a bitter taste by treating it with methylanthranilate. For the birds to eat the stained corn, these grains were placed on the floor of the living cage, and the birds were allowed to eat them for 30 min. When the red corn had a bitter taste the pigeons quickly learned to avoid it in the first 1 or 2 days.

Figure 20.4 presents results of the three tests. There were few responses to the green or silver corn in any test. Relatively higher responding to the red corn may have resulted from color generalization from the natural corn. The principal result is that responding to the red corn changes following feeding experience. The subjects increased their responding to the red corn after they had eaten red corn (test 2), and reduced responding after the aversive experience of eating bitter-tasting red corn (test 3). Thus a bird is more likely to treat a picture of "red corn" as belonging to the "edible corn group" after having had the experience of eating real red corn. On the other hand, red corn is less likely to be responded to as members of the "edible corn group" after a bird has had aversive experience of eating colored corn. In other words, this membership is not simply "perceptual" but also "functional" in the sense proposed by Lea (1984). These interactions between operant discrimination and consummatory behavior suggest that the pigeon perceived the pictures as representations of the real objects.

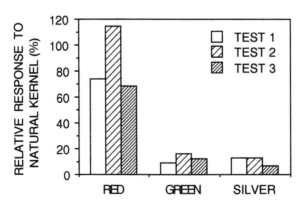

Figure 20.4 Effect of consummatory experience on discriminative behavior in the operant chamber. Responses to the colored corn were expressed relative to those made to the natural corn. Each bar indicates the mean of four subjects. Eating experience with red corn increased responding to slides of red corn (test 2) and aversive experience decreased responding (test 3). Color slides of four kinds of corn (natural, red, green, and silver) were presented in the tests. (Watanabe, unpublished data).

Vision and Cognition

Transfer between Discrimination of Real Objects and That of Their Pictures

The interaction study described above suggests a common cognitive process for perception of both real objects and their pictures. Picture-object relationships can be examined more directly, however, in a transfer experiment. Apes demonstrated successful picture-to-object transfer in a cross-modality matching paradigm (Davenport and Rogers, 1971). Cabe (1976) and Lumsden (1977), who used simple stimuli, reported object-to-photo transfer in pigeons, too. On the other hand, Gray (1974, reported by Herrnstein, 1990) found no evidence of transfer from homing experience to discrimination of photographs of the locales to which pigeons had homed.

In the following experiment, pigeons were trained with many real objects then tested with their photographs or vice versa (Watanabe, 1993). If they show transfer of discrimination, we can conclude that the pictures represent the real objects for the birds at some level, at least. In an object-to-photograph transfer experiment eight pigeons were trained to discriminate four kinds of grains (corn, pea, wheat, and buckwheat) and four kinds of junk objects (stone, twig, nut, and paper clip). These items were placed in 40 small boxes on a conveyor belt fixed in front of an operant chamber. The subjects could see the items through a transparent key on the front panel of the chamber (Watanabe, 1991). There were three tasks. The first task (food concept task) was to discriminate between food items (S+) and nonfood items (S−), the second task (nonfood concept task) was the same as the first task except that the S+ was nonfood items, and the third task (pseudoconcept task) was to make an arbitrary classification of the eight items. Thus in this third task two kinds of food and two kinds of nonfood constituted an S+ group and the S− group consisted of the other four items. After they had learned the discrimination, color-printed photographs were placed in the boxes instead of the objects. The size of the items in the photographs was identical to that of the real objects. No reinforcement was given in this transfer test. All birds that learned the two concept tasks showed good transfer (figure 20.5). The results suggest that the birds saw the pictures as representations of the real objects. On the other hand the birds that learned the pseudoconcept discrimination showed quite poor transfer. For these birds the real objects were treated differently from their pictures.

When birds were trained with the color prints then tested with the real objects, they also showed a similar tendency to transfer their discrimination (figure 20.5). The conveyor belt apparatus described above was used but the color prints of food and nonfood were presented during the training and the real objects replaced the prints in the test. The birds showed photo-to-real object transfer of the concept tasks but they did not show transfer of the pseudoconcept task.

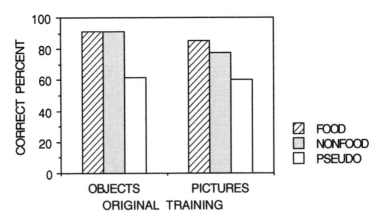

Figure 20.5 Results of transfer tests. Pigeons showed real-to-picture (left) and picture-to-real (right) transfer of a food concept and a nonfood concept discrimination but no transfer of a pseudoconcept discrimination. Correct responses were calculated by dividing the total responses to the four S+ items by the total responses to all eight items. Each bar indicates the mean of four subjects.

A two-way ANOVA indicated no significant effect of the direction of transfer (object-to-photo vs. photo-to-real), but a significant effect of type of task (food vs. nonfood vs. pseudo, $F = 19.1$, $p < 0.01$). There was a significant difference between food and pseudoconcept tasks and nonfood and pseudoconcept tasks ($t = 3.23$ and 1.96, $p < 0.01$, respectively).

These results suggest bidirectional transfer between the real objects and the photographs when the discrimination was conceptual but no transfer when the discrimination was based on an arbitrary classification. Why did the birds not show transfer when the task involved an arbitrary classification? The type of classification must be the factor that caused the difference, because the stimuli presented to the subjects were exactly the same for both concept and pseudoconcept tasks.

Some Differences between Real Object Discrimination and Picture Discrimination

Although pigeons seem to see pictures as representations of real objects in concept discrimination, there are some differences in discriminative behavior between training with real objects and with pictures. Figure 20.6 presents a comparison of generalizations after training with real objects and after that with pictures. When birds were trained to discriminate corn from stone with real objects, they showed generalization to other kinds of grains. That is, they learned a "food" concept through one pair of exemplars. However, when birds were trained on the same task with photographic slides, they did not show generalization to other grains. That is, what they learned was not a concept of "food" but a more specific concept of "corn." When the slides were used as discrim-

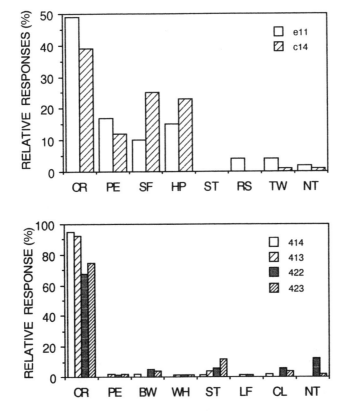

Figure 20.6 Generalizations after training with real corn (upper panel, two birds) and color slides of corn (lower panel, four birds). Test stimuli were different for the two tests. CR, corn; PE, pea; BW, buckwheat; WH, wheat; ST, stone; LF, maple leaf; CL, paper clip, NT, nut; SF, safflower, HP, hemp seed; RS, electric resistor; TW, twig. (Watanabe, unpublished data).

inative stimuli, multiple exemplars were needed to teach birds the "food" concept. The cognitive consequences of experiences with pictures and with real obejcts are different, and they have different consequences for future behavior.

CONCLUSION

A "natural concept" is usually defined, as we defined it above, in terms of human language. Sometimes an animal's conceptual behavior corresponds to the concept described by human language (for example, "people" in Herrnstein and Loveland, 1964), but sometimes they do not completely correspond (for example, "fish" in Herrnstein and de Villiers, 1980). Each species of animal relates to, or as we might say articulates with, its environment in a unique way—it has its own specific "Umwelt" (von Uexküll, 1934). It is not surprising if humans and pigeons do not always have corresponding concepts. Natural concepts such as "food" or "nonfood" consist of a set of stimuli in which each member has a similar function for a given species. Thus all pigeons should share a similar concept of food. Experience, in addition to genetic predispositions, may play a major role in establishing such concepts, but these concepts are quite different from a "pseudoconcept" or an "artificial concept" which must be established through training in an experiment. The natural concept should already have been established in the subjects when they come to the experimental chamber. Operant training with such natural concepts merely provides a tool to help us know the animal's articulation and does not lead to formation of a classification of stimuli by reinforcement. Similarly, we can teach human subjects a new concept in a so-called concept formation experiment, but such a concept differs from an everyday concept which we use in a variety of situations rather than just in a laboratory.

Furthermore, the brain regions involved in natural concept discrimination by pigeons differ from those underlying the discrimination of pseudoconcepts and of artificial patterns generated by computer graphics (Watanabe, 1991). More sensory processing seems to be necessary for the pseudoconcept and the artificial pattern discrimination.

Pigeons establish equivalence between the real objects and their pictures through a "conceptual" framework, which can be envisaged as a structure intervening between a real object and its picutre. When they learn an arbitrary classification they cannot use such a "conceptual" framework and instead have to learn each item separately. Thus, what they learn is a set of nonsense stimuli associated with reward rather than relying on the type of classification they may use outside the test chamber. There may be stimulus generalization from three-dimensional real objects to two-dimensional pictures for any stimulus, because they must share some features, but this stimulus generalization is different from the type of object-picture equivalence that is attained through the mediation of conceptual framework.

Working within the framework of a strict use of Lloyd Morgan's canon, we would have to say that the evidence that pigeons form and use concepts is still patchy. A few experiments seem to give conclusive evidence; in many others, evidence that behavior can be explained *only* as conceptually based discrimination is weak or definitely absent. In such a situation, we can never dismiss the possibility that the few apparently clear pieces of evidence are flawed in some way. But the modern approach to animal cognition bypasses Lloyd Morgan to some extent. The question to ask is not whether pigeons have been proved beyond a reasonable doubt to possess and use concepts, but whether it has proved fruitful to ask whether they do. The answer to that question is clear. The investigation of concept and picture discrimination has immeasurably extended our knowledge of the way birds discriminate the real objects which make up their visual and functional world. We confidently expect that further explorations of the mechanisms of these complicated discriminations will enrich our knowledge yet further.

REFERENCES

Bateson, P. P. G., and Chantrey, D. F. (1972). Retardation of discrimination learning in monkeys and chicks previously exposed to both stimuli. *Nature (London)* 237, 173–174.

Bhatt, R. S., and Wasserman, E. A. (1989). Secondary generalization and categorization in pigeons. *J. Exp. Anal. Behav.* 52, 213–224.

Bhatt, R. S., Wasserman, E. A., Reynolds, W. F. Jr., and Knauss, K. S. (1988). Conceptual behavior in pigeons: Categorization of both familiar and novel examples from four classes of natural and artificial stimuli. *J. Exp. Psychol.: Animal Behav. Process.* 14, 219–234.

Cabe, P. A. (1976). Transfer of discrimination from solid objects to pictures by pigeons" A test of theoretical models of pictorial perception. *Percept. Psychophysi.* 19, 545–550.

Cerella, J. (1979). Visual classes and natural categories in the pigeon. *J. Exp. Psychol.: Human Percept. Perform.* 5, 68–77.

Cerella, J. (1980). The Pigeon's analysis of pictures. *Pattern Rec.* 12, 1–6.

Cerella, J. (1982). Mechanisms of concept formation in the pigeon. In D. J. Ingle, M. A. Goodale, and R. J. W. Mansfield (Eds.), *Analysis of Visual Behavior*, pp. 241–260. MIT Press, Cambridge, MA.

Chater, N., and Heyes, C. (1992). Unpublished manuscript.

D'Amato, M. R., and Van Sant, P.(1988). The person concept in monkeys (*Cebus apella*). *J. Exp. Psychol.: Animal Behav. Process.* 14, 43–55.

Davenport, R. K., and Rogers, G. M. (1971). Perception of photographs by apes. *Behaviour* 31, 318–320.

Delius, J. D. (1992). Categorical discrimination of objects and pictures by pigeons. *Animal Learn. Behav.* 20, 301–311.

Dittrich, W. H. (1988). Wie klassifizieren Javaneraffen (*Macaca fascicularis*) natürliche Muster? *Ethology* 77, 187–208.

Dittrich, W. H., and Lea, S. E. G. (1993). Motion as a natural category for pigeons: Generalization and a feature-positive effect. *J. Exp. Anal. Behav.* 59, 115–129.

Ferster, C. B., and Skinner, B. F. (1957). *Schedules of Reinforcement*. New York: Appleton-Century-Crofts.

Fields, L., Reeve, D. F., Adams, B. J., and Verhave, T. (1991). Stimulus generalization and equivalence classes: A model for natural categories. *J. Exp. Anal. Behav.* 55, 305–312.

Herrnstein, R. J. (1985). Riddles of natural categorization. In L. Weiskrantz (Ed.), *Animal Intelligence* pp. 129–143. Oxford: Clarendon.

Herrnstein, R. J., (1990). Levels of stimulus control: A functional approach. *Cognition* 37, 133–146.

Herrnstein, R. J., and de Villiers, P. A. (1980). Fish as a natural category for people and pigeons. In G. H. Bower, (Ed), *The Psychology of Learning and Motivation*, Vol. 14, pp. 59–97. Academic Press, New York.

Herrnstein, R. J., and Loveland, D. H. (1964). Complex visual concept in the pigeon. *Science* 146, 549–551.

Herrnstein, R. J., Loveland, D. H., and Cable, C. (1976). Natural concepts in pigeons. *J. Exp. Psychol.: Animal Behav. Process.* 2, 285–302.

Holland, P. C., and Ross, R. T. (1981). Associations in serial compound conditioning. *J. Exp. Psychol.: Animal Behav. Process.* 7, 228–241.

Holland, P. C., and Straub, J. J. (1979). Differential effects of two ways of devaluing the unconditioned stimulus after Pavlovian appetitive conditioning. *J. Exp. Psychol.: Animal Behav. Process.* 5, 65–78.

Honig, W. K., and Stewart, K. E. (1988), Pigeons can discriminate locations presented in pictures. *J. Exp. Anal. Behav.* 50, 541–551.

Huber, L., and Lenz, R. (1993). A test of the linear feature model of polymorphous concept discrimination with pigeons. *Quart. J. Exp. Psychol.* In press.

Hull, C. L. (1943). *Principles of Behavior.* Appleton-Century-Crofts, New York.

Hulse, S. H., Humpal, J., and Cynx, J. (1984). Processing of rhythmic sound structures by birds. *Ann. N.Y. Acad. Sci.* 423, 407–419.

Lea, S. E. G. (1984). In what sense do pigeons learn concepts? In H. L. Roitblat, T. G. Bever, and H.S. Terrace (Eds.), *Animal Cognition*, pp. 263–276. Erlbaum, Hillsdale, NJ.

Lea, S. E. G., and Harrison, S. N. (1978). Discrimination of polymorphous stimulus sets by pigeons. *Quart. J. Exp. Psychol.* 30, 521–537.

Lea, S. E. G., and Ryan, C. M. E. (1983). Feature analysis of pigeons' acquisition of concept discrimination. In M. L. Commons, R. J. Herrnstein, and A. R. Wagner (Eds.), *Quantitative Analyses of Behavior*, Vol. 4: *Discrimination processes*, pp. 239–253. Ballinger, Cambridge, MA.

Lea, S. E. G., and Ryan, C. M. E. (1990). Unnatural concepts and the theory of concept discrimination in birds. In M. L. Commons, R. J. Herrnstein, S. Kosslyn, and D. Mumford (Eds.), *Quantitative Analyses of Behavior*, Vol, 8: *Behavioral Approaches to Pattern Recognition and Concept Formation*, pp. 165–185. Erlbaum, Hillsdale, NJ.

Lea, S. E. G., Lohmann, A., and Ryan, C. M. E. (1993). Discrimination of five-dimensional stimuli by pigeons. Limitations of feature analysis. *Quart. J. Exp. Psychol.* 46B, 19–42.

Lubow, R. E. (1974). High-order concept formation in the pigeon. *J. Exp. Anal. Behav.* 21, 475–483.

Lumsden, E. A. (1977). Generalization of an operant response to photographs and drawings/silhouettes of a three-dimensional object at various orientations. *Bull. Psychonom. Soc.* 10, 405–407.

Mackintosh, N. (1991). Perceptual and categorical learning by pigeons and people. Paper read at the meeting of the Association for the Study of Animal Behaviour, London, December.

Morgan, M. J., Fitch, M. D., Holman, J. G., and Lea, S. E. G. (1976). Pigeons learn the concept of an 'A'. *Perception* 5, 57–66.

Møller, A. P. (1985). Mixed reproductive strategy and mate guarding in a semi-colonial passerine, the swallow *Hirundo rustica. Behav. Ecol. Sociobio.* 17, 401–408.

Pearce, J. M. (1989). The acquisition of an artificial category by pigeons. *Quart. J. Exp. Psychol., Section B* 41, 381–406.

Pietrewicz, A. T., and Kamil, A. C. (1977). Visual detection of cryptic prey by blue jays (*Cyanocitta cristata*). *Science* 195, 580–582.

Poole, J., and Lander, D. G. (1971). The pigeon's concept of pigeon. *Psychonom. Sci.* 25, 157–158.

Ramsay, A. O. (1951). Familial recognition in birds. *Auk* 68, 1–17.

Real, P. G., Iannazzi, R., Kamil, A. C., and Heinrich, B. (1984). Discrimination and generalization of leaf damage by blue jays (*Cyanocitta cristata*). *Animal Learn. Behav.* 12, 202–208.

Roberts, W. A., and Mazmanian, D. S. (1988). Concept learning at different levels of abstraction by pigeons, monkeys, and people. *J. Exp. Psychol.: Animal Behav. Process.* 14, 247–260.

Ryan, C. M. E. (1982a). Concept formation and individual recognition in the domestic chicken. *Behav. Anal. Lett.* 2, 213–220.

Ryan, C. M. E. (1982b). Mechanisms of individual recognition in birds. Unpublished Master Theses, University of Exeter.

Ryan C. M. E., and Lea, S. E. G. (1990). Pattern recognition, updating, and filial imprinting in the domestic chicken (*Gallus gallus*). In M. L. Commons, R. J. Herrnstein, S. Kosslyn, S., and D. Mumford (Eds.), *Quantitative Analyses of Behavior, Vol. 8: Behavioral Approaches to Pattern Recognition and Concept Formation*, pp. 89–110. Erlbaum, Hillsdale, NJ.

Schrier, A. M., Angarella, R., and Povar, M. L. (1984). Studies of concept formation by stumptailed monkeys: Concepts humans, monkeys, and letter A. *J. Exp. Psychol.: Animal Behav. Process.* 10, 564–584.

Spence, K. W. (1936). The nature of discrimination learning in animals. *Psychol. Rev.* 43, 427–449.

Stemmer, N. (1980). Natural concepts and generalization classes. *Behav. Analyst* 3, 41–48.

Tinbergen, M. (1951). *The Study of Instict.* Oxford University Press, London.

Trillmich, F. (1976). Learning experiments on individual recognition in budgerigars (*Melopsittacus undulatus*). *Zeit. Tierpsychol.* 41, 372–395.

Vaughan, W. (1988). Formation of equivalence sets in pigeons. *J. Exp. Psychol.: Animal Behav. Process.* 14, 36–42.

Vaughan, W., and Greene, S. L. (1983). Acquisition of absolute discrimination in pigeons. In M. L. Commons, R. J. Herrnstein, and A. R. Wagner (Eds.), *Quantitative Analysis of Behavior.* Vol. 4, *Discrimination Processes*, pp. 231–238. Ballinger, Cambridge MA.

Vaughan, W., and Greene, S. L. (1984). Pigeon visual memory capacity. *J. Exp. Psychol.: Animal Behav. Process.* 10, 256–271.

von Fersen, L., and Lea, S. E. G. (1990). Category discrimination by pigeons using five polymorphous features. *J. Exp. Anal. Behav.* 54, 69–84.

von Uexküll, J. (1934). *Streifzüge durch die Umwelten von Tieren und Menschen.* Springer, Berlin.

Wasserman, E. A., Kiedinger, R. E., and Bhatt, R. S. (1988). Conceptual behavior in pigeons: Categories, subcategories, and pseudocategories. *J. Expe. Psychol.: Animal Behav. Process.* 14, 235–246.

Watanabe, S. (1988). Failure of visual prototype learning in pigeons. *Animal Learn. Behav.* 16, 147–152.

Watanabe, S. (1991). Effects of ectostriatal lesions on natural concept, pseudoconcept and artificial pattern discrimination in pigeon. *Visual Neurosci.* 6, 497–506.

Watanabe, S. (1992). Effect of lesions in the ectostriatum and Wulst on species and individual discrimination in pigeon. *Behav. Brain Res.*, 49, 197–203.

Watanabe, S. (1993). Object-picture equivalence in the pigeon: An analysis with natural concept and pseudoconcept discrimination. *Behav. Processes*, in press.

Watanabe, S., and Ito, Y. (1991). Discrimination of individuals in pigeons. *Bird Behav. 9*, 20–29.

Watanabe, S., and Tailin, J. (1993). Visual and auditory cues in conspecific discrimination learning in Bengalese finches. *J. Eth.*, in press.

Watanabe, S., Yamashita, E., and Wakita, M. (1993). Discrimination of video images of conspecific individuals in Bengalese finches. *J. Eth.*, in press.

Wittgenstein, L. (1953). *Philosophical Investigations*, 3rd ed. Basil Blackwell, Oxford.

Wright, A. A., Cook, R. G., Rivera, J. J., Sands, S. F., and Delius, J. D. (1988). Concept learning by pigeons: Matching-to-sample with trial-unique video picture stimuli. *Animal Learn. Behav. 16*, 436–444.

Yoshikubo, S. I. (1985). Species discrimination and concept formation by rhesus monkeys. *Primates 26*, 285–299.

21 Beyond Sensation: Visual Cognition in Pigeons

Jacky Emmerton and Juan D. Delius

Much research on the visual capacities of birds has focused on the ways in which they process relatively simple optical stimuli (see, e.g., Emmerton, 1983). However, birds have evolved in a complex and highly variable natural environment, and it seems unlikely that they function merely like feathered automata, reacting reflexively to the elementary dimensions of randomly encountered stimuli. Indeed, the elaborate organization of their visual systems and the complexity of their behaviors suggest that they not only make full use of the array of environmental stimuli, but extract from it information which is processed, stored, and used to guide their later behavior.

For this reason, birds, especially pigeons, are often used as subjects in studies of learning. Such research typically concentrates on the processes involved in associating stimuli with each other or with specific responses. The stimuli used in these studies have traditionally been simple, arbitrary, and easy to present under controlled laboratory conditions. In recent years, rather than asking how associations are acquired, some researchers have instead begun to explore the cognitive processes by which the properties of complex stimuli are encoded, how this stored information is further transformed, and how it might guide behavior.

Cognitive experiments often use standard conditioning techniques to control the pigeon's response. However, they differ from traditional learning experiments both with respect to the number and complexity of their stimuli, and in demanding discriminations based, not on some simple and invariant physical property of the stimulus, but on relational or abstract properties. These experiments with pigeons have demonstrated their capacity to deal with a variety of discriminations in a manner suggesting that they encode and store information about stimuli in the form of internal representations. The concept of an internal representation implies that exposure to a stimulus produces a neural trace that preserves essential characteristics of the stimulus so that these remain accessible for some variable period and can affect behavior even in the absence of the original physical stimulus. The precise nature of the neural storage mechanisms is still elusive. The encoding process, on the other hand, and the transformations that internal representations undergo are amenable to behavioral analysis, using experimental paradigms designed to examine what properties of a stimulus complex are abstracted and stored by the animal. This chapter reviews some experiments in avian visual cognition, and explores the processes involved in the internal representation of complex visual stimuli by birds.

DISCRIMINATION OF NUMEROSITY

Earlier work by Otto Koehler and his students (1935) demonstrated that birds can discriminate between stimulus arrays on the basis of the number of items they contain (e.g., groups of 4 vs. 5 seeds). However this ability seemed to operate within fairly strict numerical limits. Whereas Koehler tested his animals in seminatural situations, we used operant conditioning procedures in order to have better control of stimulus factors and to explore those numerical limits more precisely. Stimuli were varying numbers of small white dots, projected onto dark pecking keys, and pigeons were trained to respond on each trial to the key displaying the greater number of dots by reinforcing their correct choices with grain. Because the differential brightness of the groups of dots could provide cues to their numerosity, brightness was later controlled using neutral density filters. In transfer tests with novel stimuli, pigeons discriminated the new stimuli about as well as the old ones, showing that they had acquired a generalized numerical concept of "more" versus "less."

We next explored the limits of pigeons' numerical discrimination by restricting the difference between groups of dots to only a single unit, i.e., 1 vs. 2, through to 7 vs. 8 dots. As figure 21.1 shows, discrimination accuracy declined as the number of items in each group increased, so that by 7 vs. 8 dots, performance bordered on chance.

It may be a "pernicious coincidence" (Miller, 1956) but, in most species tested, numerosity discrimination breaks down when one of the displays contains the modal "magical number" of 7 items. Miller's remark originally referred to apparent limitations in processing capacity for a wide variety of tasks, including one in which human subjects rapidly and accurately reported the number of dots in a briefly presented single group of up to 6 dots, a behavior called "subitizing" (Kaufman et al., 1949). Interestingly, when we tested students with brief presentations of the same pairs of stimuli used with pigeons, their performance also fell to chance with groups of 7 vs. 8 dots. This similarity in results suggests that birds and humans might process these dot displays in similar ways. What remains at issue for any species is whether there is a specialized mechanism specifically for quantifying small numbers and, if so, what form of processing is used (e.g., serial scanning of elements in a stored image, or recognition of canonical patterns of objects: see

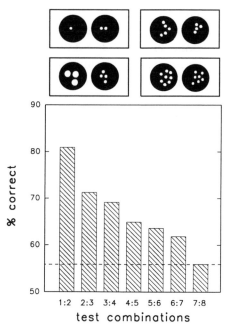

Figure 21.1 Test for the limits of numerosity discrimination. Dashed horizontal line indicates the upper limit of chance performance according to binomial statistics. Examples of stimulus pairs are shown at the top.

Miller, 1993, for a discussion of subitizing). However, whether or not birds, and indeed humans, have a limited capacity to process visual stimuli, the question still remains as to how they solve numerosity problems.

One possibility is that, even without a linguistic code, they can count, i.e., store precise information about the absolute or cardinal number of up to 7 items in a set (Davis and Memmott, 1982; Davis and Pérusse, 1988). Any stimulus group would be compared with this store, or internal representation, of absolute number and chosen if it matched. However, "counting" was unlikely in the present experiment, since the number of items per stimulus varied randomly from trial to trial and a particular stimulus group was correct only when it contained more units that the other group. Instead, our subjects probably made relative numerousness judgments (cf. Davis and Pérusse, 1988). To solve this problem, one of the stimulus displays would first have to be stored briefly, and the number of items seen in the second group then compared with this stored representation. Any capacity limitation would apply only to the short-term storage involved in the completion of a trial. Alternatively, the capacity limitation of about 7 items may be more apparent than real, and what might be discriminated is the ratio of items. Honig and Stewart (1989) showed that pigeons are capable of such a ratio discrimination when numerically larger arrays, containing mixtures of different elements, are involved.

Having tested the pigeon's capacity to discriminate "more" from "less," we next asked whether they could also order quantities of dots according to a numerical scale such that 4 > 3 > 2, for example. Birds were first trained in a conditional discrimination paradigm to distinguish the class "many" stimuli (groups of 6 or 7 elements) from the class "few" stimuli (groups of 1 or 2 elements) that were displayed on a central key. Following presentation of a "many" stimulus, pecks at a red, right-hand key were reinforced; following a "few" stimulus, pecks at a green, left-hand key were correct. During prolonged training, novel stimuli were often introduced to test acquisition of a generalized concept of "many" versus "few." Then on test trials, stimuli included not only novel exemplars of the type "few" (1 or 2 items) and "many" (6 or 7 items) but also, for the first time, stimuli comprising the intervening numerosities, 3, 4, and 5. We asked if the birds would rate these completely novel 3, 4, and 5 item stimuli as being more similar to the 6 and 7 or else to the 1 and 2 item stimuli. In these tests the birds rated novel stimuli that contained 6 or 7 elements as being of the "many" type, and new stimuli consisting of 1 or 2 items as being "few," as they had done in training. More importantly, the new numerosities, 3, 4, and 5, were serially ordered between these two extremes (figure 21.2).

These results were confirmed using a variety of control manipulations (such as altering stimulus shapes, equating brightness, etc.), none of which interfered with birds' orderly discrimination of number. All these studies indicate that pigeons are capable of abstract discriminations based on numerical quantities, an ability that might be ecologically

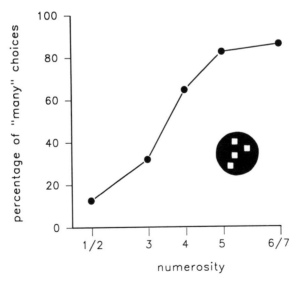

Figure 21.2 Initial test results for pigeons' serial ordering of numerosity with novel stimulus displays. Mean choices in a conditional discrimination paradigm are plotted relative to responses that would have been correct for a "many" stimulus (consisting of 6 or 7 elements). Inset shows an example of a stimulus.

useful when, during foraging, they need to make quick decisions about which food patch to choose. However, little is known about the mechanisms underlying this cognitive ability.

INTERNAL REPRESENTATIONS OF MOVEMENT PERCEPTIONS

Movement provides an important source of information about other animals in the bird's environment. This coordinated oscillatory movement has been called "biological motion" (Johansson, 1973). Pigeons can quickly learn to discriminate movement patterns (Lissajous figures), generated on an oscilloscope and consisting of either a single point of light tracing one of two cyclically variable pathways, or outline patterns resembling small wire figures rotating about a central axis (Emmerton, 1986). Various tests suggested that the animals' ability to distinguish these motion patterns could not be explained by discrimination of just a simple dimension of movement, such as a difference in overall velocity or direction. Instead, their latencies to respond to the different stimuli showed that they must have acquired internal representations of the overall patterns of movement. The starting phase of any one pattern varied randomly from trial to trial and its component phases were also repeated in a cyclical fashion, which took between 2 and 12 sec to complete. Trained birds usually responded within 1 sec of the appearance of a correct pattern, indicating that their recognition of the pattern was based on only a small part of the overall movement. This implies that they compared that part with a previously stored representation of the complete pattern when deciding whether to peck at the pattern. The ability to differentiate cyclical variations in movement could be important for the more ecologically relevant task of recognizing conspecifics, and other animals, on the basis of motion characteristics. The ability to store information about movement trajectories also makes it possible to preserve its perceptual continuity when it is briefly hidden from view. For example, a bird may be briefly occluded when it flies behind a tree. An observer that can extrapolate the animal's movement trajectory can then recognize the bird that emerges as being the same one that disappeared earlier.

An analogous situation was modeled in an experiment by Neiworth and Rilling (1987). They presented a computer-generated bar that, like a clock-hand, was rotated with constant velocity through some fixed angle. When this movement trajectory was completed and the bar stopped, the birds had to peck one of two response keys to obtain food reward. On other trials, however, the bar was "occluded," i.e., it disappeared part-way through the trajectory and then, after a delay, reappeared elsewhere as a static stimulus. From the bar's constant velocity and the delay period, it is possible to compute where it should reappear. If it reappeared in an appropriate location, the birds were reinforced for making the same response as if it had been visible throughout the delay. If it reappeared in a location inconsistent with a constant velocity of rotation, then pecks to the alternative key were reinforced. Training involved two different "visible" trajectories of bar movement, through either 135 or 180°. On the "occlusion" trials there were also two different time delays, corresponding to the correct and incorrect reappearance positions of the bar for each trajectory.

Neiworth and Rilling were not just interested in whether pigeons form an internal representation of a moving stimulus. They also asked whether birds can, in the absence of the stimulus, further transform that representation so as to extrapolate the movement of a stimulus that was no longer visible. Only then could the pigeons correctly identify how far it should have moved while it was occluded. Critical test trials involved a change in trajectories so that they ended in new locations, and corresponding novel delay periods for stimulus "occlusion." Birds still performed well on these tests so that Neiworth and Rilling concluded that pigeons have the ability to form images, i.e., they can store complex visual information in a transformable, picture-like form, or one that operates like an analog code of the physical environment.

CATEGORIZATION OF THREE-DIMENSIONAL OBJECTS

In the preceding experiments the stimuli were two-dimensional patterns. The cognitive processing that controls visually guided behavior must, however, be structured to cope with three-dimensional objects. We have recently attempted to maximize the cognitive performance of pigeons by using three-dimensional stimuli. A simultaneous presentation of several stimuli, and a closer spatial contiguity between stimuli, responses and rewards than is traditional in operant laboratories also better approximates the normal foraging situation of pigeons (Delius, 1992). Small junk objects (beads, sequins, screws, transistors, etc.), glued to a transport chain in sets of three, were successively brought into view under portholes of a horizontal platform attached to a conditioning chamber. Pecks at them were detected by shock sensors; correct choices were reinforced with grain, incorrect choices punished with darkness.

Two groups of pigeons were taught to discriminate between spherical (rewarded) and nonspherical (nonrewarded) objects, drawn from sets of either 36 or 72 different objects (exemplars). Acquisition was quite rapid (90% correct choices within 200 trials). Test trials after less than 500 training trials revealed significant discrimination (75% correct) of new sets of spherical and nonspherical stimuli, thus proving true categorization learning. The transfer to new objects by the many-exemplar group was however slightly but significantly superior to that of the few-exemplar group. The classical explanation for these findings invokes generalization gradients and decrements. The occurrence of discrimination transfer to novel objects is assumed to be based on their physical similarity with the training objects. The deficiency in transfer, in contrast, is attributed to the nonidentity between novel and familiar objects (Pearce, 1988). Within the same framework the many-exemplar subjects are expected to have a broader overall generalization gradient and thus transfer better than the few-exemplar group.

As the number of exemplars with which a subject is familiar increases, gradients should also broaden. We tested this by gradually augmenting the number of stimuli in the training set until the two groups were dealing with sets of 184 and 260 spherical and nonspherical, respectively. Despite this profusion of exemplars subjects continued to show appreciable transfer decrements. Even at a late stage about 8 reinforced presentations of initially novel stimuli were required to bring them up to the discrimination performance typical for highly familiar training objects (figure 21.3).

An alternative hypothesis proposes that the pigeons memorized their experiences with the training objects in two different ways. One involves a by-rote storage of individual stimuli. When faced with novel objects, the subjects obviously could not retrieve them from this memory store. Rather, they had to recur to another store encoding two clusters of features or properties dissociated from individual objects but corresponding to abstract concepts of spheres and nonspheres, respectively. Although these differing, so-called episodic and semantic representations of the same material are conceived as separate by theoreticians, they may nevertheless rely on closely related neural

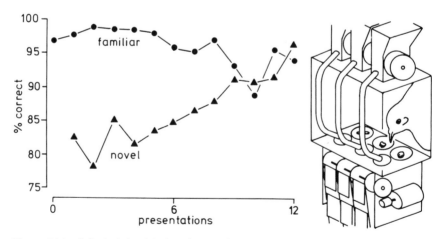

Figure 21.3 Spherical (positive) and nonspherical (negative) object discrimination by pigeons ($n = 4$). (Right) Detail of experimental apparatus. (Left) Concurrent mean discriminative performance on routine training object sets (3×54 objects; familiar) and on new test object sets (3×18 objects; novel) across successive presentations. Discrimination performance with novel stimuli reaches that with familiar stimuli on only about the ninth reinforced presentation. Modified from Delius (1992).

Emmerton & Delius: Beyond Sensation

mechanisms. The results may instead reflect two alternative retrieval strategies, the less specific one operating as a fallback strategy that sets in when the more specific one fails to trigger a behavioral routine.

The flexibility of the unspecific, semantic representation is highlighted by the result of a test in which the pigeons could choose only between nonspherical objects. They selected those having at least some attributes typical of spheres, demonstrating that they could categorize the objects in a relativistic manner, much as humans do in comparable situations. Categorization models based on neural networks relying on so-called relaxation principles are capable of precisely this performance, but they are too complex to elaborate here (see Roitblat and Fersen, 1992).

MEMORY FOR RELATIVE FAMILIARITY

As just described, pigeons responded quite differently to familiar and novel items belonging to identical stimulus classes. Is that just an accidental consequence of retrieval efforts, or does it indicate specific characteristics of memory? An experiment by Fersen and Delius (1989) suggests that a degree-of-familiarity label may be attached to each item's representation in the pigeon's episodic memory. The experiment, primarily designed to explore pigeons' visual memory capacity (cf. Vaughan and Greene, 1984), utilized a large number of different two-dimensional shapes. Of these stimuli, 100 were assigned to a positive set and 625 to a negative set. They were projected in pairs on the pecking keys of a conditioning chamber. The pigeons were rewarded with grain and punished with darkness for choosing respectively the positive or negative stimulus of these pairs. They needed as many as 9000 trials to achieve the 80% correct criterion, possibly because of the use of simple, flat shapes.

An economical way to solve this task is to memorize only the relatively few positive stimuli. Test trials in which these stimuli were paired with completely novel shapes seemed to indicate at first that the pigeons used this strategy. However, they were significantly better on these trials than on concomitant normal trials involving both positive and negative training shapes. This indicated that they somehow detected the switch from familiar to novel negative shapes. Moreover, test trials pairing negative shapes used during training with novel shapes revealed that the pigeons had in fact also memorized most of the 625 negative shapes. They avoided responding to them, preferring to peck the novel stimuli with slightly less accuracy than their discrimination performance on concurrent normal training trials (figure 21.4). Control trials in which both shapes were novel led to chance levels of performance.

The suggestion is that as the pigeons learned to recognize the individual stimuli by-rote (episodically), they also stored information about

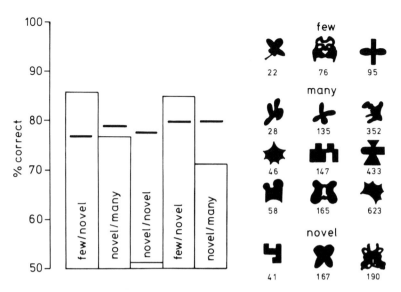

Figure 21.4 Novelty/familiarity effects in pigeons ($n = 3$) trained to discriminate between stimulus pairs assembled from 100 ("few") positive and from 625 ("many") negative shapes. (Right) Examples of stimulus shapes. (Left) Bars, discrimination performance on familiar training stimulus pairs; columns, concurrent discrimination of either "few"/novel test stimulus pairs or novel/"many" test stimulus pairs (2 series of sessions, each involving 2 × 100 test pairs) and control novel/novel stimulus pairs (one series of sessions, 100 test pairs; modified from Fersen and Delius, 1989).

how often they had seen them. During training, the few positive stimuli were seen on average every 100 trials and thus were probably labeled in memory as "very familiar" while the many negative stimuli, which were seen on average only every 625 trials, were possibly labeled as "somewhat familiar." On this familiarity–unfamiliarity continuum, novel stimuli merit the extreme label "not familiar." When stimuli of this latter kind were paired with the positive, very familiar shapes the enhanced label contrast augmented the choice accuracy beyond the normal by-rote level. When however the novel stimuli replaced the positive, very familiar stimuli, the inverse contrast with the negative shapes labeled somewhat-familiar degraded the dominant by-rote avoidance of the latter.

Meantime there is further, independent evidence that pigeons are exquisitely responsive to the novelty–familiarity of visual stimuli (Macphail and Reilly, 1989), supporting the view that pigeons may not just passively react to, but actively record, the frequency of past events. Indeed, this may be why they have some competence in judging large numerosities (Honig and Stewart, 1989). There is no doubt, incidentally, that humans keep a surprisingly precise count of the frequency of experience attached to most of the contents of episodic memory and that this information can readily be used for stimulus discrimination (Zechmeister and Nyberg, 1982).

Emmerton & Delius: Beyond Sensation

TRANSITIVE INFERENCE PERFORMANCE

In the preceding pages we espoused a cognitive view of pigeon behavior based on evidence that they store and retrieve intricate representations of experience. Now we focus on a behavior that, when it occurs in humans, has been viewed as prototypically cognitive, but that on closer examination may be explicable in terms of simpler mechanisms.

Fersen (1989) examined the performance of pigeons in a task involving what is known in classical logic as transitive inference. If premises state that A is larger than B and B is larger than C, humans concludes that A is larger than C. For pigeons, the relevant stimuli were different shapes presented on pecking keys but are referred to here by letters. During training, 5 stimuli were successively presented in four overlapping pairs A + B−, B + C−, C + D−, D + E−, where positive signifies reward and negative means punishment. These premise pairs imply the stimulus ordering A > B > C > D > E. When criterion discrimination of the individual pairs was achieved (80% choices correct), the subjects were tested for transitive inference in non-reinforced trials with the novel pair BD consisting of two stimuli that were nominally equally often rewarded and punished during training. Nevertheless, B was chosen in preference to D to the same degree as were the positive shapes of the training pairs (figure 21.5). Like young children (Bryant and Trabasso, 1971) and some primates (Gillan, 1981; McGonigle and

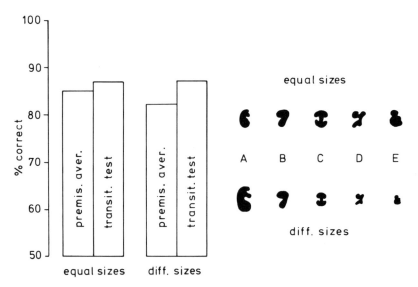

Figure 21.5 Transitive inference responding by two groups of pigeons (each $n = 4$) that discriminated equal size or different size stimuli. (Right) Stimuli employed. (Left) Mean terminal discrimination performance of the two groups on the premise stimulus pairs (AB, BC, CD, DE) and on the transitivity test pair (BD). Note the similar results for both pigeon groups. Modified from Fersen (1989).

Chalmers, 1977), pigeons seemed to behave in accordance with the B > D conclusion that derives from the premises. Indeed, the birds continued to evince analogous transitive responding when the training series was expanded to a 7 stimulus series and they were tested with 5 different novel pairings.

Classical theories assume that the solution of transitive inference problems by humans involves the application of language-couched propositions. A more modern hypothesis however supposes that the premises are integrated in memory into a linearly organized representation of the stimulus sequence, much as we have written it above. This can account for the transitivity performance of linguistically unskilled young children (Bryant and Trabasso, 1971) and offers itself as an explanation for the pigeons' transitive responding. Guided by this model, Fersen (1989) attempted to shorten the pigeons' otherwise slow acquisition of the premises (some 5000 trials) by using shapes graded in size from A (largest) to E (smallest). The pigeons could now, in principle, master the task by learning to choose the larger shape of each pair. Moreover, it could be expected that the size ordering of the stimuli would facilitate the mental linear mapping alluded to above. In the event, the subjects dealing with this paradigm proved just as slow in learning as the regular group dealing with same-sized stimuli. The former pigeons were also no more efficient in solving the presumably easier different-size BD test than were the latter ones that dealt with the more symbolic equal-size transitivity test (figure 21.5). These results indicated that the pigeons were generally not judging the test stimuli on the basis of any relational rule or, even less, sequence representation.

Prompted by this result, J. E. R. Staddon (Fersen et al., 1992) discovered that a surprisingly elementary, easily computable learning mechanism can account for the transitivity results. He proposed that stimulus A, always rewarded, accumulates the highest response eliciting value and stimulus E, always punished, the lowest one. Stimulus B, though punished when presented with A, benefits partly from A's higher values by being compounded with it. D, similarly, loses some value by being compounded with E. The result is a graded magnitude of stimulus weights with B having a higher value than D. Couvillon and Bitterman (1992) in turn suggested that this value transfer model required an unnecessary construct. Instead they pointed out that contrary to the intention of the experiment, the middle stimuli B, C, and D were not actually rewarded and punished with equal frequency. Because of the special status of the end stimuli A and E (consistently rewarded and punished respectively), subjects learn to discriminate the end pairs AB and DE more rapidly than the middle pairs. B is thus rarely punished as a member of the AB pair, which in turn facilitates learning when it is rewarded in the BC pair. D is often rewarded when a member of DE, which results in its being very often punished when it is part of the CD pair. On this basis, a very elementary learning mechanism, the so-called Luce operator, is indeed sufficient to generate the graded stimulus values required for transitive inference responding (Wynne et al., 1992). Nevertheless, value transfer mediated by a simple adjunctive classical conditioning process has been recently demonstrated so that Staddon's model is still an explanatory option (Siemann et al., 1993).

However that may be, a performance by pigeons that initially appeared prototypically cognitive, in seemingly requiring a complex representation, now appears to be based on straightforward strengthening of stimulus-response links by conditioning processes. Surprisingly, when presented with the same kind of problem disguised as a computer game, human adults appear also to deal with the task according to similar conditioning principles, even though some subjects explicitly describe the game as a transitive inference problem (Siemann and Delius, 1993; Werner et al., 1992). It is presently uncertain whether classical propositional rules or linear mapping representations are ever used by them. On the other hand, it would be premature to consider such issues as settled. Connectionist models that mediate between simple conditioning and complex representations are beginning to yield interesting explanations and predictions for transitive responding (Carmesin and Schwegler, 1993). Indeed, such models are likely to generally upset many of the current ideas about the mechanisms underlying perception and cognition, both in humans and pigeons. It is precisely because they force us to reevaluate established explanations of behavior that comparative studies are so heuristically useful.

ACKNOWLEDGMENTS

J. D. Delius thanks the Deutsche Forschungsgemeinschaft for grant support, L. von Fersen, M. Siemann, J. E. R. Staddon, and C. Wynne for collaboration, and A. Niemuth for help with the manuscript. J. Emmerton is grateful to H.-J. Knorn, A. Lohmann, and A. Niemann for assistance, and to J. Smith for help with the manuscript.

REFERENCES

Bryant, P. E., and Trabasso, T. Transitive inferences and memory in young children. *Nature (London)* 232 (1971), 456–458.

Carmesin, H. O., and Schwegler, H. Parallel versus sequential processing of relational stimulus structures. (1993), submitted.

Couvillon, P. A., and Bitterman, M. E. A conventional conditioning analysis of "transitive inference" in pigeons. *J. Exp. Psychol.: Anim. Behav. Proc.* 18 (1992), 308–310.

Davis, H., and Memmott, J. Counting behavior in animals: A critical evaluation. *Psychol. Bull.* 92 (1982), 547–571.

Davis, H., and Pérusse, R. Numerical competence in animals: Definitional issues, current evidence, and a new research agenda. *Behav. Brain Sci.* 11 (1988), 561–615.

Delius, J. D. Categorical discrimination of objects and pictures by pigeons. *Anim. Learn. Behav.* 20 (1992), 301–311.

Emmerton, J. Vision. In M. Abs (Ed.), *Physiology and Behaviour of the Pigeon*. Academic Press, London, 1983, pp. 245–266.

Emmerton, J. The pigeon's discrimination of movement patterns (Lissajous figures) and contour-dependent rotational invariance. *Perception*, 15 (1986), 573–588.

Fersen, L. von. Kognitive Prozesse bei Tauben. Ph. D. thesis, Ruhr-University, Bochum, Germany, 1989.

Fersen, L. von, and Delius, J. D. Long-term retention of many visual patterns by pigeons. *Ethology* 82 (1989), 141–155.

Fersen, L. von, Wynne, C. D. L., Delius, J. D., and Staddon, J. E. R. Transitive inference formation in pigeons. *J. Exp. Psychol.: Anim. Behav. Proc.* 17 (1992). 334–341.

Gillan, D. J. Reasoning in the chimpanzee: II. Transitive inference. *J. Exp. Psychol.: Anim. Behav. Proc.* 7 (1981), 150–164.

Honig, W. K., and Stewart, K. E. Discrimination of relative numerosity by pigeons. *Anim. Learn. Behav.* 17 (1989), 134–146.

Johansson, G. Visual perception of biological motion and a model for its analysis. *Percept. Psychophys.* 14 (1973), 201–211.

Kaufman, E. L., Lord, M. W., Reese, T. W., and Volkmann, J. The discrimination of visual number. *Am. J. Psychol.* 62 (1949), 498–525.

Koehler, O., Müller, O., and Wachholtz, R. Kann die Taube Anzahlen erfassen? *Verh. Dtsch. Zool.* 37 (1935), 39–54.

Macphail, E. M., and Reilly, S. Rapid acquisition of a novelty versus familiarity concept by pigeons (*Columba livia*). *J. Exp. Psychol.: Anim. Behav. Proc.* 15 (1989), 242–252.

McGonigle, B. O., and Chalmers, M. Are monkeys logical? *Nature (London)* 267 (1977), 694–696.

Miller, G. A. The magical number seven, plus or minus two: Some limits on our capacity for processing information. *Psychol. Rev.* 63 (1956), 81–97.

Miller, D. M. Do animals subitize? In S. T. Boysen and E. J. Capaldi (Eds.). *The Development of Numerical Competence: Animal and Human Models*. Erlbaum, Hillsdale, NJ, 1993, pp. 149–169.

Neiworth, J. J., and Rilling, M. E. A method for studying imagery in animals. *J. Exp. Psychol.: Anim. Behav. Proc.* 13 (1987), 203–214.

Pearce, M. Stimulus generalization and the acquisition of categories by pigeons. In L. Weiskrantz (Ed.), *Thought without Language*. Clarendon Press, Oxford, 1988, pp. 133–155.

Roiblat, H. L., and Fersen, L. von. Comparative cognition: Representations and processes in learning and memory. *Annu. Rev. Psychol.* 43 (1992), 671–710.

Siemann, M., and Delius, J. D. Implicit deductive responding in humans. *Naturwissenschaften* (1993), in press.

Siemann, M., Dombrowski, D., and Delius, J. D. Stimulus value transfer in visual discriminations by pigeons. (1993), in preparation.

Vaughan, W. Jr., and Greene, S. L. Pigeon visual memory capacity. *J. Exp. Psychol.: Anim. Behav. Proc.* 10 (1984), 256–271.

Werner, U. B., Koeppl, U., and Delius, J. D. Transitive Inferenz bei nicht-verbaler Auf-gabendarbietung. *Z. Exper. Angew. Psychol.* 39 (1992), 662–683.

Wynne, C. D. L., Fersen, L. von, and Staddon, J. E. R. Pigeons' inferences are transitive and the outcome of elementary conditioning principles: A response. *J. Exp. Psychol.: Anim. Behav. Proc.* 18 (1992), 313–315.

Zechmeister, E. B., and Nyberg, S. E. *Human Memory, an Introduction to Research and Theory.* Brooks/Cole, Monterey, CA, 1982.

22 Vision, Cognition, and the Avian Hippocampus

Verner P. Bingman

Among the variety of memory-related functions attributed to the hippocampal formation (see Seifert, 1983; Olton and Kesner, 1990), it is clear that for animals, the hippocampus is particularly important for memory functions regarding spatial aspects of the environment. Considerable empirical support for this position comes from two types of studies performed with laboratory rats. First, neurons have been found in the rat hippocampus that display distinct firing patterns depending on the location of an animal in a particular environment (O'Keefe and Conway, 1978; Best and Ranck, 1982; Muller et al., 1987; Muller and Kubie, 1987). Second, rats with hippocampal lesions invariably perform poorly compared to control animals in a number of spatial tasks including a water maze (Morris et al., 1982), eight-arm radial maze (Olton and Papas, 1979), and others (e.g., O'Keefe et al., 1975). Collectively, these findings can be interpreted nicely by assuming that the hippocampus functions as part of a neural representation of the environment in the form of cognitive map (O'Keefe and Nadel, 1978).

Laboratory studies with rodents have been the major source of theoretical developments regarding hippocampal function in spatial memory. However, it remains uncertain how theories derived from laboratory rodents may relate to other species and other conditions. One important issue that has not been sufficiently discussed is how ecologically relevant are laboratory rodent studies? If for ecological or evolutionary reasons the spatial behavior of rodents is not particularly well developed, or if the experimental settings in which rodents are studied lack sufficient complexity or natural significance to reveal the richness of rat's spatial ability, then the picture that is suggested by rodent laboratory work may be even more complex and differentiated then these results indicate. What is needed are field studies to complement the laboratory work. It is also imperative that other species be used if a complete understanding of the complexity of hippocampal function is to be achieved. Regarding studies examining a hippocampal role in spatial memory, experimental species should be chosen in part for the complexity of their naturally occurring spatial behavior. Presumably a species that has evolved complex spatial behavior could tell us more about the role of the hippocampus in spatial memory than a species that is a spatial "lightweight." Further, experiments should be performed under conditions that resemble those that animals normally encounter in their natural environment. Only in this way can we be certain that we are looking at hippocampal function in its appropriate evolutionary and ecological context.

Birds would seem to be one class of vertebrates particularly well suited as subjects for further investigation of hippocampal function in spatial memory. Among vertebrates, birds probably display the most sophisticated and complex forms of memory-based spatial behavior including migration, homing, and the storing and recovery of cached food. Indeed, recent studies on the role of the hippocampus in avian spatial behavior have provided new insights into understanding hippocampal function.

THE AVIAN DORSOMEDIAL FOREBRAIN AND MAMMALIAN HIPPOCAMPUS: THE QUESTION OF HOMOLOGY

If the avian hippocampal formation is to be compared to the mammalian hippocampal formation in terms of sharing certain broad functional characteristics, then it is important to consider the extent to which they share a common evolutionary ancestry. The avian dorsomedial forebrain, or hippocampal formation (HP), is a paired structure consisting of a medial hippocampus and dorsomedial parahippocampus (Karten and Hodos, 1967). Interest in the avian dorsomedial forebrain was spurred by its being identified as the homologue of the mammalian hippocampal formation (Craigie, 1935; Ariëns Kappers et al., 1936). Questions of homology are complex, particularly when functional issues are important (Campbell and Hodos, 1970). Homologous structures often have quite different functions while nonhomologous structures often share the same function. The question of homology between the avian hippocampal formation and mammalian hippocampal formation reduces to what criteria one uses for its determination. HP contains many of the cell types found in the mammalian hippocampus, including pyramidal cells (Mollá et al., 1986). However, the cytoarchitectural organization of HP, lacking distinct structures such as a dentate gyrus and Ammon's horn, clearly differs from the mammalian hippocampal formation. Embryologically, HP and the mammalian hippocampus emerge from the same portion of the developing telencephalon (Källén, 1962). HP and the mammalian hippocampus share many pathway connections, particularly with the septum, hypothalamus, brainstem monoaminergic nuclei, and telencephalic sensory processing areas, but there are also some differences in hippocampal connectivity in mammals and birds (Casini et al., 1986). An immunohistochemical analysis of the distribution of various transmitters and transmitter-related enzymes has revealed considerable similarity in the occurrence of these substances in HP and hippocampus, but their specific organization may be different (Krebs et al., 1987, 1991; Erichsen et al., 1991). HP may lack a distinct mossy fiber system (Bingman et al., 1989) and does not seem to respond to a Ca^{2+} application with an increase in NMDA receptors as does the mammalian hippocampus (Lynch and Baudry, 1984). However, HP, like the mammalian hippocampus, contains NMDA receptors (A. Reiner, personal communication), labels heavily for zinc (J. Krebs, personal communication), and displays long-term enhancement of synaptic responses (Wieraszko and Ball, 1991).

In summary, anatomical, physiological, and neurochemical evidence identifies considerable similarity between the avian dorsomedial forebrain and mammalian hippocampus. It is difficult to imagine that these similarities are a result of convergence or parallel evolution. Together with a common, broadly defined role in learning and memory, therefore, the results argue strongly for homology. However, differences in the two structures are noted—a finding consistent with 250 million years of independent evolution. It seems the challenge to researchers now is to specify along what dimensions (e.g., anatomical, neurochemical) the two structures differ and then to relate those differences to how the structures function in the context of memory and spatial behavior.

THE ROLE OF THE HIPPOCAMPUS IN NATURALLY OCCURRING SPATIAL MEMORY TASKS

The hippocampal formation has emerged as a structure critical for the performance of two naturally occurring behaviors where spatial memory plays a central role: recovery of stored seeds in some passerine species and spatial navigation in homing pigeons.

A number of bird species, foremost members of the Paridae (tits and chickadees) and Corvidae (crows and jays), show a remarkable ability to recognize the location of stored seeds and recover them, in the case of Corvids, sometimes months after they have been stored (Sherry et al., 1981; Kamil and Balda, 1985). Krushinskaya (1966), working under seminatural conditions with caged Siberian nutcrackers (*Nucifraga caryocatactes*), was the first to link HP with spatial memory. She found that when long retention intervals separated the storage of seeds from the chance to recover them, nutcrackers with HP lesions were strikingly impaired in their ability to retrieve the seeds they had stored earlier. Using a more sophisticated experimental procedure, Sherry and Vaccarino (1989) found that HP lesions impaired the ability of black-capped chickadees (*Parus atricapillus*) to recover their stored seeds. Specifically, HP lesions reduced the accuracy of cache recovery to chance, but did not reduce the amount of caching or the number of attempts to recover seeds. There was also a greater tendency to revisit already emptied cache sites. A number of studies have also shown that HP in food-storing species is larger than HP in related species that store less or not at all (e.g., Krebs et al., 1989).

The remarkable ability of homing pigeons to return home following displacement of 100 km and more from unfamiliar locations has fascinated scientist and layman for more than 2000 years. This ability is based on a complex set of navigational mechanisms that have been reviewed by Baker (1984). From what pigeons learn about certain features of their environment, it appears that they have two memory-based navigational mechanisms that are regulated in part by HP.

The pigeon uses its navigational map to home from distant, unfamiliar release sites (Papi and Wallraff, 1982). Although the details of how the navigational map works remain obscure, researchers agree it involves placing sensory information acquired at the release site into the framework of a map-like representation of the environment stored in the brain. Because the navigational map presumably permits birds to use novel sensory input encountered at unfamiliar locations to determine their position relative to home, it is perhaps the best example of a naturally occurring cognitive map in the sense of O'Keefe and Nadel (1978).

Adult, experienced homing pigeons who undergo hippocampal ablation are indistinguishable from control animals in their ability to fly off in an approximate homeward direction from distant, unfamiliar release sites (Bingman et al., 1984). These results suggest that HP is not critical for the operation of an already learned navigational map. In contrast, young, naive pigeons that undergo HP ablation before having any experience with the environment are strikingly impaired in their ability to learn a navigational map (Bingman et al., 1990). Further, adult, experienced pigeons with HP lesions are also impaired in learning a new navigational map when transferred to a new loft (Bingman and Yates, 1992). These results indicate that an intact hippocampus is necessary if homing pigeons are to learn a navigational map. Together, these results emphasize the importance of the hippocampus in learning a navigational map. Once a map is learned, however, an intact hippocampus does not appear to be essential to determine the direction home from distant, unfamiliar release sites.

When a homing pigeon returns home from a distant, unfamiliar release site, it will eventually begin to fly over familiar terrain. Once in this area, pigeons can rely on a second navigational mechanism based on landmarks that it recognizes. Given that landmark navigation is based on familiar stimuli, it is not clear under what conditions they would be used in the form of a cognitive map or a simpler type of associative map (Bingman, 1990). These types of maps correspond to the locale and taxon systems of spatial behavior, respectively, of O'Keefe and Nadel (1978).

According to the scheme of O'Keefe and Nadel (1978), locale system spatial behavior is based on the ability of an organism to build a neural representation of an environment in the form of a cognitive map. This neural representation or map could then be used by the organism to coordinate movement between locations represented on the map. Most importantly, it would allow the organism to spontaneously generate novel and efficient routes to goal locations from places within the familiar environment where it has never been before (Bingman et al., 1989). The taxon system of spatial behavior, in contrast, is based on the ability of an organism to rely on learned associations to coordinate its movements. For example, a bird may learn that from location X, where it has been on several occasions, the direction home is always toward a particular tree. The bird could then associate the direction home from location X with flying toward the tree and subsequently use the tree from location X, and only location X, to guide the trip home (Bingman et al., 1989). Although a useful spatial strategy, taxon system spatial behavior is limited to an elaboration of familiar routes and thus does not permit an organism to spontaneously generate novel routes to goal locations from places it has never been before. O'Keefe and Nadel (1978) hypothesize that the hippocampus is uniquely involved in the regulation of locale system cognitive maps

Homing pigeons given HP lesions as experienced adults fly a less direct path home and take more time to return home compared to control animals when released close to home (Bingman and Mench, 1990). These results indicate that HP is important for navigation based on familiar landmarks. Results from two other experiments suggest that HP lesion does not impair learning an association between a group of familiar landmarks and the direction home (Bingman et al., 1988), but does impair use of familiar landmarks for navigation when the landmarks are perceived from a novel location (Bingman et al., 1989). These results support the hypothesis that HP lesion disrupts familiar landmark navigation specifically in a context where they would be used in the form of a cognitive map (Bingman, 1990). Unanswered by these studies, however, is to what extent the landmark navigation deficit resulting from HP lesion can be traced to (1) memory loss of a previously learned landmark map (retrograde memory loss), (2) an impairment in the operation of a previously learned landmark map (retrieval deficit), or (3) difficulties in relearning a landmark map lost as a result of HP lesion (learning deficit). Recent research on young homing pigeons suggests that HP plays an important role in at least the learning of a landmark map (Bingman, unpublished data).

In summary, at least two distinct navigational mechanisms are used by homing pigeons to return home, both of which seem to operate under the assumptions of a cognitive map as described by O'Keefe and Nadel (1978). Importantly, the avian hippocampal formation is important for at least some aspects of both navigational systems.

LABORATORY STUDIES OF HIPPOCAMPAL FUNCTION

Experiments conducted in a natural or seminatural setting are exciting because they offer the only tangible insight into how the hippocampus may function in the real world. In addition, studying HP function in a natural environmental setting may give some clues to the ways in which evolutionary selective pressures shaped the relationship of HP and behavior. However, these studies are deficient in one obvious respect: it is difficult or impossible to specify the nature of the relevant environmental stimuli that are being processed through the hippocampus. This issue is critical because it is this sensory input that eventually results in some stored spatial representation of the environment, or accesses an already existing representation that may be used to find a seed or return home.

Given this constraint, if a bird uses vision to solve a naturally occurring spatial memory task, it is difficult to determine to what extent the hippocampus may be involved in the processing of relevant visual information by performing experiments only under field conditions. For example, unless one can move buildings, large trees, etc., it is difficult to demonstrate that homing pigeons use visual landmarks to navigate home once in familiar territory or what role the hippocampus may play in such behavior. Indeed, the only evidence suggesting that homing pigeons use vision at all in their navigation is that birds forced to wear translucent lenses, which preclude form vision, are impaired in arriving at their loft. Such birds, however, still succeed in flying toward home when released and return to the general vicinity of the loft (Schmidt-Koenig and Walcott 1978). The favored explanation for this finding is that the lenses do not impair navigational map use, which gets them close to home, but does impair their ability to rely on landmarks once near the loft. Braithwaite and Guilford (1991) also found that visual landmarks may be important for navigation.

Laboratory studies, in contrast to experiments conducted under natural conditions, have the distinct advantage of allowing the experimenter to define those aspects of the environment that are salient for a given task. It is through controlled laboratory studies that one can begin to understand more thoroughly the relationship between vision, hippocampus and cognition.

Sahgal (1984) tested HP lesioned pigeons on a Konorski pair comparison (conditional discrimination) task. In a three-key operant chamber, pigeons were exposed to a center pecking key illuminated by a color. Subsequently, two side keys were both illuminated with either the same color that illuminated the center key or a different color. The same color required the birds to peck one side key (left) for a food reward, a different color required them to peck the other side key (right). Simultaneous illumination of both the center and side keys resulted in no difference in the performance of HP ablated and control birds. HP ablated pigeons, however, displayed a performance deficit when the center key was turned off before the side keys were turned on. In other words, when the memory demands of the task were increased, HP ablated birds were impaired.

The experiment described above suggests that HP ablation in pigeons leads to a memory deficit for visual stimuli. Interpretation of the data, however, are confounded by the behavior of one HP ablated bird that performed better than any of the control animals tested. The data nonetheless link HP to the performance of a behavioral task where the salient discriminative stimuli are visual in nature.

Good (1987) used a T-maze to examine the effects of HP ablation on performance in a number of tasks. In one task, HP ablation led to a deficit in learning the reversal but not acquisition of a position discrimination task. The nature of the discriminative stimulus that defined position (e.g., proprioceptive cues, distal visual cues in the lab) was not identified in this study. A second task revealed neither an acquisition nor reversal deficit when intramaze cues, horizontal and vertical stripes, were simultaneously used as discriminative stimuli in defining the correct arm.

In a third study, birds were also examined in the acquisition of a conditional discrimination task. Colored inserts were used in the T-maze. Depending on the color of the inserts, the birds had to go left or right in the maze for a food reward. HP lesioned birds, although eventually reaching control performance levels, were slower in learning the task. This last study again links HP to a task where the salient discriminative stimuli are visual. The results of the second experiment, however, show that performance deficits following hippocampal lesions do not result just from the use of visual stimuli in a discriminative task.

Reilly and Good (1987) examined the effect of hippocampal ablation on performance in a number of operant tasks. Using a three-key chamber, they found no deficits associated with hippocampal ablation in learning a spatial alternation task, a color discrimination task, and reversal of the color discrimination task. Using a similar color discrimination and reversal task Bingman and Shimizu (unpublished data) also found no effects of HP ablations. Examining spatial alternation in a T-maze, however, Reilly and Good (1987) did observe performance deficits with hippocampal ablations. The surprising finding is that using the same basic procedure, hippocampal ablation impaired spatial alternation performance in a T-maze but not in an operant chamber.

Reilly and Good (1989), who again employed an operant chamber, found that HP ablated pigeons were impaired during autoshaping. In autoshaping, birds are conditioned to peck at a response key when it is illuminated. The illuminated pecking key is associated with the occurrence of food availability. Given that the illuminated key is the discriminative stimulus identifying the availability of food, the decision to peck or not to peck can be considered to be visually regulated. In another task that does not depend on visual discrimination, HP ablation was also found to impair performance on a differential reinforcement for low rates of responding schedule (DRL). This result conflicts with that of Reilly and Good (1987), who reported improved DRL performance following hippocampal ablation. They explain the conflicting results to be a consequence of the extensive training in other tasks received by the birds in the 1987 study.

Finally, Sherry and Vaccarino (1989) found that HP ablation in black-capped chickadees had no effect on the ability of these birds to discriminate between black and white cards to locate seeds in a seminatural setting. HP ablated birds, however, were more likely to make errors by returning to sites where they had already taken the available seed.

Summarized in table 22.1 are the experimental tasks in which hippocampal ablated pigeons have been studied under controlled laboratory conditions. The table identifies those tasks where deficits have or have not been found, and those tasks where the definitive discriminative stimuli were visual in nature. By discriminative stimuli I mean the stimuli that an animal must use to decide which of the possible set of responses will lead to a reward, e.g., if the walls are blue go right. In

Table 22.1. Effects of Hippocampal Ablation on Pigeon Behavioral Performance in Laboratory Tasks

Deficit	No Deficit
T-Maze	
Position reversal (Good, 1987)	Position discrimination (Good, 1987)
Conditional color discrimination[a] (Good, 1987)	Visual pattern discrimination and reversal[a] (Good, 1987)
Spatial alternation (Reilly and Good, 1987)	
Operant	
Delayed color conditional discrimination[a] (Sahgal, 1984)	Simultaneous color conditional discrimination[a] (Sahgal, 1984)
Autoshaping[a] (Reilly and Good, 1989)	Color discrimination and reversal[a] (Reilly and Good, 1987; Bingman and Shimizu, unpublished data)
DRL-10 sec (Reilly and Good, 1989)	Spatial alternation (Reilly and Good, 1987)
	DRL-10 sec[b] (Reilly and Good, 1987)
Seminatural	
Returns to depleted food locations[c] (Sherry and Vaccarino, 1989)	Brightness discrimination[a,c] (Sherry and Vaccarino, 1989)

[a]Tasks with visual cues as definitive discriminative stimuli.
[b]HP ablated pigeons actually performed better than controls.
[c]This experiment was performed with black-capped chickadees.

this case blue would be a discriminative stimulus that identifies a right turn as correct. A visual stimulus that simply guides a response, e.g., the alleys of a T-maze or a lighted pecking key in an operant chamber, would not be considered a discriminative stimulus. Behavioral decisions in many tasks not identified as visual, for example spatial alternation, are nonetheless probably based on visual cues. However, use of visual cues has not been demonstrated empirically in these tasks and therefore they are not identified as tasks with visual discriminative stimuli.

Examination of table 22.1 reveals a confusing pattern of results. Two points need to be made. First, there is no obvious unifying character that distinguishes tasks in which deficits are found from those where deficits are not found. Second, deficits are found in a number of tasks where behavioral decisions are made based on visual discriminative stimuli. Most importantly, the results support the hypothesis that spatial memory based on visual environmental stimuli used by food-storing birds or homing pigeons involves the hippocampus, at least under some conditions.

Based on the results from the laboratory studies using well defined behavioral procedures (table 22.1), it appears practically impossible to define with any precision the role of the hippocampus in memory processing. One problem with such studies may be that the task demands are of little ecological relevance to the animals. This may predispose either poor performance by these animals or considerable interindividual variability in performance, thus confounding any interpretations regarding structure and function. In developing laboratory studies to define better the role of the hippocampus in visual cognition, one should ideally take into account the natural history of the animal and design experiments that are ecologically relevant (e.g., Sherry and Vaccarino, 1989). This aim can still be compatible with the degree of stimulus control and precision offered by laboratory studies relying on traditional behavioral approaches. In an attempt to examine the importance of the hippocampus for spatial cognition based on visual landmarks in pigeons, I have begun an experiment intended to combine the stimulus control of operant studies with the ecological relevance of making behavioral decisions based on the spatial distribution of visual landmarks.

PERFORMANCE OF PIGEONS IN AN OPERANT LANDMARK SPATIAL RELATIONS TASK

One of the most robust findings in homing pigeons is that hippocampal ablated birds take more time to return home. A considerable amount of field evidence suggests that part of this deficit can be explained by HP birds having difficulty using familiar, presumably visual landmarks near home to localize their loft (Bingman and Mench, 1990). It is difficult in a field setting, however, to demonstrate that homing pigeons actually use these cues for navigation. It is therefore uncertain to what extent hippocampal ablation may affect the ability of homing pigeons to rely on visual landmarks. To address this issue under more controlled laboratory conditions, I have tested pigeons in an operant task where birds must rely on the relative orientation of a group of colored squares (landmarks) to determine which of four pecking keys will yield a food reward. The results to be presented are preliminary in nature, and included are only the essential features of the material and methods used.

Test Apparatus

The test apparatus was a standard pigeon operant chamber. The pecking panel (figure 22.1) contained a central, transparent acrylic plastic window. A video monitor that was used to display stimuli to the pigeons was placed behind the window. Adjacent to the four corners of the window were circular pecking keys that could be back illuminated. The entire apparatus was interfaced to a computer, which controlled all aspects of its functioning.

Behavioral Procedures

White carneaux pigeons were first taught to key-peck in an autoshaping procedure and then they learned to peck the window when a circle appeared on the monitor behind it. After being trained on an intermediate task in which only two stimulus arrays and two pecking keys were used, they were trained on the first of two spatial discrimination

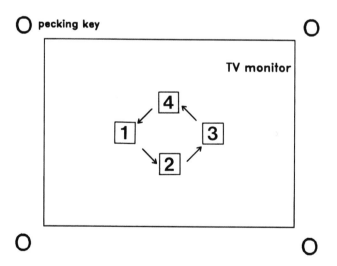

Figure 22.1 Schematic of operant chamber pecking panel used in landmark spatial relations task. The numbered squares on the TV monitor screen refer to different colors. Between trials the array of colored squares could be rotated together around an axis centered in the middle of the monitor screen.

tasks that utilized all four pecking keys. The discriminative stimulus consisted of four large squares, each 6.25 cm², that were placed symmetrically about the center of the video monitor (figure 22.1), which was located 20 cm behind the window. From trial to trial the array of colored squares could be rotated to any of four positions that were separated by 90°. For each orientation, ·a response to one of the side keys was rewarded with access to food. For example, pecking the upper left key was rewarded when the array was in position A, and pecking the lower left key was rewarded when the array was in position B, etc.

Birds were trained on this task for two sessions of 100 trials each day, 6 days a week. On each trial, the stimulus array would be presented in one of the four orientations in a quasi-random sequence. Seven pecks (FR 7) on the window would then remove the stimulus array and illuminate the four side pecking keys. One peck to the correct key was followed by food reinforcement; one peck to an incorrect key was followed by a correction procedure. Training continued until a bird performed better than 50% correct (remember 25% would be chance in this four-choice task) for three consecutive sessions. Failure to meet this criterion after 15 sessions resulted in a bird being eliminated from the study.

After training in the previous task, a bird proceeded to the final, critical experimental task. The behavioral procedure used in this task was identical to that of the previous phase. The stimuli, however, were made considerably smaller, each square was now 0.25 cm², and symmetrically clustered more centrally around the center of the video monitor (figure 22.1). Training continued until a bird achieved 70% correct or better for five consecutive sessions. Of the 12 birds tested, only 7 reached criterion in the final task.

The task described above was designed to examine the ability of birds to determine a response based on the spatial orientation of a cluster of visual landmarks. Specifically, the task was a first attempt to assess the effect of hippocampal ablation on the ability of pigeons to use the spatial relationship of visual "landmarks" to determine a response in an operant setting. Toward this end, birds were first trained preoperatively. After reaching criterion, six of seven birds were subjected to hippocampal ablation (the seventh bird served as an untreated control). Seven days later, the birds began the whole training and testing sequence again. The critical measure was a comparison of the number of preoperative and postoperative sessions to reach criterion on the last task. If the hippocampus is important for solving this task, which presumably tests some kind of spatial memory based on visual landmarks, then the postoperative performance of the birds should be impaired compared to their preoperative performance. For all experimental animals, the preoperative and postoperative landmark test arrays differed. For four birds, three of which were subjected to hippocampal lesions, the preoperative landmark array consisted of blue, red, dark green, and yellow squares on a light gray background while the postoperative array consisted of black, brown, light green, and purple squares on a yellow background. The other three birds experienced the reverse.

Summarized in figure 22.2 are the comparisons between the preoperative and postoperative performance of the experimental birds on the last experimental task. Of six HP ablated birds, five displayed poorer postoperative performance than preoperative. The one untreated control animal (V1) preformed better postoperatively. Of those birds with postoperative impairments, performance deficits ranged from three times as many sessions to about 50% more sessions to criterion. Examination of figure 22.3 reveals a strong rank correlation (Spearman $r = 0.97$) between the extent of hippocampal damage and the magnitude of the postoperative performance deficit. Indeed, the hippocampal ablated bird that performed best postoperatively was tied with another bird with the least amount of hippocampal damage (38% hippocampal damage).

Learning this task requires a bird to relate visual cues to some spatial variable. As such, the preliminary data support the idea that the pigeon hippocampus is important for at least some tasks where visual cues need to be spatially coded. The experimental design, however, does not allow one to specify what visual–spatial rule a bird may have used in solving the task. A bird may have used (1) the spatial relationship

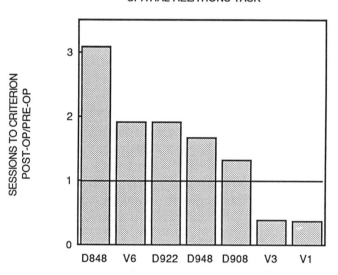

Figure 22.2 Ratio of postoperative over preoperative sessions to criterion for the experimental animals in the landmark spatial relations task. Notations along the x-axis identify the test animals. Values above the horizontal line drawn from 1 on the y-axis indicate poorer postoperative performance; values below the line indicate poorer preoperative performance. V1 was the untreated control animal; all others received hippocampal lesions.

Vision and Cognition

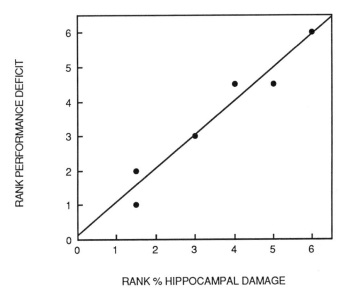

RANK % HIPPOCAMPAL DAMAGE

Figure 22.3 Correlation between extent of hippocampal damage (% total hippocampal volume destroyed) and postoperative performance deficit of the six hippocampal ablated birds. The regression line was calculated using the method of least squares. Values of 1 indicate the smallest amount of hippocampal damage and smallest performance deficit. (In the case of V3 with a rank deficit of 1, there was actually a superior post-operative performance rather than a deficit.)

among the four landmark squares (e.g., when blue is on top of the others peck upper right), (2) the walls of the video monitor as a reference (e.g., when blue is closest to the left wall, peck upper right), or (3) a particular location on the monitor as a reference (e.g., when blue is in a particular spot peck upper right). The experiment was originally designed to have a final phase where the array of colored squares was moved about the video screen to force the animals to rely on the first strategy. The birds, however, failed to learn the task when the array moved from trial to trial. In any event, whatever strategy the birds used, it had to be based on combining a visual stimulus with some spatial reference.

Any conclusion from this on-going study regarding the hippocampus must remain tentative as only one control bird has been tested, and a good correlation was also found between rank of total telecephalic lesion damage (HP plus other brain structures) and rank performance deficit (Spearman $r = 0.81$). This caution aside, there was one particularly curious finding in this experiment. The last task of the experiment differed from the previous task only in the size of the stimuli and clustering around the center of the video screen. Nonetheless, compared to their criterion performance on the large-square task, the initial performance of the birds on the small-square task was typically much poorer both pre- and postoperatively. What this suggests is that whatever strategy was employed to solve the task with large colored squares, it did not transfer readily to the last task with small colored squares. Of more interest is that there was no indication of a performance deficit following hippocampal ablation for the task with large squares. Indeed, of the six HP ablated birds, three reached criterion on the large-squared task faster postoperatively. For the large-square task there was a relatively small rank correlation between the ratio of postoperative over preoperative sessions to criterion and hippocampal lesion volume (Spearman $r = 0.56$). Together, these findings suggest that the birds used different strategies to solve the large-square and small-square tasks, and that the hippocampus was particularly important for the solution of a small-square task.

ANATOMICAL PATHWAY CONNECTIONS BETWEEN THE HIPPOCAMPUS AND VISUAL PROCESSING AREAS

If the hippocampus plays a role in the processing of visual information in the context of memory, as the behavioral data suggest, then there should be anatomical connections, whether direct or indirect, between the hippocampus and visual processing areas of the avian forebrain.

The avian Wulst is a longitudinal elevation of the avian telencephalon. Two subdivisions of the Wulst, the nucleus intercalatus of the hyperstriatum accessorium (IHA) and hyperstriatum dorsale (HD), are known to receive a projection from a retinal recipient area of the thalamus, the nucleus opticus principalis thalami (OPT, Karten et al., 1973). IHA and HD are typically identified as primary visual processing areas. HD has reciprocal connections with the parahippocampal area of the hippocampal formation (Casini et al., 1986; Shimizu et al., 1990). Further, there are numerous telecephalic regions that receive either direct or indirect projections from the primary visual processing areas (IHA, HD, and the primary telencephalic target of the tectofugal pathway, the ectostriatum) and that are connected with the hippocampus (Güntürkün, 1984; Casini et al., 1986; T. Shimizu, personal communication). These regions include the hyperstriatum accessorium, an area near the vallecula, the neostriatum frontale lateralis, and a subdivision of the archistriatum.

In experiments where hippocampal ablation led to behavioral deficits in homing pigeons (Bingman et al., 1984, 1990; Bingman and Mench, 1990) and chickadees (Sherry and Vaccarino, 1989), birds with lesions of the Wulst were used as controls and no behavioral deficits were found to result from such treatment. If, as suggested, the Wulst and targets of Wulst projections are the primary structures that interact with the hippocampus in the formation of or access to some visual spatial memories, then the absence of a deficit following Wulst lesion is somewhat paradoxical. How can these visual spatial memories which are sensitive to hippocampal ablation not also be sensitive to Wulst ablations? Inspection of the Wulst lesions in these studies, however, reveals that they never included the entire Wulst. Moreover, HD, which lies deep within the Wulst, was typically spared. It may be that those portions of the Wulst spared were sufficient to permit formation of or access to the visual spatial memories used in the behaviors studied. It should be emphasized here that if Wulst–hippocampal connections are indeed critical for visual spatial memories used by food-storing birds or homing pigeons, then complete destruction of the Wulst should lead to deficits similar to those found following hippocampal ablation.

In addition to the connections described above, the hippocampus has also been reported to share reciprocal projections with another telencephalic structure, the hyperstriatum ventrale (HV, Bradley et al., 1985). In the same study, HV was reported to receive a projection from the optic tectum, a target of retinal efferents. These connections offer an alternative pathway through which visual processing and the hippocampus may interact.

The data identify a number of possibilities through which the hippocampus and visual processing areas of the avian forebrain may influence each other. This interaction is presumably responsible for the role of the hippocampus in visual-based memories, which appear to be primarily spatial under natural conditions. The target of visual inputs to the hippocampal formation from the Wulst, in particular HD, seems to be almost exclusively the parahippocampal region.

CONCLUSIONS

The avian dorsomedial forebrain, or hippocampal formation, has been implicated in the neural regulation of spatial memories used by birds in a number of natural settings. Laboratory studies have further linked the hippocampal formation to memory function where discriminative stimuli are visual. The behavioral data suggest that the hippocampus and visual processing regions of the brain interact in some way to permit access to or formation of visual spatial memories. This hypothesis is supported by the numerous anatomical connections between the hippocampal formation and telencephalic visual processing areas. However, a number of important questions have yet to be addressed. Among these, foremost are the following: To what extent can one specify the type(s) of visual memory that involves the hippocampal formation? Can hippocampal function be primarily linked to the formation of visual memories, recall of existing memories, or the control of memory regulated motor outputs based on visual cues? What are the critical anatomical connections between visual processing areas and the hippocampal formation? How does the interrelationship of the hippocampal formation with vision and cognition in birds compare to that in other vertebrate groups? It is through the use of a research strategy that exploits the particular strengths of both field and laboratory experiments that we can best answer these questions.

REFERENCES

Ariëns Kappers, C., Huber, G., and Crosby, E. *The Comparative Anatomy of the Nervous System of Vertebrates Including Man*, Vol. 2. Macmillan, London, 1936.

Baker, R. *Bird Navigation: The Solution of a Mystery?* Hodder and Stoughton, London, 1984.

Best, P. J., and Ranck, J. B., Jr. The reliability of the relationship between hippocampal unit activity and sensory-behavioral events in the rat. *Exp. Neurol.* 75 (1982), 652–664.

Bingman, V. Spatial navigation in birds In R. Kesner and D. Olton (Eds.), *Neurobiology of Comparative Cognition*. Erlbaum, Hillsdale NJ, 1990, pp. 423–447.

Bingman, V., and Mench, J. Homing behavior of hippocampus and parahippocampus lesioned pigeons following short-distance releases. *Behav. Brain Res.* 40 (1990), 227–238.

Bingman, V., and Yates, G. Hippocampal lesions impair navigational learning in experienced homing pigeons. *Behav. Neurosci.* 106 (1992), 229–232.

Bingman, V., Bagnoli, P., Ioalé, P., and Casini, G. Homing behavior of pigeons after telencephalic ablations. *Brain Behav. Evol.* 24 (1984), 94–108.

Bingman, V., Ioalé, P., Bagnoli, P., and Casini, G. Unimpaired acquisition of spatial reference memory but impaired homing performance in pigeons following hippocampal ablation. *Behavi. Brain Res.* 27 (1988), 147–156.

Bingman, V., Bagnoli, P., Ioalé, P., and Casini, G. Behavioral and anatomical studies of the avian hippocampus. In V. Chan–Palay and C. Kohler (Eds.), *The Hippocampus, New Vistas.* (Neurology and Neurobiology, Vol. 52). Liss, New York, 1989, pp. 379–394.

Bingman, V., Ioalé, P., Casini, G., and Bagnoli, P. The avian hippocampus: Evidence for a role in the development of the homing pigeon navigational map. *Behav. Neurosci.* 104 (1990), 906–911.

Bradley, P., Davies, D., and Horn, G. Connections of the hyperstriatum ventrale of the domestic chick (*Gallus domesticus*). *J Anat.* 140 (1985), 577–589.

Braitwaite, V., and Guilford, T., Viewing familiar landscapes affects pigeon homing. *Proc. R. Soc. London* 3,245 (1991), 183–186.

Campbell, C., and Hodos, W. The concept of homology and the evolution of the nervous system. *Brain Behav. Evol.* 3 (1970), 353–367.

Casini, G., Bingman, V., and Bagnoli, P. Connections of the pigeon dorsomedial forebrain studied with WGA-HRP and 3-H proline. *J. Comp. Neurol.* 245 (1986), 454–470.

Craigie, E. The hippocampal and parahippocampal cortex of the Emu (*Dromiceius*). *J. Comp. Neurol.* 61 (1935), 563–591.

Erichsen, J., Bingman, V., and Krebs, J. The distribution of neuropeptides in the dorosomedial telencephalon of the pigeon (*Columba Livia*): A basis for regional subdivisions. *J. Comp. Neurol.* 314 (1991), 478–492.

Good, M. The effects of hippocampal-area parahippocampalis lesions on discrimination learning in the pigeon. *Behav. Brain Res.* 26 (1987), 171–184.

Güntürkün, O. Evidence for a third primary visual area in the telencephalon of the pigeon. *Brain Res.* 294 (1984), 247–254.

Källén, B. Embryogenesis of brain nuclei in the chick telencephalon. *Ergebnisse Anat. Entwicklung.* 36 (1962), 62–82.

Kamil, A. C., and Balda, R. P. Cache recovery and spatial memory in Clark's nutcrackers (*Nucifraga columbiana*). *J. Exp. Psychol.: Animal Behav. Process.* 11 (1985), 95–111.

Karten, H. J., and Hodos, W. *A Stereotaxic Atlas of the Brain of the Pigeon (Columba livia)*. The Johns Hopkins Press, Baltimore, MD, 1967.

Karten, H., Hodos, W., Nauta, W., and Revzin, A. Neural connections of the "visual wulst" of the avian telencephalon. Experimental studies in the pigeon (*Columba livia*) and owl (*Spestyto Cunicularia*). *J. Comp. Neurol.* 150 (1973), 253–278.

Krebs, J., Erichsen, J., and Bingman, V. The immunohistochemistry and cytoarchitecture of the avian hippocampus. *Soci. Neurosci. Abstr.* 13 (1987), 1125.

Krebs, J., Sherry, D., Healy, S., Perry, V., and Vaccariomo, A., Hippocampal specialization of food-storing birds. *Proc. Natl. Acad. Sci. U.S.A.* 86 (1989), 1388–1392.

Krebs, J., Erichsen, J., and Bingman, V. The distribution of choline acetyltransferase-like, glutamic acid decarboxylase-like, serotonin-like and tyrosine hydroxylase-like immuno-reactivity in the dorsomedial telencephalon of the pigeon (*Columba livia*). *J. Comp. Neurol.* 314 (1991), 467–477.

Krushinskaya, N. Some complex forms of feeding behaviour of nutcracker *Nucifraga caryocatactes,*after removal of old cortex. *Zhur. Evol. Biochim. Fisiol.* 2 (1966), 563–568.

Lynch, G., and Baudry, M. The biochemistry of memory. *Science* 224 (1984), 1057–1065.

Mollá, R., Rodriques, J., Calvet, S., and Garcia-Verdugo, J. Neuronal types of the cerebral cortex of the adult chicken, *Gallus gallus*. A Golgi study. *J. Hirnforschung* 27 (1986), 381–390.

Morris, R. G., M., Garrud, P., Rawlins, J. N. P., and O'Keefe, J. Place navigation impaired in rats with hippocampal lesions. *Nature* (London) 297 (1982), 681–683.

Muller, R. U., and Kubie, J. L. The effects of changes in the environment on the spatial firing of hippocampal complex-spike cells. *Jo. Neurosci.* 7 (1987a), 1951–1968.

Muller, R. U., Kubie, J. L., and Ranck, J. B., Jr. Spatial firing patterns of hippocampal complex-spike cells in a fixed environment. *J. Neurosci.* 7 (1987), 1935–1950.

O'Keefe, J., and Conway, D.H. Hippocampal place units in the freely moving rat: Why they fire where they fire. *Exp. Brain Res.* 31 (1978), 573–590.

O'Keefe, J., and Nadel, L. *The Hippocampus as a Cognitive Map*. Claredon Press, Oxford, 1978.

O'Keefe, J., Nadel, L., Keightley, S., and Kill, D. Fornix lesion selectively abolish place learning in the rat. *Exp. Neurol.* 48 (1975), 152–166.

Olton, D., and Kesner, R. *Neurobiology of Comparative Cognition*. Erlbaum, Hillsdale, NJ, 1990.

Olton, D., and Papas, B. Spatial memory and hippocampal function. *Neuropsychologia* 17 (1979), 669–682.

Papi, F., and Wallraff, H. *Avian Navigation*. Springer, Berlin, 1982.

Reilly, S., and Good, M. Enhanced DRL and impaired forced-choice alternation performance following hippocampal lesion in the pigeon. *Behavi. Brain Res.* 26 (1987), 185–197.

Reilly, S., and Good, M. Hippocampal lesion and associative learning in the pigeon. *Behav. Neurosci.* 103 (1989), 731–742.

Sahgal, A. Hippocampal lesion disrupt recognition memory in pigeons. *Behav. Brain Res.* 11 (1984), 47–58.

Schmidt-Koenig, K., and Walcott, C. Tracks of pigeons homing with frosted lenses. *Animal Behav.* 26 (1978), 480–486.

Seifert, W. *Neurobiology of the Hippocampus*. Academic Press, New York, 1983.

Sherry, D., and Vaccarino, A. The hippocampus and memory for food caches in black-capped chickadees. *Behav. Neurosci.* 103 (1989), 308–318.

Sherry, D. F., Krebs, J. R., and Cowie, R. J. Memory for the location of stored food in marsh tits. *Animal Behavi.* 29 (1981), 1260–1266.

Shimizu, T., Karten, H., and Cox, K. Intratelencephalic projections of the visual wulst in birds (*Columba livia*): A phaseolus vulgaris leucoagglutinin study. *Soc Neurosci. Abstr.* 16 (1990), 246.

Wieraszko, A., and Ball, G. Long-term enhancement of synaptic responses in the songbird hippocampus. *Brain Res.* 538 (1991), 102–106.

Species Index

Subject Index